Mantle Cell Lymphoma

Editor

JOHN P. LEONARD

HEMATOLOGY/ONCOLOGY CLINICS OF NORTH AMERICA

www.hemonc.theclinics.com

Consulting Editors
GEORGE P. CANELLOS
EDWARD J. BENZ Jr

October 2020 • Volume 34 • Number 5

ELSEVIER

1600 John F. Kennedy Boulevard • Suite 1800 • Philadelphia, Pennsylvania, 19103-2899

http://www.theclinics.com

HEMATOLOGY/ONCOLOGY CLINICS OF NORTH AMERICA Volume 34, Number 5
October 2020 ISSN 0889-8588, ISBN 13: 978-0-323-76312-7

Editor: Stacy Eastman
Developmental Editor: Julia McKenzie

Hematology/Oncology Clinics (ISSN 0889-8588) is published bimonthly by Elsevier Inc., 360 Park Avenue South, New York, NY 10010-1710. Months of issue are February, April, June, August, October, and December. Business and Editorial Offices: 1600 John F. Kennedy Blvd., Ste. 1800, Philadelphia, PA 19103—2899. Customer Service Office: 3251 Riverport Lane, Maryland Heights, MO 63043. Periodicals postage paid at New York, NY and at additional mailing offices. Subscription prices are $443.00 per year (domestic individuals), $876.00 per year (domestic institutions), $100.00 per year (domestic students/residents), $480.00 per year (Canadian individuals), $100.00 per year (Canadian students/residents), $1085.00 per year (Canadian institutions) $547.00 per year (international individuals), $1085.00 per year (international institutions), and $255.00 per year (international students/residents). International air speed delivery is included in all *Clinics* subscription prices. All prices are subject to change without notice. **POSTMASTER:** Send address changes to *Hematology/Oncology Clinics of North America*, Elsevier Health Sciences Division, Subscription Customer Service, 3251 Riverport Lane, Maryland Heights, MO 63043. Customer Service (orders, claims, online, change of address): Elsevier Health Sciences Division, Subscription **Customer Service, 3251 Riverport Lane, Maryland Heights, MO 63043. Tel: 1-800-654-2452 (U.S. and Canada); 314-447-8871 (outside U.S. and Canada). Fax: 314-447-8029. E-mail: journalscustomerservice-usa@elsevier.com (for print support); journalsonlinesupport-usa@elsevier.com (for online support).**

Reprints. For copies of 100 or more, of articles in this publication, please contact the Commercial Reprints Department, Elsevier Inc., 360 Park Avenue South, New York, New York 10010-1710; Tel.: 212-633-3874, Fax: 212-633-3820, E-mail: reprints@elsevier.com.

Hematology/Oncology Clinics of North America is covered in *MEDLINE/PubMed (Index Medicus), EMBASE/ Excerpta Medica, and BIOSIS.*

Contributors

CONSULTING EDITORS

GEORGE P. CANELLOS, MD
William Rosenberg Professor of Medicine, Department of Medical Oncology, Dana-Farber Cancer Institute, Boston, Massachusetts, USA

EDWARD J. BENZ Jr, MD
Professor, Pediatrics, Richard and Susan Smith Professor, Medicine, Professor, Genetics, Harvard Medical School, President and CEO Emeritus, Office of the President, Dana-Farber Cancer Institute, Boston, Massachusetts, USA

EDITOR

JOHN P. LEONARD, MD
Richard T. Silver Distinguished Professor of Hematology and Medical Oncology, Executive Vice Chair, Weill Department of Medicine, Senior Associate Dean for Innovation and Initiatives, Weill Cornell Medicine, New York, New York, USA

AUTHORS

SÍLVIA BEÀ, PhD
Institut d'Investigacions Biomèdiques August Pi i Sunyer (IDIBAPS), Hematopathology Unit, Hospital Clínic of Barcelona, University of Barcelona, Barcelona, Spain; Centro de Investigación Biomédica en Red de Cáncer, Madrid, Spain

DAVID A. BOND, MD
Assistant Professor, Division of Hematology, The Ohio State University, Columbus, Ohio, USA

ELÍAS CAMPO, MD, PhD
Institut d'Investigacions Biomèdiques August Pi i Sunyer (IDIBAPS), Hematopathology Unit, Hospital Clínic of Barcelona, University of Barcelona, Barcelona, Spain; Centro de Investigación Biomédica en Red de Cáncer, Madrid, Spain

SELINA CHEN-KIANG, PhD
Department of Pathology and Laboratory Medicine, Program in Immunology and Microbial Pathogenesis, Weill Cornell Medical College, New York, New York, USA

JONATHON B. COHEN, MD, MS
Associate Professor, Department of Hematology and Medical Oncology, Winship Cancer Institute of Emory University, Atlanta, Georgia, USA

MAURIZIO DI LIBERTO, PhD
Department of Pathology and Laboratory Medicine, Weill Cornell Medical College, New York, New York, USA

TOBY A. EYRE, MD
Honorary Senior Clinical Lecturer, Department of Haematology, Oxford University Hospitals, Oxford, United Kingdom

JONATHAN W. FRIEDBERG, MD, MMSc
James P. Wilmot Cancer Institute, University of Rochester Medical Center, Rochester, New York, USA

JORDAN GAUTHIER, MD, MSc
Assistant Professor, Clinical Research Division, Integrated Immunotherapy Research Center, Fred Hutchinson Cancer Research Center, Department of Medicine, University of Washington, Seattle, Washington, USA

DANIEL GUY, MD
Clinical Fellow, Division of Medical Oncology, Department of Medicine, Washington University School of Medicine, St Louis, Missouri, USA

XIANGAO HUANG, PhD
Department of Pathology and Laboratory Medicine, Weill Cornell Medical College, New York, New York, USA

PREETESH JAIN, MBBS, MD, DM, PhD
Department of Lymphoma/Myeloma, The University of Texas MD Anderson Cancer Center, Houston, Texas, USA

PEDRO JARES, PhD
Institut d'Investigacions Biomèdiques August Pi i Sunyer (IDIBAPS), Hematopathology Unit, Hospital Clínic of Barcelona, University of Barcelona, Barcelona, Spain; Centro de Investigación Biomédica en Red de Cáncer, Madrid, Spain

BRAD S. KAHL, MD
Professor, Division of Medical Oncology, Department of Medicine, Washington University School of Medicine, St Louis, Missouri, USA

MARCO LADETTO, MD
Struttura Complessa di Ematologia, Azienda Ospedaliera SS Antonio e Biagio e Cesare Arrigo, Alessandria, Italy

CHRISTINA LEE, MD
Clinical Fellow, Division of Hematology and Medical Oncology, Department of Medicine, Weill Cornell Medicine, New York, New York, USA

KAMI J. MADDOCKS, MD
Associate Professor, Division of Hematology, The Ohio State University, Columbus, Ohio, USA

DAVID G. MALONEY, MD, PhD
Professor, Clinical Research Division, Integrated Immunotherapy Research Center, Fred Hutchinson Cancer Research Center, Department of Medicine, University of Washington, Seattle, Washington, USA

PETER MARTIN, MD
Associate Professor, Division of Hematology and Medical Oncology, Department of Medicine, Weill Cornell Medicine, New York, New York, USA

RORY McCULLOCH, MD
Research Registrar, Department of Haematology, Peninsula Medical School, University of Plymouth, Plymouth, United Kingdom

ALBA NAVARRO, PhD
Institut d'Investigacions Biomèdiques August Pi i Sunyer (IDIBAPS), Barcelona, Spain; Centro de Investigación Biomédica en Red de Cáncer, Madrid, Spain

PRIYANKA A. POPHALI, MD
Assistant Professor, Division of Hematology, Oncology and Palliative Care, Department of Medicine, University of Wisconsin-Madison, Madison, Wisconsin, USA

CHRISTIANE POTT, MD, PhD
Second Medical Department, University Hospital Schleswig-Holstein, Campus Kiel, Kiel, Germany

THOMAS D. RODGERS Jr, MD
James P. Wilmot Cancer Institute, University of Rochester Medical Center, Rochester, New York, USA

JASON T. ROMANCIK, MD
Hematology and Oncology Fellow, Department of Hematology and Medical Oncology, Winship Cancer Institute of Emory University, Atlanta, Georgia, USA

JIA RUAN, MD, PhD
Division of Hematology and Medical Oncology, Meyer Cancer Center, Weill Cornell Medicine, New York, New York, USA

SIMON RULE, MD
Professor of Clinical Haematology, Department of Haematology, Peninsula Medical School, University of Plymouth, Plymouth, United Kingdom

RITA TAVAROZZI, MD
Struttura Complessa di Ematologia, Azienda Ospedaliera SS Antonio e Biagio e Cesare Arrigo, Alessandria, Italy

GITA THANARAJASINGAM, MD
Assistant Professor of Medicine, Division of Hematology, Department of Medicine, Mayo Clinic, Rochester, Minnesota, USA

KEVIN WANG, BS
Department of Pathology and Laboratory Medicine, Weill Cornell Medical College, New York, New York, USA

MICHAEL WANG, MD
Director of Mantle Cell Lymphoma Research Program, Department of Lymphoma/Myeloma, The University of Texas MD Anderson Cancer Center, Houston, Texas, USA

THOMAS E. WITZIG, MD
Consultant, Hematology Mayo Clinic Rochester, Professor of Medicine, Mayo Clinic Alix School of Medicine, Associate Director of Translational Research, Mayo Clinic Cancer Center, Rochester, Minnesota, USA

Contents

> Mantle cell lymphoma (MCL) is a mature B-cell neoplasm with heteroge-
> neous clinical behavior molecularly characterized by the constitutive over-
> expression of cyclin D1 and deregulation of different signaling pathways.
> SOX11 expression determines an aggressive phenotype associated with
> accumulation of many chromosomal alterations and somatic gene muta-
> tions. A subset of patients with the SOX11-negative leukemic non-nodal
> MCL subtype follows an initial indolent clinical evolution and may not
> require treatment at diagnosis, although eventually may progress to an
> aggressive disease. We discuss the genetic and molecular alterations
> with impact on the cancer hallmarks that characterize the lymphomagen-
> esis of the 2 MCL subtypes.

> Cell cycle dysregulation caused by aberrant cyclin D1 and CDK4 expres-
> sion is a major determinant for proliferation of cancer cells in mantle cell
> lymphoma (MCL). Inhibition of CDK4/6 induces G1 arrest of MCL cells in
> patients, appearing to deepen and prolong the clinical response to partner
> agents. This article reviews aberrations of cell cycle genes in MCL cells
> and clinical trials of CDK4/6 inhibitors for MCL. Integrative longitudinal
> functional genomics is discussed as a strategy to discover genomic
> drivers for resistance in cancer cells and cancer-immune interactions
> that potentially contribute to the clinical response to palbociclib combina-
> tion therapy in MCL.

> Mantle cell lymphoma, despite its common derivation from a t(11;14) er-
> ror that occurs in a naïve B-cell leading to overexpression of cyclin D1
> protein, is characterized by substantial heterogeneity in biology and
> clinical outcome. Unlike other non-Hodgkin lymphoma types, it is
> more common in men. Clinical presentation patterns vary from nodal
> to splenomegaly with leukemia to gastrointestinal involvement. Biolog-
> ical variability is linked to tumor cell proliferation. Increased mono-
> cyte/macrophages and their associated proinflammatory cytokines are
> associated with inferior outcomes. These clues mandate that new treat-
> ments should target signal pathways that contribute to these adverse
> outcomes.

Mantle cell lymphoma (MCL) is a biologically heterogeneous disease, and patients may experience a clinical course ranging from indolent to very aggressive. Observational studies suggest that a subset of patients can be safely observed for a period of months to years from initial diagnosis without adversely impacting their outcomes. However, identification of candidates for the "watch and wait" approach remains challenging because selection criteria are not well-defined. Studies that prospectively stratify patients on the basis of MCL biology and disease risk will be informative, and patients with indolent MCL may be ideal candidates for frontline clinical trials exploring novel therapies.

Limited-stage (stage I–II) mantle cell lymphoma (MCL) is rarely encountered. There is no standard approach to treatment and available data to guide management decisions mainly are retrospective studies. A thorough staging evaluation, including positron emission tomography/computed tomography, bone marrow biopsy, and gastrointestinal evaluation, should be completed because disseminated disease is common. Radiation therapy is effective for local control, and, although prolonged remission can be achieved, distant relapses are common and there are insufficient data to say that patients can be cured using this treatment. This article reviews literature pertaining to management of patients with limited-stage MCL and discusses approach to treatment.

Mantle cell lymphoma is an incurable B-cell malignancy. Treatment of young fit patients is particularly challenging, because careful consideration should be made when building a long-term treatment strategy that would provide longer remissions and increase patients' quality of life. Most young fit patients achieve long remissions with a combination of immunochemotherapy containing rituximab and high-dose cytarabine, followed by high-dose chemotherapy and autologous stem-cell transplantation. The addition of maintenance therapy with rituximab following autologous stem-cell transplantation prolongs the time to relapse and increases overall survival. Despite an intensive approach, late relapses are common and are usually treated with novel agents.

With a median age of 65 years, mantle cell lymphoma affects predominantly older patients with comorbidities. Initial treatment of older patients is not standardized but traditionally includes chemoimmunotherapy regimens that are not curative. Incorporation of maintenance strategy after induction and introduction of novel agents have expanded access to effective treatment options and improved survival outcome. Ongoing randomized studies comparing induction regimens and maintenance strategies are expected to further define the role of novel agents and combinations in the initial treatment of older patients with mantle cell lymphoma.

Several biological and clinical features have been recognized in mantle cell lymphoma (MCL). In recent years, the minimal residual disease (MRD) has been extensively investigated and is now considered as one of the strongest clinical predictors in this lymphoma. This article reviews methods used for the assessment of MRD in MCL and discusses their strengths and weaknesses. In addition, it examines the MRD contribution to the biology knowledge of MCL and the development of effective strategies for its management, including the possibility of personalized treatment based on MRD response.

The Bruton tyrosine kinase inhibitors (BTKi), acalabrutinib, ibrutinib, and zanubrutinib, are all approved in the United States for the treatment of relapsed mantle cell lymphoma (MCL). BTKi as a class have become the preferred therapy for most of the patients with relapsed MCL, and ongoing clinical trials are evaluating whether combining BTKi with other targeted agents may deepen response and further improve outcomes. Emerging evidence supports the efficacy of BTKi-containing combinations as front-line treatment, and clinical studies to define the role of this class of drugs for newly diagnosed patients with MCL are in progress.

In this review, we explore insights into the pathophysiology of Bruton tyrosine kinase inhibitor (BTKi) resistance in mantle cell lymphoma, and consider potential therapeutic targets. We review the possible clinical benefits of giving BTKis alongside other novel therapies, and evaluate clinical data for treatment strategies post BTKi progression that may help guide current practice. We conclude by considering future approaches, including the potential role of chimeric antigen receptor T-cell therapy.

Blastoid and pleomorphic mantle cell lymphoma (MCL) are among the worst prognostic, aggressive histology, high-risk variants of MCL, and, in this article, they are presented as blastoid MCL. Blastoid MCL have not been systematically studied, probably due to their rarity. De novo blastoid MCLs have superior outcomes compared with transformed MCL.

Compared with classic MCL, extranodal involvement (mainly skin, central nervous system), frequent relapses, and inferior responses to conventional chemoimmunotherapy, BTK inhibitors and venetoclax are frequent in blastoid MCL. KTE-X19 induces excellent response in blastoid MCL. Combinations with novel agents are actively investigated. This article presents a comprehensive review on blastoid MCL in 2020.

Mantle cell lymphoma (MCL) accounts for fewer than 10% of non-Hodgkin lymphoma. There is a high initial response rate to chemotherapy and rituximab, but a nearly universal risk of relapse. Allogeneic hematopoietic cell transplantation (allo-HCT) provides one of the only curative options. We review the role of allo-HCT for relapsed and refractory (R/R) MCL and discuss a novel promising approach using autologous chimeric antigen receptor-engineered T (CAR-T) cells. We review preliminary safety and efficacy data of 2 pivotal trials investigating the use of CD19-targeted CAR-T cells for R/R MCL after ibrutinib failure and discuss potential timing of these approaches.

Mantle cell lymphoma (MCL) is a unique lymphoma that is heterogeneous in its clinical course, and lacks consensus treatment approaches. It is often treated with immunochemotherapy at diagnosis and chronic therapies in relapse. Despite significant advances in therapy, MCL remains incurable. Maintaining patients' health-related quality of life (HRQOL) is an important treatment goal. Assessment of HRQOL elucidates the impact of an illness and its treatment on patients' lives. This review highlights the relevance of HRQOL assessment in MCL, evaluates existing evidence, current knowledge gaps and challenges in HRQOL assessment, and defines future directions for improving HRQOL evaluation in MCL patients.

Survival for patients with mantle cell lymphoma has improved dramatically over the last 2 decades owing to a better understanding of disease biology and the development of more effective treatment regimens for patients with untreated and relapsed disease. With these advancements, we are now poised to ask questions that challenge old treatment strategies, use new technologies, and improve our understanding of disease heterogeneity. This article focuses on questions that we believe will drive the future of mantle cell lymphoma treatment. Although not an exhaustive list, we review current literature, ongoing studies, and provide expert opinion on future trial design.

HEMATOLOGY/ONCOLOGY
CLINICS OF NORTH AMERICA

SERIES OF RELATED INTEREST

Surgical Oncology Clinics of North America
https://www.surgonc.theclinics.com/

THE CLINICS ARE AVAILABLE ONLINE!
Access your subscription at:
www.theclinics.com

HEMATOLOGY/ONCOLOGY CLINICS OF NORTH AMERICA

FORTHCOMING ISSUES

December 2020
Systemic Amyloidosis due to Monoclonal Immunoglobulins
Raymond L. Comenzo, Editor

February 2021
Melanoma
F. Stephen Hodi, Editor

April 2021
Myeloproliferative Neoplasms
Ronald Hoffman, Ross Levine, John Mascarenhas, and Raajit Rampal, Editors

RECENT ISSUES

August 2020
Follicular Lymphoma
Jonathan W. Friedberg, Editor

June 2020
Blastic Plasmacytoid Dendritic Cell Neoplasm
Andrew A. Lane, Editor

April 2020
Myelodysplastic Syndromes
David P. Steensma, Editor

ISSUES OF RELATED INTEREST

Surgical Oncology Clinics of North America
https://www.surgonc.theclinics.com

THE CLINICS ARE AVAILABLE ONLINE!
Access your subscription at
www.theclinics.com

Preface

Mantle Cell Lymphoma: Biologic Insights to Bedside Impact

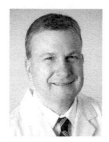

John P. Leonard, MD
Editor

Since the recognition of mantle cell lymphoma (MCL) as a distinct entity within B-cell non-Hodgkin lymphoma, progress in the evolution of treatment has occurred at a pace perhaps more rapid than any other lymphoma subtype. Better diagnostic and prognostic tools extending from cytogenetics, immunohistochemistry (SOX11, Ki-67), and assessment of p53 status have augmented clinical assessments (such as the Mantle Cell International Prognostic Index) to define heterogeneity among MCL patients. While chemotherapy-based treatment has long been a mainstay of management, novel agents targeting the cell cycle, Bruton's Tyrosine Kinase (BTK), and new immune-based approaches have undoubtedly improved patient outcomes. We now know that a subset of patients can be monitored expectantly ("watch and wait"), while others can do reasonably well with standard chemoimmunotherapy alone or in combination with high-dose chemotherapy and autologous stem cell transplant consolidation with rituximab (anti-CD20) maintenance treatment. Minimal residual disease (MRD) assessment can help to identify more and less favorable prognostic groups, and ongoing trials are evaluating whether interventions based on MRD status can help to optimize the therapeutic strategy. Several BTK inhibitors are now Food and Drug Administration approved and used primarily in the relapsed disease setting, where they frequently can provide multiyear remissions. Efficacy seems comparable among agents, though there are relatively minor distinctions in the side-effect profile. Whether BTK inhibitor should be used as single agents (eg, in sequential use followed by other drugs) or in concurrent combinations remains an important research question. In this generally incurable disease situation, where treatments clearly improve progression-free survival but have less significant overall survival benefits, the quality of life that patients experience on therapy is an essential factor in therapeutic choice. Unfortunately, at this point the effective use of quality-of-life metrics to compare across agents and regimens over time is yet to have a major role in guiding treatment.

Hematol Oncol Clin N Am 34 (2020) xiii–xiv
https://doi.org/10.1016/j.hoc.2020.07.001
0889-8588/20/© 2020 Published by Elsevier Inc.

Once patients have disease progressive beyond a BTKi, the prognosis tends to be less favorable, and a variety of regimens are used, including chemotherapy, Bcl-2 inhibitors, lenalidomide, and stem cell transplant. Several novel agents are under study, including chimeric antigen receptor T-cell approaches with evidence of early efficacy. In this issue, leading clinical and laboratory researchers in the MCL field provide a state-of-the-art review of the latest understanding of disease biology and new treatment developments. With close collaboration among investigators in the laboratory and the clinic, and carefully designed trials, I expect that we will continue to see progress for patients with MCL and added clarity around optimal therapeutic approaches and sequencing.

John P. Leonard, MD
Weill Department of Medicine
Weill Cornell Medicine
1300 York Avenue
New York, NY 10021, USA

E-mail address:
jpleonar@med.cornell.edu

Molecular Pathogenesis of Mantle Cell Lymphoma

Alba Navarro, PhD[a,b], Sílvia Beà, PhD[a,b,c], Pedro Jares, PhD[a,b,c], Elías Campo, MD, PhD[a,b,c],*

KEYWORDS

- Mantle cell lymphoma • CCND1 • SOX11 • Molecular pathogenesis
- Gene mutations • Genome instability • Cancer hallmarks

KEY POINTS

- Cryptic translocations of IG enhancers near *CCND1, CCND2,* and *CCND3* represent an alternative mechanism to the t(11;14) as an initial oncogenic event in MCL.
- The leukemic non-nodal MCL subtype displays different clinicobiological features and better outcome than conventional MCL.
- SOX11 is an oncogenic transcription factor highly expressed in conventional MCL with a relevant role in its pathogenesis, but its regulation is poorly understood.
- Next generation sequencing studies have provided new insights into the molecular MCL pathogenesis and have helped to refine the MCL cancer hallmarks.

INTRODUCTION

Mantle cell lymphoma (MCL) is a B-cell neoplasm characterized by the expansion of mature B cells frequently coexpressing CD5 that tend to widely spread in bone marrow, blood, lymphoid tissues, and extranodal sites. The tumor cells carry the t(11;14) (q13;q32) that leads to the constitutive overexpression of cyclin D1. In spite of this common initial oncogenic event, the tumors follow a very heterogeneous biological behavior, indicating that other molecular mechanisms drive the evolution of the disease. The identification of 2 MCL subtypes, conventional and leukemic non-nodal, with different molecular characteristics and clinical manifestations may explain, in part, the diversity of the tumor. Recent genomic and molecular studies have expanded our perspective on the cell of origin and pathogenesis of these MCL subtypes. In this review, we address new findings on the MCL pathogenesis and the 2

[a] Institut d'Investigacions Biomèdiques August Pi i Sunyer (IDIBAPS), Rosselló, 149-153, Barcelona 08036, Spain; [b] Centro de Investigación Biomédica en Red de Cáncer, Madrid, Spain; [c] Hematopathology Unit, Hospital Clínic of Barcelona, University of Barcelona, Villarroel 170, Barcelona 08036, Spain
* Corresponding author. Hematopathology Unit, Hospital Clínic of Barcelona, Villarroel 170, Barcelona 08036, Spain.
E-mail address: ecampo@clinic.cat

Hematol Oncol Clin N Am 34 (2020) 795–807
https://doi.org/10.1016/j.hoc.2020.05.002
0889-8588/20/© 2020 Elsevier Inc. All rights reserved.

hemonc.theclinics.com

molecular subtypes that may assist in the interpretation of the clinical diversity of these tumors.

TRANSLOCATION T(11;14) AND OVEREXPRESSION OF CYCLIN D1

The t(11;14) (q13;q32) is considered the primary oncogenic event in MCL development, virtually present in all cases, that juxtaposes CCND1 at 11q13 with the IGH regulatory region leading to a constitutive overexpression of cyclin D1. The translocation occurs at the pro/pre-B stage of differentiation during the V(D)J recombination process and is mediated by recombination activating gene enzymes.[1] The levels of cyclin D1 could be further increased by secondary rearrangements at the 3′ of the gene or point mutations in the 3′ untranslated region that create stable truncated cyclin D1 messenger RNAs (mRNAs).[2] This cyclin D1 overexpression may deregulate the G1/S cell cycle transition and promote the malignant transformation of B cells. Beyond its well-characterized role in cell cycle, a number of growing evidences implicate cyclin D1 in additional cellular processes including transcriptional regulation by interacting with transcription factors, chromatin-remodeling elements, and histone-modifying enzymes.[3,4] Cyclin D1 may also directly participate in DNA damage response and apoptosis regulation.[5,6] Interestingly, cyclin D1 binds to a high number of active promoters and interacts with the transcription machinery leading to a global transcriptome down-modulation in neoplastic lymphoid cells,[7]

VARIANT CCND1 TRANSLOCATIONS AND EXPRESSION IN MANTLE CELL LYMPHOMA

A small subset of MCL cases show CCND1 rearrangement with IgK or IgL light chain resulting in variant translocations t(2;11) (p11;q13)[8] and t(11;22) (q13;q11.2),[9] respectively, that determine similar cyclin D1 dysregulation. Intriguingly, recent studies have reported a minor subset of MCL that expresses cyclin D1 protein and high mRNA levels but CCND1 rearrangements are not detected when evaluated by conventional cytogenetics or fluorescence in situ hybridization (FISH) using fusion or break-apart probes. Whole-genome sequencing (WGS) or FISH using custom bacterial artificial clones-labeled probes have detected that these cases carry cryptic rearrangements of IgK or IgL enhancers with CCND1 gene which may be responsible for the cyclin D1 upregulation. The clinical and pathologic features of this small subgroup of patients are similar to conventional MCL, suggesting that they correspond to the same molecular entity.[10,11] This finding is in line with the identification by WGS of cryptic insertions of MYC into the IGH locus in IG-MYC negative Burkitt lymphoma cases,[12] or the detection of cryptic rearrangements involving MYC and BCL2 in high-grade B-cell lymphomas.[13]

CYCLIN D1–NEGATIVE MANTLE CELL LYMPHOMA

A particular subset of cases with the same MCL morphology and phenotype lack cyclin D1 expression and t(11;14) translocation (cyclin D1⁻ MCL).[14–16] These tumors have also similar gene expression profile, secondary chromosomal alterations, and clinical behavior as cyclin D1⁺ MCL, suggesting that they correspond to the same disease.[15–17] These cases should be distinguished from the uncommon MCL carrying the t(11;14) in which the cyclin D1 expression is not detected by immunohistochemistry due to mutations in the C-terminal domain of CCND1 or the presence of CCND1b as the only expressed isoform that renders the protein undetectable by current antibodies used in the pathology diagnostic routine.[18]

Initial FISH studies identified chromosomal rearrangements fusing *CCND2* with IG loci (IgH, IgK, or IgL) in 55% of cyclin D1⁻ MCL.[15] However, the primary oncogenic event remained elusive in a substantial fraction of these cases. More recently, next generation sequencing (NGS) studies and FISH with custom probes have found the insertion of a small IgK region including its enhancer near *CCND3* (16%) or *CCND2* (7%), leading to cyclin D3 or cyclin D2 overexpression, respectively. Similar cryptic insertions involving the IgL-enhancer in the vicinity of *CCND3* associated with cyclin D3 overexpression have been also detected in a subset of cyclin D1⁻ MCL. Overall, 23% of the cyclin D1⁻ MCL cases showed an Ig light chain enhancer hijacking as initial oncogenic event.[19]

SOX11: A KEY ONCOGENIC FACTOR

SOX11 is a transcription factor that plays an important oncogenic role in MCL pathogenesis through its impact in B-cell differentiation, tumor microenvironment interactions, cell cycle control, and apoptosis.[20,21] SOX11 is not expressed in normal lymphoid cells or other mature B-cell lymphomas with the exception of 25% to 50% of Burkitt lymphoma, but it is highly expressed in conventional MCL, including cyclin D1⁻MCL.[17] Hence, SOX11-nuclear staining is a useful tool in the differential diagnosis of MCL and other small B-cell neoplasias. SOX11 may contribute to MCL pathogenesis by the constitutive activation of PAX5, a master regulator of B-cell development, that blocks terminal B-cell differentiation and promotes tumor growth.[21] Another SOX11 direct regulated target is BCL6, an essential element for B-cell development and maintenance of follicular germinal centers (GC). SOX11 may block BCL6 expression preventing the entrance of MCL cells in the GC.[20] The transgenic mouse model (Eμ-SOX11-EGFP) developed by Kuo and colleagues[22] shows hyperactivation of pBTK and other molecules of the B-cell receptor (BCR) signaling pathway driving tumor development. Moreover, SOX11 regulates interactions of MCL cells with the microenvironment inducing angiogenesis through PDGFA[23] and promoting tumor cell migration, adhesion, and cell proliferation by upregulating CXCR4 and FAK.[24] Accordingly, treatment in vitro of MCL cells with FAK inhibitors could overcome ibrutinib resistance.[25]

In spite of the relevant role of SOX11 in MCL the mechanisms leading to its specific upregulation in this lymphoma are not well understood. Recent studies have suggested that SOX11 expression in these cells could be mediated by epigenetic mechanisms that alter the 3-dimensional configuration of chromatin bringing together a distant active enhancer region with the promoter of the gene.[26]

MANTLE CELL LYMPHOMA MOLECULAR SUBTYPES: DISTINCT PATHOGENIC PATHWAYS

The initial translocation t(11;14) (q13;q32) may be followed by 2 distinct pathogenic pathways resulting in 2 subtypes of tumors with different biological behavior. The most common subtype is the conventional MCL (cMCL), that derives from a cell that does not enter into the follicular GC and carry no or a limited number of IGHV somatic mutations (**Fig. 1**).[27] The second subtype, leukemic non-nodal MCL (nnMCL), derives from a cell that has gone through the GC acquiring IGHV somatic mutations.[28] These 2 subtypes have different cellular origin, a naïve-like B-cell for cMCL and an experienced GC memory-like B cell for nnMCL. This idea is supported by the observation that both subtypes retain the DNA methylation pattern of their normal cellular counterparts.[26,28]

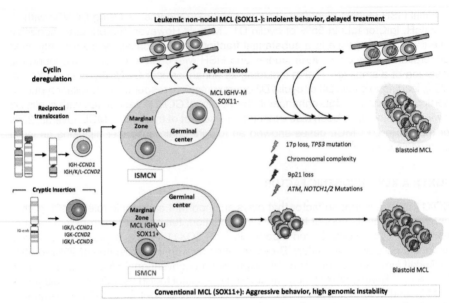

Fig. 1. MCL molecular subtypes. The naïve B-cell with cyclin deregulation may evolve into 2 distinct molecular subtypes with different molecular and clinicopathological characteristics.

Although cMCL and nnMCL share similar global gene expression profiles, they differ in some genetic and molecular characteristics. cMCL cases overexpress SOX11, are genetically unstable and tend to accumulate many chromosomal alterations. Clinically, patients with cMCL usually have generalized lymphadenopathy at diagnosis and follow an aggressive clinical course.[29,30] Contrarily, nnMCL present an initial indolent disease that may be stable for long periods of time. Patients have leukemic involvement with minimal lymphadenopathy and later on may develop splenomegaly.[31–35] These cases might benefit of a careful observation management without negatively impacting their outcome.[36–39] Although nnMCL cells initially harbor few or no chromosomal alterations besides the t(11;14), they may evolve over time acquiring TP53 mutation, 17p loss and increased genome instability that confer a dismal prognosis.[34] Recently, a 16-gene assay on the NanoString platform (L-MCL16 assay) has been used to classify patients with leukemic involvement into cMCL or nnMCL subgroups and, in combination with genomic complexity and TP53 alterations, predict patients' outcome.[35]

FROM EARLY LESIONS TO AN OVERT LYMPHOMA

The oncogenic steps from the early CCND1 rearrangement to the development of an overt lymphoma are not well known. The detection of cells carrying the t(11;14) in the peripheral blood of 8% of healthy individuals suggests that not all the cells acquiring the initial translocation will evolve into a malignant lymphoma.[36] These clones may persist for long latency periods before evolving into a malignant neoplasm as supported by the observation of a simultaneous MCL with the same clonal origin in the recipient and donor 12 years after an allogeneic bone marrow transplantation.[37]

Cyclin D1–positive cells are occasionally found in the inner mantle zone of reactive lymphoid follicles, a situation now known as in situ mantle cell neoplasia (ISMCN) (see **Fig. 1**). These in situ lesions are usually identified incidentally and sometimes in association with other lymphomas.[38,39] Although some of these cases may affect different territories the patients have a long-term follow-up without developing progressive disease in the absence therapeutic intervention. The proportion of ISMCN that may develop an overt lymphoma is not well known but seems very low.[40] However, some patients with these lesions may have already a disseminated MCL at diagnosis and therefore they should be explored carefully to rule out this situation (see **Fig. 1**).

THE HALLMARKS OF CANCER IN MANTLE CELL LYMPHOMA

The concept of cancer hallmarks helped to dissect the malignant phenotypes that are associated with specific physiologic circuits dysregulated during the oncogenic process.[41] The order in which the different neoplasias acquire their hallmarks capabilities and their contribution during oncogenesis depends on the type of tumor. In MCL, the t(11;14) translocation responsible of cyclin D1 dysregulation would represent the initial acquisition of a sustained proliferative signaling. However, this event is not sufficient to explain the MCL pathogenesis. Secondary genetic alterations would reinforce the proliferation dysregulation and promote the acquisition of additional hallmarks relevant to MCL lymphomagenesis (**Fig. 2**).

Sustaining Proliferative Signaling and Growth Suppressors Evasion

An essential feature of tumor cells is their capacity for continuous proliferation together with the ability to circumvent the constrain proliferation promoted by tumor suppressors under cell stress conditions. In MCL, the initial dysregulation of cyclin D1 may promote G1/S phase transition through the binding of the cyclin to CDK4, followed by RB1 phosphorylation, and subsequent E2F release. Besides this initial alteration, secondary genetic events also impact directly in cell cycle control affecting mainly 2 pathways INK4A/CDK4/RB1 and ARF/MDM2/TP53. The 12q13 amplification (20%) may led to CDK4 overexpression that would further promote cell cycle dysregulation.[42] Interestingly, the inhibition of CDK4 can be a reliable mechanism to overcome the ibrutinib resistance in MCL patients.[43] The 9p21 deletion (25%), involving the *CDKN2A*, is one of the most frequent genetic alteration in MCL. *CDKN2A* gene encodes for p16 (*INK4A*), a cyclin-dependent kinase inhibitor that specifically inhibits CDK4 and CDK6 keeping RB1 active, and for p14 (*ARF*), a E3 ubiquitin-protein ligase that stabilize p53 by interacting with MDM2 preventing its degradation.[42] Alternatively, few MCL cases with wild-type *CDKN2A* show *BMI1* (10q13) amplification and overexpression which act as a transcriptional repressor of the *CDKN2A* locus.[44] Inactivation of *CDKN2A* is associated with an unfavorable prognosis in MCL patients and is related to aggressive variants.[45] Similarly, inactivation of *RB1* by mutations and homozygous deletion, although uncommon, occurs mainly in aggressive cases.[46] Other genetic alterations targeting cell cycle–related genes that might confer increased proliferation rates are *MYC* amplification and translocation,[44,47] and deletions of *CUL4A* and *ING1* (13q34).[48]

The high number of genetic alterations that potentially dysregulate cell cycle in MCL underscores the relevance of this hallmark in MCL pathogenesis. Moreover, its relevance is supported by the fact that the best predictor of patient survival in MCL is a proliferation gene expression signature that may integrate the multiple genetic alterations dysregulating cell cycle and may now be reliably determined in formalin fixed paraffin embedded tissues (MCL35 proliferation assay).[49,50]

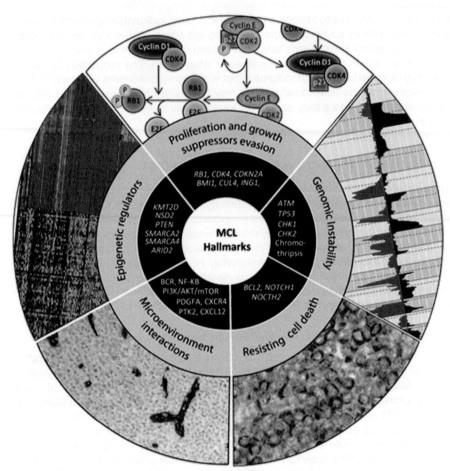

Fig. 2. MCL hallmarks. The conceptual framework encompasses many different cellular functions that transform normal cells into malignant cancer cells. All the related pathways involved in MCL pathogenesis may be globally grouped into 5 main hallmarks.

Genomic Instability

Cancer cells have a tendency to accumulate genetic alterations and increased genomic instability, a hallmark of many tumors. MCL is one of the B-cell malignancies with highest degree of genomic instability. More than 90% of the MCL cases display highly altered genomes, with gains/amplifications and homozygous/heterozygous losses, as well as other non-recurrent chromosomal rearrangements. Losses in 1p, 6q, 8p, 9p, 9q, 10p, 11q, 13q, and 17p and gains in 3q, 7p, 8q, 10p, 15q, and 18q are the most frequent chromosomal alterations identified in MCL.[51] The high number of chromosome alterations in MCL cells is consistent with the fact that the 2 most common mutated genes are *ATM* (40%–50%) and *TP53* (21%–45%), both involved in DNA damage response. *ATM* alterations, including mutations and 11q deletions, are considered early events but do not correlate with prognosis, despite being related to increased chromosomal instability.[52] Downregulation of *CHK2* and *CHK1*, 2 critical serine-threonine kinases involved in signal transduction during DNA damage response, may constitute another mechanism to promote chromosome instability in a limited number of MCL cases.[53] *TP53* is frequently inactivated by point mutations and 17p13 deletion, compromising the p53-mediated cell cycle arrest, apoptosis, and senescence as response to DNA damage. *TP53* alterations are identified at similar proportion in cMCL and nnMCL. Additionally, the increased number of chromosomal imbalances, *TP53* mutations, and global genetic instability are associated with blastoid variants and worse clinical outcome in MCL patients.[35,54–56]

Resisting Cell Death

The evasion of apoptotic cell death, considered a natural barrier to cancer development, is a key hallmark of cancer cells. In MCL, dysregulation of the anti-apoptotic protein BCL2 mainly by amplifications or mRNA overexpression is described in 3% to 17% of cases. Upregulation of other proteins of the BCL-family, like BCLX, as well as occasional biallelic loss of the proapoptic *BCL2L11* (2q13) have been also observed.[57] In the past decade, several reports have described recurrent gain-of-function truncating mutations in *NOTCH1* (5%–14%) and *NOTCH2* (5%) associated with blastoid variants and dismal prognosis.[58,59] NOTCH pathway is one of the most evolutionary conserved signaling cascades across species that regulates cell death but also cell proliferation and activates specific differentiation programs.[60] NOTCH signaling regulates, directly or indirectly through MYC, a gene signature consisting of BCR signaling, RNA metabolism and chromatin/transcriptional modulation. Clinically, NOTCH targeted approaches may be a therapeutic option for a subset of patients.[61]

Modulation of Tumor Microenvironment Interactions

Normal B-cell maturation involves somatic recombination and mutation of the IGHV genes that encode the antigen binding domains of the BCR. The observation of restricted repertoires of IGHV genes in MCL, called BCR IG stereotypy, highlights the antigen selection and BCR signaling pathway as important hallmark for MCL pathogenesis.[62] Additionally, constitutive activation of the BCR signaling pathway has a key role promoting survival and proliferation of the malignant B cells. Although the specific mechanisms involved in this deregulation are not well understood, different BCR associated kinases including tyrosine protein kinase (LYN), spleen tyrosine kinase (SYK),[63] and especially Bruton's tyrosine kinase (BTK) are considered therapeutic targets due to their constitutive activation or amplification in MCL. In this context, the oral covalent inhibitor of BTK ibrutinib, shows durable single-agent efficacy in MCL cases.[64] Recently, in the MCL-0208 trial, high expression levels of a 6-gene BCR signature (*AKT3, BCL2, BTK, CD79B, PIK3CD*, and *SYK*) was associated with shorter progression-free survival and OS.[65]

The constitutive activation of PI3K/AKT and NF-κB signaling pathways also play a relevant role in MCL pathogenesis. Activated PI3K/AKT/mTOR components target a wide range of downstream processes in MCL, including angiogenesis but also cell survival, growth, and protein synthesis. Activation of downstream kinases such as SYK and *PI3KCA* amplification may cause activation if this pathway and can determine the therapeutic potential of small molecule inhibitors.[66] The activation of the canonical NF-κB pathway directly correlates with increased tumor proliferation and inferior survival in MCL.[67] The NF-κB activation can be mediated by different alterations, mainly by inactivating mutations or deletions in negative regulators as *TNFAIP3/A20*,[68] *TRAF2, BIRC3, NFKBIE*, and *CARD11*. *NFKBIE* deletions are associated with poor outcome,[69] meanwhile *TRAF2* and *BIRC3* mutations are associated with resistance to ibrutinib therapies in MCL.[63] The antiapoptotic proteins BCL-2, BCL-X$_L$, XIAP and cFLIP, are also NF-κB targets highly expressed in MCL.[70,71]

In addition, during tumor progression the ability to sprout new blood vessels must be kept intact. Experimental studies have shown that SOX11 expression is associated with an angiogenic switch trough platelet-derived growth factor subunit A (PDGFA) activation and is characterized by increased expression of angiogenic-related signatures and vascularization.[23,72] Interestingly, SOX11 directly regulates CXCR4 and PTK2 conferring a protective microenvironment-related signature in SOX11+ MCL cases. CXCR4 and CXCL12 overexpression enhance FAK activation promoting MCL cell migration and adhesion facilitating the crosstalk with the stromal cells that confers survival and drug resistance to MCL cells.[24]

Epigenetic Dysregulation

Epigenetic dysregulation can promote malignant cellular transformation and is considered a hallmark for a large number of different neoplasms. In the past years, the characterization of whole tumor cell methylomes confirmed the critical role that DNA methylation plays in MCL tumorigenesis and it was identified as a dynamic process prone to be altered on neoplastic transformation. In MCL cells, an increased DNA methylation burden, defined as the number of methylation changes acquired by tumor cells, is associated with worse clinical outcome and higher number of driver mutations.[26] Moreover, the genomic analysis of MCL has revealed that epigenetic modulators are recurrent altered targets. The most frequently mutated epigenetic modifier in MCL is *KMT2D* (17%–23%), a regulator of transcriptional and posttranslational processes of which mutations may impact on the outcome of patients.[55] Mutations in the catalytic domain of the *NSD2* are also found in cMCL and are associated with overexpression of signatures related to proliferation and cell cycle, as well as with global chromatin methylation driving oncogenic reprogramming in other lymphoid malignancies.[73,74] Recently, *NSD2* has been described to mediate dimethylation of PTEN and facilitate its recruitment into DNA-damage sites contributing to the repair of DNA double strand breaks.[75] Moreover, alterations in SWI-SNF chromatin-remodeling complexes, including *SMARCA4* mutations (5%–12%) or deletions involving *SMARCA2* (9p24) or *ARID2* (12q12) confer resistance to ibrutinib and venetoclax.[76] Other dysregulated epigenetic modifiers are *KMT2C* (5%–16%), *BMI1* (6%–12%), and *TET2* (5%–12%). Finally, mutations targeting regulators of transcription such as *MEF2B* (3%–7%) or post-transcription *UBR5* (7%–18%) are also recurrently found in MCL.[58,77]

SUMMARY

The translocation t(11;14) is the genetic hallmark of MCL, although cryptic rearrangements of Ig regulatory regions could be an alternative oncogenic mechanism in a minor subgroup of patients. Interestingly this Ig enhancer hijacking phenomenon is found recurrently in MCL cyclin D1$^-$ cases with cyclin D2 or cyclin D3 overexpression. MCL is considered one of the most aggressive lymphomas. However, a small subset of cases may follow an initial indolent clinical course without need of treatment. The presence of IGHV somatic mutations, leukemic expression in the absence of lymphadenopathies, as well as low number of genomic alterations are characteristics that differentiate nnMCL from cMCL cases. The dysregulation of cyclin D1, although considered the primary oncogenic event, is not enough for malignant transformation of B-cell clones. In this sense, additional somatic genetic alterations affecting genes involved in many cancer hallmarks, like cell cycle control (*CDKN2A*, CDK4, and

RB1), DNA damage response (*TP53, ATM, CDKN2A,* and *MYC*), epigenetic modulation (*KMT2D, SMARCA4,* and *NSD2*) and NF-κB signaling pathways (*BIRC3, NFKBIE,* and *TNFAIP3*) among others, may impact MCL lymphomagenesis. In addition, SOX11 seems to collaborate with cyclin D1 in MCL pathogenesis, regulating a complex transcriptional program and enhancing the aggressiveness of the tumor. The better understanding of MCL pathogenesis generated by the use of NGS technologies and the integration of multidisciplinary research, from molecular biology and pathology to the clinic, has revealed new potential management strategies for the treatment of aggressive MCL.

ACKNOWLEDGMENTS

This work was supported by research funding from Fondo de Investigaciones Sanitarias, Instituto de Salud Carlos III (PI17/01061 to S. Beà), National Institutes of Health "Molecular Diagnosis, Prognosis, and Therapeutic Targets in Mantle Cell Lymphoma" (P01CA229100 to E. Campo); Spanish Ministerio de Ciencia, Innovación y Universidades (RTI2018-094274-B-I00 to E. Campo; Generalitat de Catalunya Suport Grups de Recerca AGAUR (2017-SGR-1142 to E. Campo). E. Campo is an Academia Researcher of the "Institució Catalana de Recerca i Estudis Avançats (ICREA)" of the Generalitat de Catalunya. This work was mainly developed at the Center Esther Koplowitz (CEK), Barcelona, Spain. The authors are grateful to Sílvia Ruiz for their technical and logistic assistance.

REFERENCES

1. Kuppers R, La-Favera R. Mechanisms of chromosomal translocations in B cell lymphomas. Oncogene 2001;20(40):5580–94.
2. Wiestner A, Tehrani M, Chiorazzi M, et al. Point mutations and genomic deletions in CCND1 create stable truncated cyclin D1 mRNAs that are associated with increased proliferation rate and shorter survival. Blood 2007;109(11):4599–606.
3. Aggarwal P, Vaites LP, Kim JK, et al. Nuclear cyclin D1/CDK4 kinase regulates CUL4 expression and triggers neoplastic growth via activation of the PRMT5 methyltransferase. Cancer Cell 2010;18(4):329–40.
4. Bienvenu F, Jirawatnotai S, Elias JE, et al. Transcriptional role of cyclin D1 in development revealed by a genetic-proteomic screen. Nature 2010;463(7279): 374–8.
5. Jirawatnotai S, Hu Y, Livingston DM, et al. Proteomic identification of a direct role for cyclin d1 in DNA damage repair. Cancer Res 2012;72(17):4289–93.
6. Beltran E, Fresquet V, Martinez-Useros J, et al. A cyclin-D1 interaction with BAX underlies its oncogenic role and potential as a therapeutic target in mantle cell lymphoma. Proc Natl Acad Sci U S A 2011;108(30):12461–6.
7. Albero R, Enjuanes A, Demajo S, et al. Cyclin D1 overexpression induces global transcriptional downregulation in lymphoid neoplasms. J Clin Invest 2018;128(9): 4132–47.
8. Wlodarska I, Meeus P, Stul M, et al. Variant t(2;11)(p11;q13) associated with the IgK-CCND1 rearrangement is a recurrent translocation in leukemic small-cell B-non-Hodgkin lymphoma. Leukemia 2004;18(10):1705–10.
9. Marrero WD, Cruz-Chacon A, Cabanillas F. Mantle Cell Lymphoma with t(11;22) (q13;q11.2) an indolent clinical variant? Leuk Lymphoma 2018;59(10):2509–11.
10. Peterson JF, Baughn LB, Ketterling RP, et al. Characterization of a cryptic IGH/ CCND1 rearrangement in a case of mantle cell lymphoma with negative CCND1 FISH studies. Blood Adv 2019;3(8):1298–302.

11. Fuster C, Martin-Garcia D, Balague O, et al. Cryptic insertions of the immuno-globulin light chain enhancer region near CCND1 in t(11;14)-negative mantle cell lymphoma. Haematologica 2019. https://doi.org/10.3324/haematol.2019.237073.

12. Wagener R, Bens S, Toprak UH, et al. Cryptic insertion of MYC exons 2 and 3 into the IGH locus detected by whole genome sequencing in a case of MYC-negative Burkitt lymphoma. Haematologica 2020;105(4):e202–5.

13. Hilton LK, Tang J, Ben-Neriah S, et al. The double-hit signature identifies double-hit diffuse large B-cell lymphoma with genetic events cryptic to FISH. Blood 2019;134(18):1528–32.

14. Seto M. Cyclin D1-negative mantle cell lymphoma. Blood 2013;121(8):1249–50.

15. Salaverria I, Royo C, Carvajal-Cuenca A, et al. CCND2 rearrangements are the most frequent genetic events in cyclin D1(-) mantle cell lymphoma. Blood 2013;121(8):1394–402.

16. Fu K, Weisenburger DD, Greiner TC, et al. Cyclin D1-negative mantle cell lymphoma: a clinicopathologic study based on gene expression profiling. Blood 2005;106(13):4315–21.

17. Mozos A, Royo C, Hartmann E, et al. SOX11 expression is highly specific for mantle cell lymphoma and identifies the cyclin D1-negative subtype. Haematologica 2009;94(11):1555–62.

18. Iaccarino I, Afify L, Aukema SM, et al. t(11;14)-positive mantle cell lymphomas lacking cyclin D1 (CCND1) immunostaining because of a CCND1 mutation or exclusive expression of the CCND1b isoform. Haematologica 2018;103(9):e432–5.

19. Martin-Garcia D, Navarro A, Valdes-Mas R, et al. CCND2 and CCND3 hijack immunoglobulin light-chain enhancers in cyclin D1(-) mantle cell lymphoma. Blood 2019;133(9):940–51.

20. Palomero J, Vegliante MC, Eguileor A, et al. SOX11 defines two different sub-types of mantle cell lymphoma through transcriptional regulation of BCL6. Leuke-mia 2016;30(7):1596–9.

21. Vegliante MC, Palomero J, Perez-Galan P, et al. SOX11 regulates PAX5 expres-sion and blocks terminal B-cell differentiation in aggressive mantle cell lym-phoma. Blood 2013;121(12):2175–85.

22. Kuo P-Y, Jatiani SS, Rahman AH, et al. SOX11 augments BCR signaling to drive MCL-like tumor development. Blood 2018;131(20):2247–55.

23. Palomero J, Vegliante MC, Rodriguez ML, et al. SOX11 promotes tumor angio-genesis through transcriptional regulation of PDGFA in mantle cell lymphoma. Blood 2014;124(14):2235–47.

24. Balsas P, Palomero J, Eguileor A, et al. SOX11 promotes tumor protective micro-environment interactions through CXCR4 and FAK regulation in mantle cell lym-phoma. Blood 2017;130(4):501–13.

25. Rudelius M, Rosenfeldt MT, Leich E, et al. Inhibition of focal adhesion kinase over-comes resistance of mantle cell lymphoma to ibrutinib in the bone marrow micro-environment. Haematologica 2018;103(1):116–25.

26. Queiros AC, Beekman R, Vilarrasa-Blasi R, et al. Decoding the DNA Methylome of Mantle Cell Lymphoma in the Light of the Entire B Cell Lineage. Cancer Cell 2016;30(5):806–21.

27. Jares P, Colomer D, Campo E. Molecular pathogenesis of mantle cell lymphoma. J Clin Invest 2012;122(10):3416–23.

28. Navarro A, Clot G, Royo C, et al. Molecular subsets of mantle cell lymphoma defined by the IGHV mutational status and SOX11 expression have distinct biologic and clinical features. Cancer Res 2012;72(20):5307–16.

29. Fernandez V, Salamero O, Espinet B, et al. Genomic and gene expression profiling defines indolent forms of mantle cell lymphoma. Cancer Res 2010; 70(4):1408–18.

30. Ek S, Dictor M, Jerkeman M, et al. Nuclear expression of the non B-cell lineage Sox11 transcription factor identifies mantle cell lymphoma. Blood 2008;111(2): 800–5.

31. Espinet B, Ferrer A, Bellosillo B, et al. Distinction between asymptomatic monoclonal B-cell lymphocytosis with cyclin D1 overexpression and mantle cell lymphoma: from molecular profiling to flow cytometry. Clin Cancer Res 2014;20(4): 1007–19.

32. Martin P, Chadburn A, Christos P, et al. Outcome of deferred initial therapy in mantle-cell lymphoma. J Clin Oncol 2009;27(8):1209–13.

33. Orchard J, Garand R, Davis Z, et al. A subset of t(11;14) lymphoma with mantle cell features displays mutated IgVH genes and includes patients with good prognosis, nonnodal disease. Blood 2003;101(12):4975–81.

34. Royo C, Navarro A, Clot G, et al. Non-nodal type of mantle cell lymphoma is a specific biological and clinical subgroup of the disease. Leukemia 2012;26(8):6.

35. Clot G, Jares P, Gine E, et al. A gene signature that distinguishes conventional and leukemic nonnodal mantle cell lymphoma helps predict outcome. Blood 2018;132(4):413–22.

36. Lecluse Y, Lebailly P, Roulland S, et al. (11;14)-positive clones can persist over a long period of time in the peripheral blood of healthy individuals. Leukemia 2009; 23:1190–3.

37. Christian B, Zhao W, Hamadani M, et al. Mantle cell lymphoma 12 years after allogeneic bone marrow transplantation occurring simultaneously in recipient and donor. J Clin Oncol 2010;28(27):459–60.

38. Carvajal-Cuenca A, Sua LF, Silva NM, et al. In situ mantle cell lymphoma: Clinical implications of an incidental finding with indolent clinical behavior. Haematologica 2012;97(2):270–8.

39. Swerdlow SH, Campo E, Pileri SA, et al. The 2016 revision of the World Health Organization classification of lymphoid neoplasms. Blood 2016;127(20):2375–90.

40. Karube K, Scarfo L, Campo E, et al. Monoclonal B cell lymphocytosis and "in situ" lymphoma. Semin Cancer Biol 2014;24:3–14.

41. Hanahan D, Weinberg RA. Hallmarks of cancer: the next generation. Cell 2011; 144(5):646–74.

42. Hernandez L, Bea S, Pinyol M, et al. CDK4 and MDM2 gene alterations mainly occur in highly proliferative and aggressive mantle cell lymphomas with wild-type INK4a/ARF locus. Cancer Res 2005;65(6):2199–206.

43. Chiron D, Di LM, Martin P, et al. Cell-cycle reprogramming for PI3K inhibition overrides a relapse-specific C481S BTK mutation revealed by longitudinal functional genomics in mantle cell lymphoma. Cancer Discov 2014;4(9):1022–35.

44. Bea S, Ribas M, Hernandez JM, et al. Increased number of chromosomal imbalances and high-level DNA amplifications in mantle cell lymphoma are associated with blastoid variants. Blood 1999;93(12):4365–74.

45. Hoster E, Rosenwald A, Berger F, et al. Prognostic value of Ki-67 index, cytology, and growth pattern in mantle-cell lymphoma: results from randomized trials of the european mantle cell lymphoma network. J Clin Oncol 2016;34:1386–94.

46. Pinyol M, Bea S, Pla L, et al. Inactivation of RB1 in mantle-cell lymphoma detected by nonsense-mediated mRNA decay pathway inhibition and microarray analysis. Blood 2007;109(12):5422–9.

47. Hu Z, Medeiros LJ, Chen Z, et al. Mantle cell lymphoma with MYC rearrangement: a report of 17 patients. Am J Surg Pathol 2017;41(2):216–24.

48. Hartmann EM, Campo E, Wright G, et al. Pathway discovery in mantle cell lymphoma by integrated analysis of high-resolution gene expression and copy number profiling. Blood 2010;116(6):953–61.

49. Rosenwald A, Wright G, Wiestner A, et al. The proliferation gene expression signature is a quantitative integrator of oncogenic events that predicts survival in mantle cell lymphoma. Cancer Cell 2003;3(2):185–97.

50. Scott DW, Abrisqueta P, Wright GW, et al. New molecular assay for the proliferation signature in mantle cell lymphoma applicable to formalin-fixed paraffin-embedded biopsies. J Clin Oncol 2017;35(15):1668–77.

51. Salaverria I, Zettl A, Bea S, et al. Specific secondary genetic alterations in mantle cell lymphoma provide prognostic information independent of the gene expression-based proliferation signature. J Clin Oncol 2007;25(10):1216–22.

52. Camacho E, Hernandez L, Hernandez S, et al. ATM gene inactivation in mantle cell lymphoma mainly occurs by truncating mutations and missense mutations involving the phosphatidylinositol-3 kinase domain and is associated with increasing numbers of chromosomal imbalances. Blood 2002;99(1):238–44.

53. Tort F, Hernandez S, Bea S, et al. Checkpoint kinase 1 (CHK1) protein and mRNA expression is downregulated in aggressive variants of human lymphoid neoplasms. Leukemia 2005;19(1):112–7.

54. Delfau-Larue MH, Klapper W, Berger F, et al. High-dose cytarabine does not overcome the adverse prognostic value of CDKN2A and TP53 deletions in mantle cell lymphoma. Blood 2015;126(5):604–11.

55. Ferrero S, Rossi D, Rinaldi A, et al. KMT2D mutations and TP53 disruptions are poor prognostic biomarkers in mantle cell lymphoma receiving high-dose therapy: a FIL study. Haematologica 2019. https://doi.org/10.3324/haematol.2018.214056.

56. Eskelund CW, Dahl C, Hansen JW, et al. TP53 mutations identify younger mantle cell lymphoma patients who do not benefit from intensive chemoimmunotherapy. Blood 2017;130(17):1903–10.

57. Bea S, Salaverria I, Armengol L, et al. Uniparental disomies, homozygous deletions, amplifications, and target genes in mantle cell lymphoma revealed by integrative high-resolution whole-genome profiling. Blood 2009;113(13):3059–69.

58. Bea S, Valdes-Mas R, Navarro A, et al. Landscape of somatic mutations and clonal evolution in mantle cell lymphoma. Proc Natl Acad Sci U S A 2013;110(45):18250–5.

59. Kridel R, Meissner B, Rogic S, et al. Whole transcriptome sequencing reveals recurrent NOTCH1 mutations in mantle cell lymphoma. Blood 2012;119(9):1963–71.

60. Kopan R, Ilagan MXG. The canonical Notch signaling pathway: unfolding the activation mechanism. Cell 2009;137(2):216–33.

61. Silkenstedt E, Arenas F, Colom-Sanmarti B, et al. Notch1 signaling in NOTCH1-mutated mantle cell lymphoma depends on Delta-Like ligand 4 and is a potential target for specific antibody therapy. J Exp Clin Cancer Res 2019;38(1):446.

62. Hadzidimitriou A, Agathangelidis A, Darzentas N, et al. Is there a role for antigen selection in mantle cell lymphoma? Immunogenetic support from a series of 807 cases. Blood 2011;118(11):3088–95.

63. Hershkovitz-Rokah O, Pulver D, Lenz G, et al. Ibrutinib resistance in mantle cell lymphoma: clinical, molecular and treatment aspects. Br J Haematol 2018; 181(3):306–19.
64. Wang ML, Rule S, Martin P, et al. Targeting BTK with ibrutinib in relapsed or refractory mantle-cell lymphoma. N Engl J Med 2013;369(6):507–16.
65. Bomben R, Ferrero S, D'Agaro T, et al. A B-cell receptor-related gene signature predicts survival in mantle cell lymphoma: results from the Fondazione Italiana Linfomi MCL-0208 trial. Haematologica 2018;103(5):849–56.
66. Psyrri A, Papageorgiou S, Liakata E, et al. Phosphatidylinositol 3'-kinase catalytic subunit alpha gene amplification contributes to the pathogenesis of mantle cell lymphoma. Clin Cancer Res 2009;15(18):5724–32.
67. Balaji S, Ahmed M, Lorence E, et al. NF-kappaB signaling and its relevance to the treatment of mantle cell lymphoma. J Hematol Oncol 2018;11(1):83.
68. Honma K, Tsuzuki S, Nakagawa M, et al. TNFAIP3/A20 functions as a novel tumor suppressor gene in several subtypes of non-Hodgkin lymphomas. Blood 2009; 114(12):2467–75.
69. Mansouri L, Noerenberg D, Young E, et al. Frequent NFKBIE deletions are associated with poor outcome in primary mediastinal B-cell lymphoma. Blood 2016; 128(23):2666–70.
70. Pham LV, Tamayo AT, Yoshimura LC, et al. Inhibition of constitutive NF-kappa B activation in mantle cell lymphoma B cells leads to induction of cell cycle arrest and apoptosis. J Immunol 2003;171(1):88–95.
71. Roue G, Perez-Galan P, Lopez-Guerra M, et al. Selective inhibition of IkappaB kinase sensitizes mantle cell lymphoma B cells to TRAIL by decreasing cellular FLIP level. J Immunol 2007;178(3):1923–30.
72. Petrakis G, Veloza L, Clot G, et al. Increased tumour angiogenesis in SOX11-positive mantle cell lymphoma. Histopathology 2019;75(5):704–14.
73. Oyer JA, Huang X, Zheng Y, et al. Point mutation E1099K in MMSET/NSD2 enhances its methyltranferase activity and leads to altered global chromatin methylation in lymphoid malignancies. Leukemia 2014;28(1):198–201.
74. Valdes-Mas R, Bea S, Puente DA, et al. Estimation of copy number alterations from exome sequencing data. PLoS One 2012;7(12):e51422.
75. Zhang J, Lee Y-R, Dang F, et al. PTEN methylation by NSD2 controls cellular sensitivity to DNA damage. Cancer Discov 2019;9(9):1306–23.
76. Agarwal R, Chan YC, Tam CS, et al. Dynamic molecular monitoring reveals that SWI-SNF mutations mediate resistance to ibrutinib plus venetoclax in mantle cell lymphoma. Nat Med 2019;25(1):119–29.
77. Meissner B, Kridel R, Lim RS, et al. The E3 ubiquitin ligase UBR5 is recurrently mutated in mantle cell lymphoma. Blood 2013;121(16):3161–4.

Cell Cycle Dysregulation in Mantle Cell Lymphoma
Genomics and Therapy

Kevin Wang, BS[a,1], Xiangao Huang, PhD[a,1],
Maurizio Di Liberto, PhD[a], Selina Chen-Kiang, PhD[b,*]

KEYWORDS

- Mantle cell lymphoma • Palbociclib • Ibrutinib • CDK4 • Cyclin D1 • Rb • p16[INK4a]

KEY POINTS

- Deletions and amplifications of genes controlling cell cycle progression through early G1 are frequent in mantle cell lymphoma (MCL) cells.
- Targeting CDK4/6 with palbociclib appears to deepen and prolong the clinical response to ibrutinib in MCL.
- CDK4/6 inhibition may modulate tumor-immune interaction in MCL.
- Longitudinal functional genomics of patient specimens represents the best approach to discover resistant biomarkers for CDK4/6 inhibitor therapy.

INTRODUCTION

A hallmark of mantle cell lymphoma (MCL) is aberrant cyclin D1 expression in tumor cells due to a t(11;14) (q13;q32) chromosomal translocation (**Fig. 1**A, **Table 1**),[1] which places the *CCND1* genes (encoding cyclin D1) under the control of the immunoglobulin heavy chain enhancer.[2–5] Constitutive cyclin D1 expression in MCL cells is aberrant because normal mature human B cells express only cyclin D2 or cyclin D3 but no cyclin D1.[6] It accelerates the assembly of an active cyclin D–cyclin-dependent kinase 4 (CDK4) complex that drives cell cycle progression through early G1 by phosphorylating Rb and subsequently releasing E2Fs from phosphorylated Rb (CDK6 is barely expressed in MCL cells). In turn, E2Fs transcriptionally regulate genes that promote cell cycle progression through S (*CCNA2*, *PCNA*, and *TK1*), G2-M (*CDK1*), and cell division as well as a multitude of other genes that modulate cellular functions, such as

[a] Department of Pathology and Laboratory Medicine, 1300 York Avenue, C316, New York, NY 10065, USA; [b] Department of Pathology and Laboratory Medicine, Program in Immunology and Microbial Pathogenesis, Weill Cornell Medical College, 1300 York Avenue, Room C316, New York, NY 10065, USA
[1] Authors contributed equally.
* Corresponding author.
E-mail address: sckiang@med.cornell.edu

Hematol Oncol Clin N Am 34 (2020) 809–823
https://doi.org/10.1016/j.hoc.2020.05.003
0889-8588/20/© 2020 Elsevier Inc. All rights reserved.

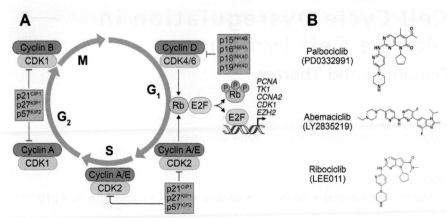

Fig. 1. (*A*) A schema of the mammalian cell cycle. When released from Rb after it is phosphorylated by cyclin D1–CDK4, E2F1 directly activates the transcription of *CCNA2* (encoding cyclin A), *TK1* (encoding thymidine kinase), *PCNA* (encoding proliferating cell nuclear antigen), *CDK1* (encoding cyclin-dependent kinase I), and *EZH2* (encoding EZH2), among other target genes. (*B*) Three oral small molecule reversible CDK4/6 inhibitors.

EZH2[7] (see **Fig. 1**A). To ensure that the cell cycle progresses as programmed, the CDK4/6 activity is subject to negative control by 4 physiologic inhibitors (p16^{INK4a}, p15^{INK4b}, p18^{INK4c}, and p19^{INK4d}) (see **Fig. 1**A).

Following the discovery of *CCND1* translocation, Dreyling and colleagues[8] provided the first evidence that the Rb-p16^{INK4a} axis plays an important role in MCL biology. Fluorescence in situ hybridization (FISH) demonstrated that *CDKN2A* (encoding p16^{INK4a}) and *RB1* (encoding Rb) frequently were deleted (41%) in primary MCL cells and that deletion of *CDKN2A*, but not *RB1*, correlated with proliferation as determined by Ki67 expression (see **Table 1**). Based on gene expression profiling, it was further suggested that deletions of the *INK4a/ARF* locus determine the tumor proliferation rate and survival in synergy with the abundance of cyclin D1 mRNA.[9] Ki67 then was shown to be a prognostic indicator for the patients treated with immunochemotherapy in MCL.[10] Collectively, these findings provide a strong rationale to control proliferation of MCL cells by inhibiting CDK4/6, especially in progression disease. Clinical trials targeting CDK4/6 in combination therapy in recurrent MCL have shown promise, but more needs to be done to fully understand the underpinnings and identify resistant biomarkers. To advance precision medicine–based cell cycle therapy, this article reviews genomic aberrations and functions of key cell cycle genes in MCL cells as well as clinical trials of CDK4/6 inhibitors for MCL. Integrative longitudinal functional genomics is discussed as a strategy to discover genomic drivers for resistance in tumor cells and tumor-immune interactions that potentially contribute to the clinical response to palbociclib combination therapy for MCL.

GENOMIC ABERRATIONS IN KEY CELL CYCLE GENES IN MANTLE CELL LYMPHOMA CELLS
G0–G1

The primary cause for aberrant cyclin D1 expression in MCL is the signature t(11;14)(q13;q32) chromosomal translocation[1] (**Fig. 1**, see **Table 1**). Amplification and mutations of *CCND1*, however, also contribute to cyclin D1 overexpression associated with poor prognosis. For example, truncating deletions and point mutations in the

Table 1
Genomic alterations in cell cycle genes in primary mantle cell lymphoma cells

Gene (Protein)	Locus	Genomic Alterations	Method	References
CCND1	11q13.3	t(11;14) (q13;q32) translocation, causing cyclin D1 overexpression	Southern blot, PCR, Sanger sequencing	Williams et al,[1] 1993
		Deletions in 3'-UTR in 7 of15 cases, creating stable truncated mRNAs	qPCR	Wiestner et al,[11] 2007
		Point mutations in proximal 3'-UTR in 3 of 15 cases, creating stable truncated mRNAs via premature polyadenylation	Cycle sequencing	Wiestner et al,[11] 2007
		Nonsynonymous SNVs in 17 of 90 samples in 5'-UTR or exon 1	Sanger sequencing	Kridel et al,[16] 2012
		Mutations in 10 of 29 cases, most in exon 1, and more common in SOX11⁻ and/or IGHV-mutated MCL	WES	Bea et al,[17] 2013
		Mutations in 19 of 102 cases (26 nonsynonymous, all in exon 1)	Targeted sequencing	Meissner et al,[15] 2013
		Missense mutations in 9 of 56 cases	WES	Zhang et al,[12] 2014
		Mutations in 15 of 176 cases	NGS, Sanger sequencing	Eskelund et al,[14] 2017
		Missense mutations in 3 of 16 cases	WES	Yang et al,[13] 2018
		Mutations in 2 of 24 cases, all in nonresponders to ibrutinib-venetoclax therapy	WES, WGS, targeted sequencing	Agarwal et al,[18] 2019
CCND2	12p13.32	Rearrangements of Ig light chain enhancer regions in 43 of 56 CCND1⁻ cases, associated with overexpression	FISH	Martin-Garcia et al,[19] 2019
CCND3	6p21.1	Rearrangements of Ig light chain enhancer regions in 9/56 CCND1⁻ cases, associated with overexpression	WGS, WES, Sanger sequencing , FISH	Martin-Garcia et al,[19] 2019
CDK4	12q14.1	12q gains in 9 of 45 cases, associated with CDK4 amplification in 5 of 6 such cases	CGH	Bea et al,[21] 1999
		Copy number gains in 4 of 69 cases, all in highly proliferative blastoid MCL	qPCR	Hernandez et al,[20] 2005
		Monoallelic deletions in 2 of 129 cases, gain in 8 cases	qPCR, MLPA	Delfau-Larue et al,[25] 2015

(continued on next page)

Table 1
(continued)

Gene (Protein)	Locus	Genomic Alterations	Method	References
CDKN2A (p16[INK4a])	9p21.3	Deletions in 15 of 37 cases (9 hemizygous, 6 homozygous)	FISH	Dreyling et al,[8] 1997
		Deletions in 3 of 24 cases (2 homozygous), all associated with aggressive MCL	Southern blot	Pinyol et al,[23] 1997
		A148T mutation in 1 of 21 cases	PCR-SSCP	Pinyol et al,[23] 1997
		Deletions in 18 of 85 cases, more common in proliferative MCLs	qPCR	Rosenwald et al,[9] 2003
		Deletions in 3 of 15 cases	Microarray	Fernandez et al,[24] 2010
		Recurrent homozygous deletions, but no mutations	WES	Bea et al,[17] 2013
		Deletions in 34 of 134 cases (19 monoallelic, 15 biallelic), associated with poor prognosis	qPCR, MLPA	Delfau-Larue et al,[25] 2015
		Deletions in 35 of 176 cases, associated with poor prognosis	ddPCR	Eskelund et al,[14] 2017
		Deletions in 15 of 68 cases, associated with shorter OS	Sanger sequencing, WES, SNP microarray	Clot et al,[26] 2018
		Missense mutations in 1 of 16 cases	WES	Yang et al,[13] 2018
		Deletions in 20 of 42 *CCND1*⁻ cases (11 homozygous)	Array CGH, CNV assay	Martin-Garcia et al,[19] 2019
RB1	13q14.2	Hemizygous deletions in 15 of 37 cases (9 also with *CDKN2A* deletion)	FISH	Dreyling et al,[8] 1997
		13q14 homozygous deletions in 12 of 32 cases	CGH	Pinyol et al,[27] 2007
		13q14 deletion in 1 of 1 case on ibrutinib relapse	WES	Chiron et al,[22] 2014
		Mutations in 6 of 56 cases (3 frameshift, 2 missense, 1 nonsense)	WES	Zhang et al,[12] 2014
		Deletions in 34 of 131 cases (33 monoallelic, 1 biallelic), gain in 1 case, associated with shorter OS	qPCR, MLPA	Delfau-Larue et al,[25] 2015

Gene	Locus	Description	Method	Reference
CDK2	12q13.2	Monoallelic deletion in 1 of 116 cases, gain in 8 cases	qPCR, MLPA	Delfau-Larue et al,[25] 2015
CDKN1A (p21^Waf1^)	6p21.2	S31R mutation in 1 of 23 cases	PCR-SSCP	Pinyol et al,[23] 1997
CDKN1B (p27^Kip1^)	12p13.1	Monoallelic deletions in 13 of 109 cases, gain in 3 cases, associated with shorter OS	qPCR, MLPA	Delfau-Larue et al,[25] 2015
AURKA	20q13.2	Homozygous P311 polymorphisms in 3 of 58 cases	PCR-RFLP	Camacho et al,[28] 2006
TTK (Mps1)	6q14.1	Hemizygous deletions in 6 of 26 cases	qPCR	Camacho et al,[28] 2006

This table lists only reported CNVs, mutations, translocations, and rearrangements of key cell cycle genes in MCL cells; cell cycle genes without reported alterations are not listed.

Abbreviations: Array CGH, array comparative genomic hybridization; copy number variation analysis, quantitative polymerase chain reaction Taqman assay; Cycle sequencing, double-strand direct sequencing; ddPCR, droplet-digital PCR; Ig, immunoglobulin; MLPA, multiplex ligation-dependent probe amplification; NGS, next-generation sequencing; OS, overall survival; PCR-RFLP, restriction fragment length polymorphism polymerase chain reaction; PCR-SSCP, single-strand conformation polymorphism polymerase chain reaction; SNP, single-nucleotide polymorphism; WGS, whole-genome sequencing.

3'-UTR region increase the stability of *CCND1* mRNAs.[11] Numerous other studies have identified mutations of *CCND1*,[11–14] often missense, particularly in exon 1.[15–17] In a recent clinical trial of ibrutinib in combination with venetoclax, *CCND1* mutations were seen exclusively in nonresponders.[18] In cyclin D1–negative MCL cells, rearrangements of immunoglobulin light chain genes with *CCND2* or *CCND3* led to their overexpression.[19]

Although cyclin D1 alone has no enzymatic activity, its overexpression promotes early G1 progression by accelerating the assembly of the active cyclin D1–CDK4 complexes in MCL cells This is further fueled by amplifications of *CDK4*,[20,21] which has been associated with tumorigenesis and worsened prognosis in some cases. No deleterious mutations in CDK4 have been reported so far. Nor have there been reports of genomic alterations in *CDK6*, which is marginally expressed in primary MCL cells.[22]

Conversely, *CDKN2A* encoding p16[INK4a] frequently is deleted in MCL cells, especially in aggressive diseases with poorer outcomes.[8,9,13,14,17,19,23–26] Although missense mutations have been detected in rare cases,[13,23] hemizygous or homozygous deletions are the dominant genomic alterations in *CDKN2A*. This results in impaired G1 cell cycle control. Similarly, deletions, but not mutations, are the key alterations in *RB1*,[8,12,22,25,27] resulting in unbridled transcriptional activation of E2Fs and downstream genes to reprogram both the cell cycle and cellular function.

G1–S

Further along the cell cycle, a mutation in *CDKN1A* encoding p21[Waf1], which inhibits various cyclin-CDK complexes in particular CDK2, but not CDK4 or CDK6, has been identified.[27] Copy number gains in *CDK2* and hemizygous deletions in *CDKN1B* also were shown to be associated with shorter overall survival.[25] *CDKN1B* encodes p27[Kip1], an inhibitor of CDK2–cyclin E(A) that promotes G1 to S transition as well as CDK1–cyclin A(B) for progression through G2 (see **Fig. 1A**).

G2–M

Homozygous polymorphisms in *AURKA* (encoding Aurora-A) and hemizygous deletions in *TTK* (encoding hMPS1) important for the spindle checkpoint and centrosome regulation have been identified,[28] although their role in genetic predispositions to lymphoma remains to be clarified.

Overall, the multitude of genomic alterations identified across cell cycle components can individually and collectively contribute to cell cycle dysregulation in MCL cells. Clustering of amplifications (*CDK4*) and deletions (*CDKN2A*, *RB1*) in genes that regulate G1 cell cycle progression and the association of these copy number variations (CNVs) with poorer outcomes further support targeting CDK4 in MCL.

GENOMIC ABERRATIONS IN *ATM*, *TP53*, *MYC*, AND *BTK* IN MANTLE CELL LYMPHOMA

ATM and *TP53* are among the most frequently mutated and deleted genes in MCL cells. *ATM*, encoding a serine/threonine kinase that activates the DNA damage checkpoint in response to double-strand breaks, is mutated and deleted at a high frequency in MCL cells.[15,17,18,29,30] Although its prognostic value has not been consistently significant, inactivating alterations due to truncation or missense mutations involving its PI3K domain have been shown to correlate with increased chromosomal instability.[31] *TP53* encodes the well-defined tumor suppressor protein p53 that commonly is disrupted in human cancer. Likewise, mutations and deletions of *TP53* in MCL are frequent, many of which have been associated with poor prognosis and shorter survival.[15,17,18,22,25,29] Moreover, amplifications and deletions in *MDM2* encoding a p53-interacting protein and negative regulator have been reported,[25,32] and alteration of *MDM2* along with *CDK4* occurred mainly in highly proliferative MCL with wild-type INK4a/ARF locus.[20] A mutation in *GTSE1*, a p53-binding protein and G2/M checkpoint regulator, also was identified.[22]

The proto-oncogene *MYC* is a prominent driver for lymphomagenesis. Burkitt-type 8q24 *MYC* translocation is frequent in MCL with blastoid features, and amplifications of *MYC* also contributed to elevated c-Myc expression, increased proliferation, and poor outcomes.[33–35]

BTK is central to B-cell development and MCL survival. A C481S BTK mutation was identified in MCL cells of patients who progressed after a durable response to the BTK inhibitor ibrutinib but not in those with primary resistance or transient responses to ibrutinib.[22] This BTK mutation apparently led to enhanced activation of both BTK and PI3K/AKT in vivo.[22] Although infrequent in MCL, BTK^{C481S} was detected in a separate ibrutinib-relapsed patient.[36] Finally, *PIK3CA* was shown to be amplified in MCL cells,[37] leading to overactivation of the PI3K/AKT/mTOR pathway that attenuates apoptosis and augments proliferation. These genomic alterations are likely to compound the aberrations in genes that directly control the cell cycle in MCL for cell cycle dysregulation and poorer outcomes.

TARGETING CDK4/6 IN MANTLE CELL LYMPHOMA

Three oral small molecule reversible CDK4/6 inhibitors have been approved by the Food and Drug Administration (FDA) (see **Fig. 1**B) for treatment of breast cancer, in which cyclin D1 and CDK4 frequently are overexpressed. Palbociclib (PD 0332991), the first selective CDK4/6 inhibitor,[38] is highly specific for cyclin D–CDK4 based on a KINOMEScan against 468 serine-threonine kinases, including lipid kinases (Di Liberto M, Huang X, Chen-Kiang S. Targeting CDK4/6, unpublished data, 2020) whereas abemaciclib (LY2835214) appeared significantly less selective.[39] The specificity of ribociclib (LEE011)[40] is not yet available.

Palbociclib was shown to inhibit CDK4/6 and induce early G1 cell cycle arrest in primary human myeloma cells *ex vivo*[41] and suppress tumor growth in xenografts of various human cancer cell lines in severe combined immunodeficiency mice[41–44] and in immunocompetent mouse models of multiple myeloma[45] and T-cell acute leukemia.[46] Mechanistically, induction of prolonged early G1 arrest (*pG1*) by sustained CDK4/6 inhibition not only arrested the cell cycle but also restricted the expression of genes programmed for early G1 only.[47] This caused an imbalance in gene expression that reprogrammed cancer cells for killing by diverse clinically relevant agents,[41,45,47] including inhibitors of PI3K and BTK in primary MCL cells *ex vivo*[22,48] and in animal models. Collectively, these preclinical studies provide compelling evidence for targeting CDK4/6 in human cancer.

PALBOCICLIB

In the first disease-specific single-agent clinical trial, palbociclib not only inhibited CDK4/6 and induced early G1 arrest initially in all patients with previously treated MCL but also elicited clinical responses with tumor regression in some patients, as indicated in preclinical studies[49] (**Table 2**). In this multicenter phase Ib study of 17 patients, an objective response was observed in 3 patients (18%) including 1 complete response (CR) and 2 partial responses (PRs), in addition to 7 patients with stable disease (SD). Although the median progression-free survival (PFS) was 4 months, responding patients experienced a duration of response (DOR) of 18 months or

Table 2
Summary of CDK 4/6 inhibitor clinical trials in mantle cell lymphoma

Agent (s)	Specificity	Design	No. of Patients	Results	References
Palbociclib	CDK4, CDK6	Phase Ib, multicenter	17	ORR 18% (CR 6%) PFS 4 mo	Leonard et al,[49] 2012
Palbociclib + bortezomib	CDK4, CDK6	Phase I, single-center	19	ORR 24% (CR 6%) SD 30%	Martin et al,[50] 2019
Palbociclib + ibrutinib	CDK4, CDK6	Phase I, multicenter	27	ORR 67% (CR 37%) 2-y PFS 59% 2-y OS 61%	Martin et al,[51] 2019
Palbociclib + ibrutinib	CDK4, CDK6	Phase II, multicenter	61 (estimated)	Pending	NCT03478514
Abemaciclib	CDK4, CDK6	Phase II, multicenter	22	ORR 23% (CR 0%)	Morschhauser et al,[55] 2014
Ribociclib	CDK4, CDK6	Phase I, multicenter	7 MCL (132 total)	ORR 0% SD 0%	Infante et al,[56] 2016
AT7519M	CDK1, CDK2 CDK4, CDK5 CDK9	Phase II, multicenter	12	ORR 27% (PR 18%) mDOR 4.5 mo	Seftel et al,[57] 2017
Voruciclib	CDK1, CDK4, CDK6, CDK9	Phase Ib, multicenter	84 (estimated, including MCL)	Pending	NCT03547115

Abbreviations: mDOR, median DOR; OS, overall survival.

greater. Dual immunohistochemical staining and ^{18}F-fluorothymidine positron emission tomography imaging further confirmed that palbociclib inhibited CDK4/6 and induced G1 arrest in MCL cells.

Tumor regression in responding patients, particularly in 1 patient with a CR for more than 30 months, was in line with a mechanistic link between palbociclib-induced prolonged early G1 arrest and cell death observed in preclinical studies.[47] As the first disease-specific clinical trial of a selective CDK4/6 inhibitor, it laid the groundwork for future studies of CDK4/6 in MCL as well as cancers of solid tissue origin, such as breast cancer.

PALBOCICLIB IN SEQUENTIAL COMBINATION WITH BORTEZOMIB

Leveraging the selectivity of palbociclib, a phase I dose escalation study of palbociclib in sequential combination with bortezomib in patients with previously treated MCL was designed to capitalize on bortezomib killing of MCL cells during palbociclib-induced pG1 as well as synchronous transition of G1-arrested cells into S phase after cessation of palbociclib.[50] Bortezomib was administered at a reduced dose (1 mg/m^2) during dose escalation of palbociclib with only 4 days of overlap (days 8–11), which potentially minimizes the combined toxicity. Of the 7 patients treated at the optimal dose combination, 4 remained progression-free for greater than 12 months, including 1 patient with a CR that has lasted for more than 7 years while remaining on single-agent palbociclib (see **Table 2**).

This single-center phase I study demonstrated that selective inhibition of CDK4/6 in sequential combination with reduced-dose bortezomib is biologically active and tolerable in previously treated MCL. Only 1 patient progressed while receiving treatment and this patient subsequently achieved a PR in response to ibrutinib,[51] suggesting that the mechanisms mediating clinical responses to palbociclib and ibrutinib are distinct. The maintenance of a durable CR by palbociclib alone after 6 cycles of palbociclib + bortezomib further invokes palbociclib as a potential maintenance treatment after achieving a CR to palbociclib-based combination therapy.

PALBOCICLIB IN COMBINATION WITH IBRUTINIB

Ibrutinib is a standard of care for MCL.[52] Approximately half of all patients progressed on treatment during the first year, and this often is associated with a more aggressive disease.[53] Induction of pG1 by CDK4/6 inhibition had been shown to overcome ibrutinib resistance in primary human MCL cells expressing the wild-type BTK,[22] in part by inactivating NF-κB as well as PI3K through up-regulation of a negative regulator, PIK3IP1, in palbociclib-induced pG1.[22,48]

On this basis, a multiple institutional clinical trial was undertaken to test if inhibition of CDK4/6 could deepen and prolong the clinical response to ibrutinib while assessing the tolerability. This phase I study of palbociclib + ibrutinib in 27 patients with previously treated MCL demonstrated a CR rate of 37% and median PFS of 25.6 months,[51] which appear better than might be expected based on studies of single-agent ibrutinib, despite a comparable objective response rate (ORR) of 67%.[54] Among 7 patients with a Ki67 higher than 30%, 5 responded, including 3 patients with a CR. Among 7 patients with a high MIPI, 4 responded, including 1 with a CR.[50] The combination had an acceptable safety profile, with a dose-limiting toxicity of grade 3 rash that resulted in discontinuation in 2 patients taking the highest does of palbociclib (125 mg) (see **Table 2**).

The observed activity was consistent with the hypothesis that induction of pG1 by CDK4/6 inhibition could deepen and prolong the clinical response to ibrutinib, including MCL patients with a high Ki67 and MIPI. A multicenter, phase II study to further characterize the efficacy of this combination regimen, along with longitudinal functional genomics to identify genomic drivers for resistance to palbociclib and ibrutinib is under way (see **Table 2**).

OTHER CDK4/6 INHIBITORS

Abemaciclib, a broad-spectrum oral CDK4/6 inhibitor, is under study in a single-arm phase II trial for patients with previously treated MCL. Preliminary results in 22 patients treated with abemaciclib showed that 5 patients achieved PR (23%) and 9 patients had SD.[55] Despite comparable clinical activity, the adverse effects (diarrhea, nausea, and vomiting) differ considerably from those of palbociclib, potentially due to inhibition of off target serine-threonine kinases besides CDK4 and CDK6. How these features of abemaciclib might contribute to the clinical outcome, tolerability, and durability in combination therapy remain to be determined.

Ribociclib is the third oral FDA-approved CDK4/6 inhibitor for treatment of metastatic breast cancer. A total of 7 patients with MCL were enrolled in a large phase I trial involving patients with a variety of previously treated solid tumors and lymphomas. As expected, myelosuppression was the primary dose-limiting toxicity. There were no responses among the patients with MCL.[56]

AT7519M is an inhibitor of CDKs 1, 2, 4, 5, and 9. In a phase II single-agent study for patients with previously treated chronic lymphocytic leukemia and MCL, the ORR in 12 MCL patients was 27%, with 2 patients achieving PR (18%) with a DOR of 4.5 months; 6 patients (55%) had SD, including 1 patient who subsequently met PR criteria 9 months after discontinuation of AT7519M with no other therapy. AT7519M had a favorable toxicity profile, with only 2 grade 3 nonhematologic adverse events.[57]

Voruciclib, a potent inhibitor of CDK9, CDK4, CDK6, and CDK1, is being studied in a phase Ib trial in patients with previously treated B-cell malignancies, including an MCL cohort.[58] CDK9 is not a classic cell cycle regulator. It is a transcription factor regulating *MCL1* (an antiapoptotic member of the BCL2 family) and *MYC*, among other targets. Voruciclib potentially may block cell proliferation by inhibiting CDK4, CDK6, and CDK1 and impair cell survival by down-regulating MCL1. Its therapeutic window depends on how inhibiting multiple CDKs can be translated into a clinical response and the tolerability and durability of this broad-spectrum CDK inhibitor.

DISCUSSION

The cell cycle is directional and exquisitely controlled by the balance between positive and negative regulators (see **Fig. 1**A). Cyclin D1 overexpression in MCL cells alone is insufficient to subvert the cell cycle program, because cyclin D has no enzymatic activity. It predisposes MCL cells, however, to aggressive proliferation and poorer outcome by accelerating the formation of an active cyclin D–CDK4 complex that drives G1 progression. This is exacerbated further by loss of the CDK4/6 inhibitor p16^{IN4a} due to deletions of *CDKN2a* or increased CDK4 as a consequence of gene amplification, each associated with worsened outcome[8,21] (see **Table 1**). Genomic analyses using various methods, including unbiased whole-exome sequencing (WES), have validated these early studies and established CNV in genes directly regulating the cell cycle (see **Table 1**) as the driver for cell cycle dysregulation in MCL.

The advent of selective CDK4/6 inhibitors has made it possible to target the cell cycle in mechanism-based clinical trials. Data emerging from 3 completed clinical trials of palbociclib are consistent with the hypothesis that induction of prolonged early G1 arrest by CDK4/6 inhibition not only prevents proliferation of MCL cells but also reprograms them for a deeper and more durable clinical response to the partner drug, including patients with high Ki67 and high MIPI. Durable CR was observed in 1 patient treated with palbociclib for 30 months[49]; in 1 patient for more than 7 years while on treatment with palbociclib alone after 6 cycles of palbociclib + bortezomib[50]; and in 10 patients (37%) in the palbociclib + ibrutinib clinical trial,[51] for 3 to 5.5 years while on therapy as of 4/2020 (Di Liberto M, Huang X, Chen-Kiang S. Targeting CDK4/6, unpublished data). Rb, the substrate of CDK4/6, is necessary but insufficient for a clinical response to palbociclib therapy. Although preliminary, these findings reinforce the potential of targeting CDK4/6, and the critical importance of defining the mechanisms that discriminate sensitivity from resistance to targeting CDK4/6 in MCL.

Longitudinal integrated analysis of whole-transcriptome sequencing (WTS) and WES of MCL cells isolated from sequential specimens from individual patients before, during, and after treatment represents the best approach to address this question. Such a longitudinal integrated analysis in a single-agent ibrutinib therapy has led to the discovery of a relapse-specific C418S BTK mutation in MCL.[22] The ongoing longitudinal functional genomics of palbociclib combination therapies (Di Liberto M, Huang X, Chen-Kiang S. Targeting CDK4/6, unpublished) should shed light on the genomic drivers for resistance to targeting CDK4/6 and BTK. They also could illuminate genes and signaling pathways that are programmed in G1 arrest to maintain a durable clinical response and advance the selection and sequencing of a partner drug(s) with a CDK4/6 inhibitor in combination therapy.

Inhibition of CDK4/6 is not limited to disease or cell lineage, suggesting that the immune landscape and tumor-immune interactions are likely to be dynamically regulated by CDK4/6 inhibition and contribute to the clinical response. Consistent with this possibility, CDK4/6 inhibition has been shown to promote cytotoxic T-cell–mediated clearance of tumor cells in patient-derived mouse model of breast cancer[59]; increase the infiltration of $CD4^+$ and $CD8^+$ T cells as well as the levels of T_H1 cytokines in a mouse model of lung cancer[60]; and repress a tumor resistance program associated with T-cell exclusion and immune evasion as determined by single-cell RNA sequencing in melanoma tumors.[61] Collectively, these studies illustrate the tumor-extrinsic mechanisms by which CDK4/6 inhibitors may enhance antitumor immunity in solid tumors. It will be important to see if these promising preclinical data are recapitulated in lymphoma and translate into better efficacy in patients.

Integrating longitudinal single-cell RNA-sequencing with WTS and WES of purified MCL cells from the phase II palbociclib-ibrutinib clinical trial present an ideal strategy to investigate tumor-immune interactions in the context of a clinical response and shed light on the therapeutic potential of dual CDK4/6 and immune checkpoint inhibition in MCL.

CONTRIBUTIONS

(1) Conception and design: all authors; (2) provision of study materials or patients: all authors; (3) collection and assembly of data: all authors; (4) data analysis and interpretation: all authors; (5) Manuscript writing: all authors; and (6) Final approval of manuscript: all authors.

ACKNOWLEDGMENTS

The authors thank Nicole Zhao for a critical reading of this article and helpful suggestions. This study was supported in part by a Translational Research Grants from V Foundation, United States, (S. Chen-Kiang, M. Di Liberto), NIH/NCI RO1CA18894, United States, (S. Chen-Kiang), MCL-RI Award (MCL7001-18) from The Leukemia &

Lymphoma Society, United States, to S. Chen-Kiang. Funding for this project has been provided by the Sarah Cannon Fund at the HCA Foundation (S. Chen-Kiang, X. Huang, M. Di Liberto), and NIH/NCI P01CA21427401, United States, (S. Chen-Kiang, X. Huang, M. Di Liberto).

CONFLICTS OF INTEREST

The authors have no conflicts of interest to declare.

REFERENCES

1. Williams ME, Swerdlow SH, Meeker TC. Chromosome t(11;14)(q13;q32) breakpoints in centrocytic lymphoma are highly localized at the bcl-1 major translocation cluster. Leukemia 1993;7:1437–40.

2. Bosch F, Jares P, Campo E, et al. PRAD-1/cyclin D1 gene overexpression in chronic lymphoproliferative disorders: a highly specific marker of mantle cell lymphoma. Blood 1994;84:2726–32.

3. de Boer CJ, van Krieken JH, Kluin-Nelemans HC, et al. Cyclin D1 messenger RNA overexpression as a marker for mantle cell lymphoma. Oncogene 1995; 10:1833–40.

4. Ott MM, Helbing A, Ott G, et al. bcl-1 rearrangement and cyclin D1 protein expression in mantle cell lymphoma. J Pathol 1996;179:238–42.

5. Rosenberg CL, Wong E, Petty EM, et al. PRAD1, a candidate BCL1 oncogene: mapping and expression in centrocytic lymphoma. Proc Natl Acad Sci U S A 1991;88:9638–42.

6. Bretz J, Garcia J, Huang X, et al. Noxa mediates p18INK4c cell-cycle control of homeostasis in B cells and plasma cell precursors. Blood 2011;117:2179–88.

7. Kent LN, Leone G. The broken cycle: E2F dysfunction in cancer. Nat Rev Cancer 2019;19:326–38.

8. Dreyling MH, Bullinger L, Ott G, et al. Alterations of the cyclin D1/p16-pRB pathway in mantle cell lymphoma. Cancer Res 1997;57:4608–14.

9. Rosenwald A, Wright G, Wiestner A, et al. The proliferation gene expression signature is a quantitative integrator of oncogenic events that predicts survival in mantle cell lymphoma. Cancer Cell 2003;3:185–97.

10. Determann O, Hoster E, Ott G, et al. Ki-67 predicts outcome in advanced-stage mantle cell lymphoma patients treated with anti-CD20 immunochemotherapy: results from randomized trials of the European MCL Network and the German Low Grade Lymphoma Study Group. Blood 2008;111:2385–7.

11. Wiestner A, Tehrani M, Chiorazzi M, et al. Point mutations and genomic deletions in CCND1 create stable truncated cyclin D1 mRNAs that are associated with increased proliferation rate and shorter survival. Blood 2007;109:4599–606.

12. Zhang J, Jima D, Moffitt AB, et al. The genomic landscape of mantle cell lymphoma is related to the epigenetically determined chromatin state of normal B cells. Blood 2014;123:2988–96.

13. Yang P, Zhang W, Wang J, et al. Genomic landscape and prognostic analysis of mantle cell lymphoma. Cancer Gene Ther 2018;25:129–40.

14. Eskelund CW, Dahl C, Hansen JW, et al. TP53 mutations identify younger mantle cell lymphoma patients who do not benefit from intensive chemoimmunotherapy. Blood 2017;130:1903–10.

15. Meissner B, Kridel R, Lim RS, et al. The E3 ubiquitin ligase UBR5 is recurrently mutated in mantle cell lymphoma. Blood 2013;121:3161–4.

16. Kridel R, Meissner B, Rogic S, et al. Whole transcriptome sequencing reveals recurrent NOTCH1 mutations in mantle cell lymphoma. Blood 2012;119:1963–71.

17. Bea S, Valdes-Mas R, Navarro A, et al. Landscape of somatic mutations and clonal evolution in mantle cell lymphoma. Proc Natl Acad Sci U S A 2013;110: 18250–5.

18. Agarwal R, Chan YC, Tam CS, et al. Dynamic molecular monitoring reveals that SWI-SNF mutations mediate resistance to ibrutinib plus venetoclax in mantle cell lymphoma. Nat Med 2019;25:119–29.

19. Martin-Garcia D, Navarro A, Valdes-Mas R, et al. CCND2 and CCND3 hijack immunoglobulin light-chain enhancers in cyclin D1(-) mantle cell lymphoma. Blood 2019;133:940–51.

20. Hernandez L, Bea S, Pinyol M, et al. CDK4 and MDM2 gene alterations mainly occur in highly proliferative and aggressive mantle cell lymphomas with wild-type INK4a/ARF locus. Cancer Res 2005;65:2199–206.

21. Bea S, Ribas M, Hernandez JM, et al. Increased number of chromosomal imbalances and high-level DNA amplifications in mantle cell lymphoma are associated with blastoid variants. Blood 1999;93:4365–74.

22. Chiron D, Di Liberto M, Martin P, et al. Cell-cycle reprogramming for PI3K inhibition overrides a relapse-specific C481S BTK mutation revealed by longitudinal functional genomics in mantle cell lymphoma. Cancer Discov 2014;4:1022–35.

23. Pinyol M, Hernandez L, Cazorla M, et al. Deletions and loss of expression of p16INK4a and p21Waf1 genes are associated with aggressive variants of mantle cell lymphomas. Blood 1997;89:272–80.

24. Fernandez V, Salamero O, Espinet B, et al. Genomic and gene expression profiling defines indolent forms of mantle cell lymphoma. Cancer Res 2010;70: 1408–18.

25. Delfau-Larue MH, Klapper W, Berger F, et al. High-dose cytarabine does not overcome the adverse prognostic value of CDKN2A and TP53 deletions in mantle cell lymphoma. Blood 2015;126:604–11.

26. Clot G, Jares P, Gine E, et al. A gene signature that distinguishes conventional and leukemic nonnodal mantle cell lymphoma helps predict outcome. Blood 2018;132:413–22.

27. Pinyol M, Bea S, Pla L, et al. Inactivation of RB1 in mantle-cell lymphoma detected by nonsense-mediated mRNA decay pathway inhibition and microarray analysis. Blood 2007;109:5422–9.

28. Camacho E, Bea S, Salaverria I, et al. Analysis of Aurora-A and hMPS1 mitotic kinases in mantle cell lymphoma. Int J Cancer 2006;118:357–63.

29. Greiner TC, Dasgupta C, Ho VV, et al. Mutation and genomic deletion status of ataxia telangiectasia mutated (ATM) and p53 confer specific gene expression profiles in mantle cell lymphoma. Proc Natl Acad Sci U S A 2006;103:2352–7.

30. Schaffner C, Idler I, Stilgenbauer S, et al. Mantle cell lymphoma is characterized by inactivation of the ATM gene. Proc Natl Acad Sci U S A 2000;97:2773–8.

31. Camacho E, Hernandez L, Hernandez S, et al. ATM gene inactivation in mantle cell lymphoma mainly occurs by truncating mutations and missense mutations involving the phosphatidylinositol-3 kinase domain and is associated with increasing numbers of chromosomal imbalances. Blood 2002;99:238–44.

32. Hartmann E, Fernandez V, Stoecklein H, et al. Increased MDM2 expression is associated with inferior survival in mantle-cell lymphoma, but not related to the MDM2 SNP309. Haematologica 2007;92:574–5.

33. Setoodeh R, Schwartz S, Papenhausen P, et al. Double-hit mantle cell lymphoma with MYC gene rearrangement or amplification: a report of four cases and review of the literature. Int J Clin Exp Pathol 2013;6:155–67.

34. Felten CL, Stephenson CF, Ortiz RO, et al. Burkitt transformation of mantle cell lymphoma. Leuk Lymphoma 2004;45:2143–7.

35. Au WY, Horsman DE, Viswanatha DS, et al. 8q24 translocations in blastic transformation of mantle cell lymphoma. Haematologica 2000;85:1225–7.

36. Jain P, Kanagal-Shamanna R, Zhang S, et al. Long-term outcomes and mutation profiling of patients with mantle cell lymphoma (MCL) who discontinued ibrutinib. Br J Haematol 2018;183:578–87.

37. Psyrri A, Papageorgiou S, Liakata E, et al. Phosphatidylinositol 3'-kinase catalytic subunit alpha gene amplification contributes to the pathogenesis of mantle cell lymphoma. Clin Cancer Res 2009;15:5724–32.

38. Fry DW, Harvey PJ, Keller PR, et al. Specific inhibition of cyclin-dependent kinase 4/6 by PD 0332991 and associated antitumor activity in human tumor xenografts. Mol Cancer Ther 2004;3:1427–38.

39. Gelbert LM, Cai S, Lin X, et al. Preclinical characterization of the CDK4/6 inhibitor LY2835219: in-vivo cell cycle-dependent/independent anti-tumor activities alone/ in combination with gemcitabine. Invest New Drugs 2014;32:825–37.

40. Rader J, Russell MR, Hart LS, et al. Dual CDK4/CDK6 inhibition induces cell-cycle arrest and senescence in neuroblastoma. Clin Cancer Res 2013;19: 6173–82.

41. Baughn LB, Di Liberto M, Wu K, et al. A novel orally active small molecule potently induces G1 arrest in primary myeloma cells and prevents tumor growth by specific inhibition of cyclin-dependent kinase 4/6. Cancer Res 2006;66:7661–7.

42. Marzec M, Kasprzycka M, Lai R, et al. Mantle cell lymphoma cells express predominantly cyclin D1a isoform and are highly sensitive to selective inhibition of CDK4 kinase activity. Blood 2006;108:1744–50.

43. Wang L, Wang J, Blaser BW, et al. Pharmacologic inhibition of CDK4/6: mechanistic evidence for selective activity or acquired resistance in acute myeloid leukemia. Blood 2007;110:2075–83.

44. Finn RS, Dering J, Conklin D, et al. PD 0332991, a selective cyclin D kinase 4/6 inhibitor, preferentially inhibits proliferation of luminal estrogen receptor-positive human breast cancer cell lines in vitro. Breast Cancer Res 2009;11:R77.

45. Menu E, Garcia J, Huang X, et al. A novel therapeutic combination using PD 0332991 and bortezomib: study in the 5T33MM myeloma model. Cancer Res 2008;68:5519–23.

46. Sawai CM, Freund J, Oh P, et al. Therapeutic targeting of the cyclin D3:CDK4/6 complex in T cell leukemia. Cancer Cell 2012;22:452–65.

47. Huang X, Di Liberto M, Jayabalan D, et al. Prolonged early G(1) arrest by selective CDK4/CDK6 inhibition sensitizes myeloma cells to cytotoxic killing through cell cycle-coupled loss of IRF4. Blood 2012;120:1095–106.

48. Chiron D, Martin P, Di Liberto M, et al. Induction of prolonged early G1 arrest by CDK4/CDK6 inhibition reprograms lymphoma cells for durable PI3Kdelta inhibition through PIK3IP1. Cell Cycle 2013;12:1892–900.

49. Leonard JP, LaCasce AS, Smith MR, et al. Selective CDK4/6 inhibition with tumor responses by PD0332991 in patients with mantle cell lymphoma. Blood 2012;119: 4597–607.

50. Martin P, Ruan J, Furman R, et al. A phase I trial of palbociclib plus bortezomib in previously treated mantle cell lymphoma. Leuk Lymphoma 2019. https://doi.org/10.1080/10428194.2019.1612062:1-5.

51. Martin P, Bartlett NL, Blum KA, et al. A phase 1 trial of ibrutinib plus palbociclib in previously treated mantle cell lymphoma. Blood 2019;133:1201–4.
52. Wang ML, Rule S, Martin P, et al. Targeting BTK with ibrutinib in relapsed or refractory mantle-cell lymphoma. N Engl J Med 2013;369:507–16.
53. Martin P, Maddocks K, Leonard JP, et al. Postibrutinib outcomes in patients with mantle cell lymphoma. Blood 2016;127:1559–63.
54. Rule S, Dreyling M, Goy A, et al. Outcomes in 370 patients with mantle cell lymphoma treated with ibrutinib: a pooled analysis from three open-label studies. Br J Haematol 2017;179:430–8.
55. Morschhauser F, Bouabdallah K, Stilgenbauer S, et al. Clinical Activity of Abemaciclib (LY2835219), a Cell Cycle Inhibitor Selective for CDK4 and CDK6, in Patients with Relapsed or Refractory Mantle Cell Lymphoma. Blood 2014;124:3067.
56. Infante JR, Cassier PA, Gerecitano JF, et al. A phase I study of the cyclin-dependent kinase 4/6 inhibitor ribociclib (LEE011) in patients with advanced solid tumors and lymphomas. Clin Cancer Res 2016;22:5696–705.
57. Seftel MD, Kuruvilla J, Kouroukis T, et al. The CDK inhibitor AT7519M in patients with relapsed or refractory chronic lymphocytic leukemia (CLL) and mantle cell lymphoma. A Phase II study of the Canadian Cancer Trials Group. Leuk Lymphoma 2017;58:1358–65.
58. Dey J, Deckwerth TL, Kerwin WS, et al. Voruciclib, a clinical stage oral CDK9 inhibitor, represses MCL-1 and sensitizes high-risk Diffuse Large B-cell Lymphoma to BCL2 inhibition. Sci Rep 2017;7:18007.
59. Goel S, DeCristo MJ, Watt AC, et al. CDK4/6 inhibition triggers anti-tumour immunity. Nature 2017;548:471–5.
60. Deng J, Wang ES, Jenkins RW, et al. CDK4/6 inhibition augments antitumor immunity by enhancing T-cell activation. Cancer Discov 2018;8:216–33.
61. Jerby-Arnon L, Shah P, Cuoco MS, et al. A cancer cell program promotes T cell exclusion and resistance to checkpoint blockade. Cell 2018;175:984–97.e4.

What Is Responsible for Heterogeneity in Mantle Cell Lymphoma Biology and Outcomes?

Thomas E. Witzig, MD

KEYWORDS

- Cell proliferation • *TP53* mutation • Cytokines • Minimal residual disease
- Metabolomics

KEY POINTS

- Clinical presentations of mantle cell lymphoma vary between nodal, splenic/leukemia, tonsil, gastrointestinal tract, and rarely leptomeningeal.
- Blastoid morphology and pleomorphic tumor cell morphology are adverse prognostic factors.
- Tumor cell proliferation rates vary widely, with high defined as KI-67 greater than 30%.
- Genomic alterations in p53 (deletions or mutations) predict a lower chemotherapy response and shorter survival.
- Increased monocytes/macrophages and their associated proinflammatory cytokines are found in a subset of mantle cell lymphoma patients and predict inferior outcomes.

INTRODUCTION

Mantle cell lymphoma (MCL) accounts for approximately 8% of all non-Hodgkin lymphoma (NHL) cases. Some physicians consider MCL to be incurable; actually, MCL is always treatable but not reliably curable. As is evident from the overall survival (OS) curves in the stem cell transplant era with 15-year to 20-year follow-up,[1,2] there are very-long-term survivors without relapse. Unfortunately, the progression-free survival (PFS) curves from most studies show a steady relapse and death rate throughout the first 5 years, with a slower downward trajectory that never completely flattens out. Why do some patients do well and others not? Despite a characteristic t(11;14) translocation in tumor cells that leads to cyclin D1 overexpression in nearly all MCL cases, there is remarkable clinical and biological heterogeneity (summarized in **Table 1**) in

Conflict of Interest: None.
Hematology Mayo Clinic Rochester, Mayo Clinic Alix School of Medicine, Mayo Clinic Cancer Center, 200 Southwest 1st Street, Rochester, MN 55905, USA
E-mail address: witzig.thomas@mayo.edu

Hematol Oncol Clin N Am 34 (2020) 825–835
https://doi.org/10.1016/j.hoc.2020.06.001
0889-8588/20/© 2020 Elsevier Inc. All rights reserved.

the disease. Understanding this heterogeneity is important for clinical care and also for development of therapies that target the most aggressive forms of the disease.

DIFFERENCES IN CLINICAL PRESENTATION
Age, Sex, Comorbidities, and Heredity

For unclear reasons, the incidence of MCL is more common in men. In a study of risk factors in 557 patients, the median age was 62 years, and 76% were men.[3] In a recent registry study in Sweden, where 1385 patients diagnosed with MCL between 2000 to 2014 were studied, 73% (1009/1385) were male. MCL also is a disease of older adults, with median age in that series of 71 years (22–96 years).[4] The biological reasons for these sex and age differences remain unclear. The fitness of the patient also varies, and poor performance status is an adverse prognostic factor in the MCL International Prognostic Index (MIPI) score.[5–7] Using the Charlson Comorbidity Index, 44% had some comorbidities with 28% severe comorbidities.[4] Age and comorbidities are important and they factor greatly in the decision to consider a patient transplant eligible. Because the OS of MCL patients is long, with a pattern of continuous slow relapse, the impact of MCL on patients is much different if they are 50 years old compared with 80 years old at diagnosis. Only age and performance status are factors in the MIPI; sex is not. There is a mild effect of heredity, with the risk of MCL twice as high in men with a first-degree relative with a blood cancer.[3]

Diet

The diet of patients varies widely and is influenced by culture and location. Diet offers another potential actionable risk factor that could contribute to MCL disease heterogeneity. Unfortunately, there are few data about the importance of diet on the risk of MCL or its prognosis. In a study by Holtan and colleagues,[8] 4% (24/603) of cases were MCL and they were not commented on specifically. When evaluating all NHL cases versus controls, the NHL risk was higher for patients who consumed diets low in antioxidant foods in general and vegetables specifically. In another study of diffuse large B-cell lymphoma (DLBCL) or follicular lymphoma (FL) risk, a similar association was found—those patients who ate more vegetables had a lower risk of being diagnosed with lymphoma.[9] Finally, in the large study of risk of NHL by Chang and colleagues,[10] there were no reported MCL cases. This is likely due to the fact that this study only included women and they have a lower rate of MCL.

Table 1
Laboratory features associated with variable outcome in mantle cell lymphoma

	Adverse	Favorable
Ki-67 cell proliferation	≥30% (high rate)	<30% (low rate)
Pathology	Blastoid, pleomorphic	Classic
SOX11	Nonexpression	Expression
Cyclin D1	Nonexpression	Expression
TP53	Deletion or mutation	No deletion or mutation
KMT2D (MLL2)	Mutation	No deletion or mutation
Lactate dehydrogenase	High	Normal
Blood AMC	>500 cells/µL	<500 cells/µL
MRD at end of therapy	If MRD positive after therapy	Negative after therapy
sIL-2R, IL-8, and MIP1a		

In patients already diagnosed with NHL (DLBCL, FL, or chronic lymphocytic leukemia/small lymphocytic lymphoma), patients consuming a high intake of vegetables (especially cruciferous vegetables) had a superior survival.[11] It is likely that these data also apply to MCL, but this cannot be stated with certainty.

Patterns of Clinical Presentation

There are a variety of clinical presentation patterns of MCL, summarized in **Fig. 1**.

- Nodal: lymph node enlargement in the neck, axilla, abdomen, and inguinal nodal groups is a common presentation. These nodes can be measured on physical examination or on positron emission tomography (PET)/computed tomography (CT). If the nodes are bulky, they can produce lymphedema of an extremity

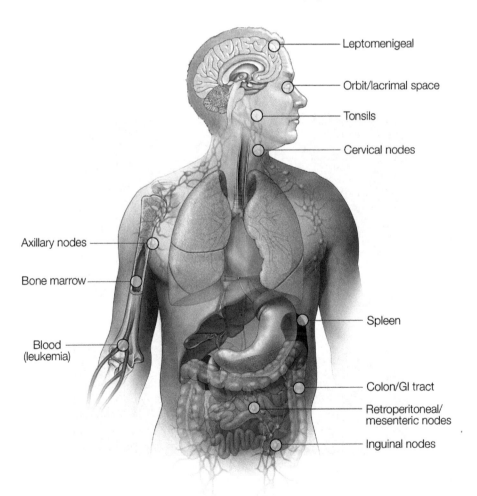

Clinical Presentation of Mantle Cell Lymphoma

- Leptomenigeal
- Orbit/lacrimal space
- Tonsils
- Cervical nodes
- Axillary nodes
- Bone marrow
- Spleen
- Blood (leukemia)
- Colon/GI tract
- Retroperitoneal/mesenteric nodes
- Inguinal nodes

Fig. 1. Patterns of presentation of MCL. (Used with permission of Mayo Foundation for Medical Education and Research, all rights reserved.)

(usually the legs), compression of a ureter leading to hydronephrosis, or obstruction of the biliary tree leading to jaundice.

- Splenomegaly: some patients present with splenomegaly (**Fig. 2**) and a leukemic phase. Why some patients develop massive splenomegaly and others do not is unknown. The splenomegaly can produce significant cytopenia, abdominal discomfort, early satiety, and weight loss. These patients often have minimal lymphadenopathy but a prominent leukemic phase with cells that are SOX11 negative.[12,13] In these cases, diagnostic tests can be performed on a blood sample. Splenectomy typically is not performed unless the spleen size has an impact on the delivery of chemotherapy. In a study in the prerituximab era, splenectomy improved cytopenia in 69% of patients.[14]
- Tonsillar: enlargement of the tonsils from MCL is an uncommon, but important pattern of presentation that is easy for clinicians to miss. These patients typically report abnormal swallowing or sleep-disordered breathing. Any patients with markedly enlarged tonsils and MCL should be evaluated for obstructive sleep apnea, especially if they have daytime sleepiness or excessive snoring. The symptoms typically resolve with successful treatment, or, rarely, tonsillectomy is required.
- Gastrointestinal: MCL can involve the small or large bowel. In the colon, MCL may take the form of polyps that often are asymptomatic and are discovered on routine screening colonoscopy.

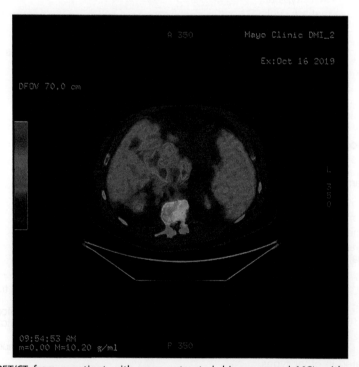

Fig. 2. PET/CT from a patient with new, untreated, biopsy-proved MCL with prominent splenomegaly and a platelet count of 33 x 10(9)/L. The platelet count increased to 213 x 10(9)/L postsplenectomy. Also note the prominent lymphadenopathy and the variability of the FDG-uptake (standard uptake value) between the very FDG-avid mesenteric nodes and the mild uptake in the spleen and liver. This image shows the ability of the PET/CT to detect involvement in the spine and more FDG-avid areas of the spleen.

- Leptomeningeal: involvement of the leptomeninges is unusual at initial presentation but it can appear in the later stages of the disease. Any cranial nerve abnormalities or other neurologic symptoms should be evaluated with a magnetic resonance image and cerebrospinal fluid evaluation.[15]
- Symptoms: patients may present with symptoms related to the sites of involvement, discussed previously. In addition, they may have systemic symptoms, such as fevers, night sweats, and weight loss (B symptoms).

HETEROGENEITY IN LABORATORY FEATURES

- Tumor morphology: by light microscopy, there are 3 types of MCL—classic, blastoid, and pleomorphic.[16] Blastoid and pleomorphic types represent only 10% of the cases and are associated with a high Ki-67 (high proliferation) rate. The overall prognosis is poor but no specific therapeutic programs for these types have been developed.[16]
- Tumor cell cyclin D1 expression: a majority of cases express cyclin D1 by immunohistochemistry; however, cyclin D1–negative cases do occur.[17] In these cases, the cells may express another cyclin protein, such as D2 or D3.
- Tumor cell SOX11 expression: sex-determining region Y-box 11 (SOX11) is a gene located on chromosome 2 and is involved in embryonic neurogenesis. SOX11 protein typically is expressed in classic MCL and it is a useful marker for cases that are cyclin D1 negative.[18] A small number of MCL cases, however, are SOX11 negative. These cases typically have mutated immunoglobulin genes; present with a leukemic, non-nodal phase; and have a shorter survival than SOX11 positive cases.[7,19]
- Tumor cell proliferation rate—Ki-67: the t(11;14) (q13;q32) is the hallmark cytogenetic abnormality of MCL. This translocation involves the *CCND1* gene and the immunoglobulin heavy chain on 14q32. This leads to cyclin D1 protein overexpression. It is understandable that cell proliferation is disrupted in MCL tumors given the nature of this translocation. Using Ki-67 staining on formalin-fixed paraffin-embedded samples, the prognosis can be predicted. Patients with highly proliferative tumors (Ki-67 >30%) have an inferior prognosis.[20,21] Because most tumors have the translocation, there must be other mechanisms as to why this important proliferative variability exists. There also is heterogeneity within tumor sites in the same patient.
- Tumor cell mutations: mutations occur frequently in MCL tumors. Using whole-exome sequencing, *ATM*, *CCND1*, and *TP53* are among the most frequently mutated genes in MCL.[22] *ATM* was the most common (41% of cases) and, when these mutations were found, the tumors typically were SOX11 positive; no *ATM* mutations were found in the SOX11-negative cases.[22] In contrast, *CCND1* mutations were more common in the SOX11 negative cases. The histone methyltransferase *MLL2* (*KMT2D*) is located on chromosome 12q13.12[23] and was mutated in 18% (4/29) of primary tumors; *TP53* mutations were detected in 28% with no preference for SOX11 status. The global mutational burden was low, at 1.2 per megabase. No mutations in genes that commonly are mutated in other types of NHL, such as *MYD88*, *CARD11*, *EZH2*, and *SF3B1*, were detected. A second study by Zhang and colleagues[24] studied 56 cases and also found *ATM*, *CCND1*, *MLL2*, and *TP53* the most commonly mutated. *MYC* was not mutated in any cases of MCL. Eskelund and colleagues[2] described a similar analysis on the bone marrow from patients who participated on the Nordic trials of chemoimmunotherapy for MCL; 51% of 176 samples had a

mutation documented with 19% of cases carrying more than 1 mutated gene. *ATM* again was the most frequently (27% of cases) mutated gene; *TP53* mutations were found in 11% and were associated with other known adverse prognostic factors in MCL—namely, blastoid morphology, high MIPI index, and high Ki-67% ($\geq$30%). *TP53*-mutated cases had a median OS of only 1.8 years compared with a median of 12.7 years for *TP53*-unmutated cases (P<.0001). The investigators also reported that 14% had *KMT2D* mutations but these were not predictive of outcome in this MCL cohort. Ferrero and colleagues[25] recently correlated mutations found in bone marrow CD19$^+$ cells from 190 patients with MCL to outcome of treatment on the MCL0208 phase III trial; 28% of patients had tumors with a high Ki-67 score and 8% were blastoid variant. The investigators used a targeted resequencing approach that focused on genes previously described to be mutated in MCL. Using this panel, 70% of patients had at least 1 mutation. *KMT2D* mutations were found in only 12% of cases (an additional 1.6% had deletions of *KMT2D*). For *TP53*, mutations were documented in 8% and deletions in 13% for a total of 16.6% of cases having at least 1 of the *TP53* abnormalities. Only *KMT2D* and *TP53* mutations along with 17p deletions were adverse prognostic factors.[25] *ATM* mutations were the most common mutation detected at 42% but they were not predictive of relapse or OS. The investigators then added these mutation results to the standard MIPI score to form the MIPI–genetic index (MIPI-g); 70% of patients were low risk (0 points), 22% intermediate (1–2 points), and 8% high risk ($\geq$3 points). The PFS rates at 4 years were 72%, 42%, and 12% for the low-risk, intermediate-risk, and high-risk MIPI-g groups, respectively. The corresponding OS rates for those same 3 groups were 95%, 66%, and 45%, respectively.

- Blood involvement—minimal residual disease (MRD): virtually all patients with MCL have detectable tumor cells in the blood at diagnosis by 4-color flow cytometry (FC) or molecular techniques.[26] Thus, at the baseline timepoint there really is no heterogeneity in this factor in MCL. The level of involvement, however, differs and correlates with disease stage, elevated lactate dehydrogenase, histologic bone marrow infiltration, and MIPI prognostic index.[26] In the recently conducted E1411 study (NCT01415752), MRD was studied with 2 methods: a next-generation sequencing (NGS) MRD assay (clonoSEQ; Adaptive Biotechnologies, Seattle, Washington) that uses multiplex PCR followed by NGS to detect malignant cells based on their patient-specific and tumor-specific DNA rearrangements of IgH, V-J, D-J, and IgK/L loci; and, an 8-color FC technique that detects tumor cells based on their immunophenotype at a level of 1×10^4 (**Fig. 3**).[27] Both methods detected clonal cells at baseline in more than 90% of cases. After 3 cycles of bendamustine/rituximab-based induction, MRD negativity rates were 89% by NGS analysis of blood versus 87% by FC in the blood. The patients who achieved a negative MRD status (by either NGS or FC) at this timepoint had a median PFS of 58.9 months, whereas the median PFS for those MRD positive by NGS or FC were only 26.9 months and 29.9 months, respectively. Thus, achieving a negative MRD status is clinically important and is a marker of tumor sensitivity to whatever regimen is being tested. The underlying biological mechanisms of why some tumors are resistant (and hence persist in the blood) is unknown; however, these MRD-positive cases offer an opportunity for further research into MCL resistance. The use of MRD status at end of induction is used as an eligibility factor in the ongoing US National Clinical Trials Network trial EA4151 (NCT03267433), where patients who are MRD negative

FLOW CYTOMETRIC ASSAY for MRD in CD5-POSITIVE B-CELL LYMPHOPROLIFERATIVE DISORDERS

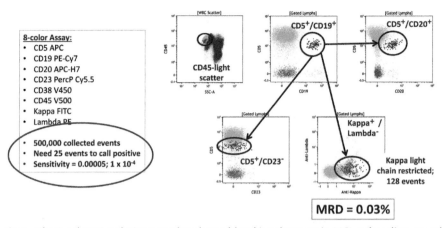

8-color Assay:
- CD5 APC
- CD19 PE-Cy7
- CD20 APC-H7
- CD23 PercP Cy5.5
- CD38 V450
- CD45 V500
- Kappa FITC
- Lambda PE

- 500,000 collected events
- Need 25 events to call positive
- Sensitivity = 0.00005; 1 x 10^{-4}

Kappa light chain restricted; 128 events

MRD = 0.03%

Fig. 3. The 8-color FC technique used to detect blood involvement in MCL at baseline or end of therapy. Using this technique, patients who are MRD positive at end of therapy have a shorter time to progression.

at end of induction are randomized to rituximab maintenance with or without autologous stem cell transplant.

The other factor in the complete blood cell count at the time of diagnosis of MCL that is somewhat useful is the absolute monocyte count (AMC). Monocytes can be suppressive to the immune system in patients with lymphoma[28]; thus, conceivably, the more monocytes, the worse the prognosis. Indeed, 2 reports demonstrate that an AMC greater than 500 at diagnosis predicts for inferior PFS and OS.[29,30]

- Blood gamma globulin levels: hypogammaglobulinemia is rare (3%) at baseline.[31] This can lead to infections and the requirement for intravenous immunoglobulin prophylaxis but has not been determined to be a prognostic factor.
- Blood cytokines: serum cytokines also are a source of variability in MCL patients. In a study of serum from 88 untreated and 20 relapsed MCL patients, the cytokine levels were compared with controls and the MIPI score.[32] Compared with controls without MCL, interleukin (IL)-12, interferon-inducible protein (IP)-10, soluble IL (sIL)-2Rα, monokine induced by gamma interferon (MIG), IL-1RA, IL-8, macrophage inflammatory protein (MIP)-1α, and MIP-1β (all $P<.05$) were elevated in MCL patients. Of these elevated cytokines, sIL-2Rα, IL-8, MIG, MIP-1α, and MIP-1β were predictive of inferior event-free survival. sIL-2Rα, IL-8, and MIP-1β were independent of MIPI score; only sIL-2Rα was associated with OS after adjustment for MIPI. In the relapsed MCL patient group, the only significantly elevated plasma cytokines that predicted EFS were sIL-2Rα and IL-8. Elevated blood levels of sIL-2Rα and the proinflammatory cytokines IL-8 and MIP-1β are adverse prognostic factors in MCL and independent of the MIPI score. IL-8 (CXCR8) is a proinflammatory and proangiogenic chemokine made by a variety of cells, including macrophages. The macrophage inflammatory proteins MIP-1α (CCL-3) and MIP-1β (CCL-4) also are proinflammatory and have a potential role in the pathophysiology of MCL. These monocyte/macrophage cytokines may relate to the adverse prognosis of the AMC, as discussed previously.

Stool Microbiome

There have been limited studies on the gut microbiome (GMB) in patients with MCL. A study by Montassier and colleagues[33] of 28 patients with NHL undergoing autologous stem cell transplant included 5 MCL patients. In all 28, those with a GMB that was less diverse had a higher likelihood of a bloodstream infection after transplant. Reduced diversity after myelosuppressive chemotherapy also was shown for NHL patients going through SCT.[34] Studies are needed on many more MCL patients to learn the impact of the GMB on side effects and outcome. Given the GI involvement with MCL in some patients, it will be interesting to learn if the GMB differs in MCL patients with or without gut involvement.

Metabolomics of Mantle Cell Lymphoma Tumors

Tumor metabolism is the net result of all of the changes in a cell that result it in becoming malignant.[35] Understanding how the metabolomics of NHL cells compare with normal cells helps focus on the most important abnormalities to target. Studies of metabolism on MCL have been conducted primarily on patient-derived MCL cell lines.[36] At rest, these MCL cells had high rates of glycolysis, glutaminolysis, and oxidative pentose phosphate pathway activities. Ibrutinib treatment inhibited these metabolic activities in ibrutinib-sensitive lines, less so in those poorly responsive to ibrutinib. The addition of glutaminase inhibitors led to cytotoxicity in the ibrutinib-insensitive lines. Early metabolic markers of response to ibrutinib in vitro was a drop in lactate and alanine.[36] Ibrutinib-resistant lines tended to shift their metabolism to oxidative phosphorylation.[37] These studies need to be performed on clinical samples from MCL patients on specific regimens to further translate this to practice.

DIFFERENCES IN TUMOR IMAGING

- PET/CT—MCL is considered a fluorodeoxyglucose (FDG)-avid NHL.[38,39] Just as there is heterogeneity in tumor cell proliferation as measured by Ki-67, there also is variability in FDG uptake between patients and even within the same patient (see **Fig. 2**). This FDG avidity in MCL, as detected by PET, offers insight into the disease and is consistent with the molecular biology, cell proliferation, and metabolomics data, discussed previously. In FL, PET/CT detects bone and soft tissue sites of involvement better than standard CT and is an independent predictor of outcome.[40] This type of analysis has not been reported for untreated MCL. Initial PET/CT scans in MCL are always positive and the results of end of treatment PET/CT predicts PFS.[41] Functional imaging with PET/CT offers a valuable, as yet underutilized, window into the metabolism of MCL that may prove useful in rapidly determining the effects of new agents on the hypermetabolism of MCL tumors.

SUMMARY

MCL is a disease with a common cytogenetic abnormality but with a variety of presentations and outcome. The most important of the diverse presentations are the adverse consequences of blastoid morphology, TP53 deletions and mutations, and their link with high proliferative tumors. As new therapies are developed, studies need to report the differential results within these categories and features so that specific types of therapies can be tailored to the tumor biology. Stool microbiome studies are likely to offer further insights into the disease, especially in those patients who present with prominent gastrointestinal tract involvement.

REFERENCES

1. Eskelund CW, Kolstad A, Jerkeman M, et al. 15-year follow-up of the Second Nordic Mantle Cell Lymphoma trial (MCL2): prolonged remissions without survival plateau. Br J Haematol 2016;175(3):410–8.
2. Eskelund CW, Dahl C, Hansen JW, et al. TP53 mutations identify younger mantle cell lymphoma patients who do not benefit from intensive chemoimmunotherapy. Blood 2017;130(17):1903–10.
3. Smedby KE, Sampson JN, Turner JJ, et al. Medical history, lifestyle, family history, and occupational risk factors for mantle cell lymphoma: the InterLymph Non-Hodgkin Lymphoma Subtypes Project. J Natl Cancer Inst Monogr 2014; 2014(48):76–86.
4. Glimelius I, Smedby KE, Eloranta S, et al. Comorbidities and sex differences in causes of death among mantle cell lymphoma patients - A nationwide population-based cohort study. Br J Haematol 2020;189(1):106–16.
5. Hoster E, Dreyling M, Klapper W, et al. A new prognostic index (MIPI) for patients with advanced-stage mantle cell lymphoma. Blood 2008;111(2):558–65.
6. Geisler CH, Kolstad A, Laurell A, et al. The mantle cell lymphoma international prognostic index (MIPI) is superior to the International Prognostic Index (IPI) in predicting survival following intensive first-line immunochemotherapy and autologous stem cell transplantation (ASCT). Blood 2010;115(8):1530–3.
7. Nordstrom L, Sernbo S, Eden P, et al. SOX11 and TP53 add prognostic information to MIPI in a homogenously treated cohort of mantle cell lymphoma - a Nordic Lymphoma Group study. Br J Haematol 2014;166(1):98–108.
8. Holtan SG, O'Connor HM, Fredericksen ZS, et al. Food-frequency questionnaire-based estimates of total antioxidant capacity and risk of non-Hodgkin lymphoma. Int J Cancer 2012;131(5):1158–68.
9. Thompson CA, Habermann TM, Wang AH, et al. Antioxidant intake from fruits, vegetables and other sources and risk of non-Hodgkin's lymphoma: the Iowa Women's Health Study. Int J Cancer 2010;126(4):992–1003.
10. Chang ET, Canchola AJ, Clarke CA, et al. Dietary phytocompounds and risk of lymphoid malignancies in the California Teachers Study cohort. Cancer Causes Control 2011;22(2):237–49.
11. Han X, Zheng T, Foss F, et al. Vegetable and fruit intake and non-Hodgkin lymphoma survival in Connecticut women. Leuk Lymphoma 2010;51(6):1047–54.
12. Molina TJ, Delmer A, Cymbalista F, et al. Mantle cell lymphoma, in leukaemic phase with prominent splenomegaly. A report of eight cases with similar clinical presentation and aggressive outcome. Virchows Arch 2000;437(6):591–8.
13. Matutes E, Parry-Jones N, Brito-Babapulle V, et al. The leukemic presentation of mantle-cell lymphoma: disease features and prognostic factors in 58 patients. Leuk Lymphoma 2004;45(10):2007–15.
14. Yoong Y, Kurtin PJ, Allmer C, et al. Efficacy of splenectomy for patients with mantle cell non-Hodgkin's lymphoma. Leuk Lymphoma 2001;42(6):1235–41.
15. Chihara D, Asano N, Ohmachi K, et al. Ki-67 is a strong predictor of central nervous system relapse in patients with mantle cell lymphoma (MCL). Ann Oncol 2015;26(5):966–73.
16. Dreyling M, Klapper W, Rule S. Blastoid and pleomorphic mantle cell lymphoma: still a diagnostic and therapeutic challenge! Blood 2018;132(26):2722–9.
17. Fu XQ, Chou GX, Kwan HY, et al. Inhibition of STAT3 signalling contributes to the antimelanoma action of atractylenolide II. Exp Dermatol 2014;23(11):855–7.

18. Mozos A, Royo C, Hartmann E, et al. SOX11 expression is highly specific for mantle cell lymphoma and identifies the cyclin D1-negative subtype. Haematologica 2009;94(11):1555–62.

19. Nygren L, Baumgartner Wennerholm S, Klimkowska M, et al. Prognostic role of SOX11 in a population-based cohort of mantle cell lymphoma. Blood 2012; 119(18):4215–23.

20. Determann O, Hoster E, Ott G, et al. Ki-67 predicts outcome in advanced-stage mantle cell lymphoma patients treated with anti-CD20 immunochemotherapy: results from randomized trials of the European MCL Network and the German Low Grade Lymphoma Study Group. Blood 2008;111(4):2385–7.

21. Hoster E, Rosenwald A, Berger F, et al. Prognostic Value of Ki-67 index, cytology, and growth pattern in mantle-cell lymphoma: results from randomized trials of the european mantle cell lymphoma network. J Clin Oncol 2016;34(12):1386–94.

22. Bea S, Valdes-Mas R, Navarro A, et al. Landscape of somatic mutations and clonal evolution in mantle cell lymphoma. Proc Natl Acad Sci U S A 2013; 110(45):18250–5.

23. Froimchuk E, Jang Y, Ge K. Histone H3 lysine 4 methyltransferase KMT2D. Gene 2017;627:337–42.

24. Zhang J, Jima D, Moffitt AB, et al. The genomic landscape of mantle cell lymphoma is related to the epigenetically determined chromatin state of normal B cells. Blood 2014;123(19):2988–96.

25. Ferrero S, Rossi D, Rinaldi A, et al. KMT2D mutations and TP53 disruptions are poor prognostic biomarkers in mantle cell lymphoma receiving high-dose therapy: a FIL study. Haematologica 2020;105(6):1604–12.

26. Pott C, Hoster E, Delfau-Larue MH, et al. Molecular remission is an independent predictor of clinical outcome in patients with mantle cell lymphoma after combined immunochemotherapy: a European MCL intergroup study. Blood 2010; 115(16):3215–23.

27. Smith M, Jegede O, Parekh S, et al. Minimal residual disease (MRD) assessment in the ECOG1411 randomized phase 2 trial of front-line bendamustine-rituximab (BR)-Based Induction Followed By Rituximab (R) ± Lenalidomide (L) Consolidation for Mantle Cell Lymphoma (MCL). Blood 2019;134(Supplement_1):751.

28. Lin Y, Gustafson MP, Bulur PA, et al. Immunosuppressive CD14+HLA-DR(low)/-monocytes in B-cell non-hodgkin lymphoma. Blood 2011;117(3):872–81.

29. Porrata LF, Ristow K, Markovic SN. Absolute monocyte count at diagnosis and survival in mantle cell lymphoma. Br J Haematol 2013;163(4):545–7.

30. von Hohenstaufen KA, Conconi A, de Campos CP, et al. Prognostic impact of monocyte count at presentation in mantle cell lymphoma. Br J Haematol 2013; 162(4):465–73.

31. Casulo C, Maragulia J, Zelenetz AD. Incidence of hypogammaglobulinemia in patients receiving rituximab and the use of intravenous immunoglobulin for recurrent infections. Clin Lymphoma Myeloma Leuk 2013;13(2):106–11.

32. Sonbol MB, Maurer MJ, Stenson MJ, et al. Elevated soluble IL-2Ralpha, IL-8, and MIP-1beta levels are associated with inferior outcome and are independent of MIPI score in patients with mantle cell lymphoma. Am J Hematol 2014;89(12): E223–7.

33. Montassier E, Al-Ghalith GA, Ward T, et al. Pretreatment gut microbiome predicts chemotherapy-related bloodstream infection. Genome Med 2016;8(1):49.

34. Montassier E, Gastinne T, Vangay P, et al. Chemotherapy-driven dysbiosis in the intestinal microbiome. Aliment Pharmacol Ther 2015;42(5):515–28.

35. Ricci JE, Chiche J. Metabolic reprogramming of non-Hodgkin's B-cell lymphomas and potential therapeutic strategies. Front Oncol 2018;8:556.
36. Lee SC, Shestov AA, Guo L, et al. Metabolic detection of bruton's tyrosine kinase inhibition in mantle cell lymphoma cells. Mol Cancer Res 2019;17(6):1365–77.
37. Zhang L, Yao Y, Zhang S, et al. Metabolic reprogramming toward oxidative phosphorylation identifies a therapeutic target for mantle cell lymphoma. Sci Transl Med 2019;11(491).
38. Barrington SF, Mikhaeel NG, Kostakoglu L, et al. Role of imaging in the staging and response assessment of lymphoma: consensus of the International Conference on Malignant Lymphomas Imaging Working Group. J Clin Oncol 2014; 32(27):3048–58.
39. Cheson BD, Fisher RI, Barrington SF, et al. Recommendations for initial evaluation, staging, and response assessment of Hodgkin and non-Hodgkin lymphoma: the Lugano classification. J Clin Oncol 2014;32(27):3059–68.
40. St-Pierre F, Broski SM, LaPlant BR, et al. Detection of extranodal and spleen involvement by FDG-PET imaging predicts adverse survival in untreated follicular lymphoma. Am J Hematol 2019;94(7):786–93.
41. Lamonica D, Graf DA, Munteanu MC, et al. 18F-FDG PET for measurement of response and prediction of outcome to relapsed or refractory mantle cell lymphoma therapy with bendamustine-rituximab. J Nucl Med 2017;58(1):62–8.

Watch and Wait in Mantle Cell Lymphoma

Christina Lee, MD, Peter Martin, MD*

KEYWORDS

- Mantle cell lymphoma • Indolent • Deferred treatment • Observation
- Non-Hodgkin lymphoma

KEY POINTS

- Observational studies suggest that a subset of patients with mantle cell lymphoma (MCL) can safely defer therapy at the time of initial diagnosis without negatively impacting long-term outcomes.
- Predictors of the "watch and wait" approach include asymptomatic presentation, good performance status, nonnodal disease, normal lactate dehydrogenase, and low Ki67.
- The presence of negative prognosticators including diffuse adenopathy, high-risk MCL International Prognostic Index score, *TP53* mutation, and complex karyotype alone should not exclude an asymptomatic patient from a period of initial observation.
- Further study is required to identify the most appropriate candidates for treatment deferral in MCL to avoid unnecessary toxicities while maximizing survival and quality of life.

INTRODUCTION

Mantle cell lymphoma (MCL) can have a heterogeneous clinical course ranging from indolent to very aggressive disease. The 2016 revision of the World Health Organization classification divided MCL into two major subtypes based on distinct molecular features: classical MCL and leukemic nonnodal MCL.[1] Classical MCL is usually composed of *IGHV*-unmutated or minimally mutated B cells that express the transcription factor SOX11, exhibits a higher degree of genomic instability, and involves lymph nodes and other extranodal sites.[2] In contrast, leukemic nonnodal MCL, which is typically SOX11-negative, is thought to arise from B cells that are germinal center-experienced because of *IGHV* somatic hypermutation.[3,4] It usually involves the peripheral blood, bone marrow, and spleen and is generally associated with an indolent

Funding: This work was funded by a Conquer Cancer Foundation of ASCO/Frist Family Endowed Young Investigator Award in honor of Howard A. Burris, III, MD (C. Lee) and a Leukemia & Lymphoma Society Mantle Cell Lymphoma Research Initiative Award (P. Martin).
Division of Hematology and Medical Oncology, Department of Medicine, Weill Cornell Medicine, 1305 York Avenue, 7th Floor, New York, NY 10065, USA
* Corresponding author.
E-mail address: pem9019@med.cornell.edu

disease course. *In situ* mantle cell neoplasia and primary gastrointestinal tract MCL also seem to be more clinically indolent variants.[5,6]

Risk stratification of newly diagnosed patients with MCL is primarily based on the MCL International Prognostic Index (MIPI), which uses the patient's age, Eastern Cooperative Oncology Group (ECOG) performance status (PS), lactate dehydrogenase (LDH) level, and white blood cell count to categorize into low-, intermediate-, and high-risk disease.[7] In addition, the proportion of cells expressing Ki67, cytogenetic abnormalities, and some recurrent genetic mutations (ie, *TP53* and *CDKN2A*) may also assist with predicting more aggressive disease.[8–12] Although these prognostic factors are well-established in patients with MCL treated with chemoimmunotherapy, they have not been validated to prospectively identify patients with indolent disease or to drive therapeutic decisions, including when to initiate treatment. Intensive chemoimmunotherapy induction regimens followed by consolidation with autologous stem cell transplantation (ASCT) have shown to improve overall survival (OS) in MCL, but these approaches are not curative and are associated with substantial acute and long-term toxicity.[13] Because a subset of patients have an indolent presentation, this may lead to overtreatment and unnecessary toxicities over potentially long periods of time.

This review evaluates the available evidence for expectant monitoring, or "watch and wait," in MCL, focusing on the clinical and biologic characteristics of the patients who were initially observed compared with those who received upfront systemic therapy and the associated outcomes.

PREDICTORS AND OUTCOMES OF DEFERRED THERAPY IN MANTLE CELL LYMPHOMA

We previously described our experience at Weill Cornell with deferred therapy, defined as a period of 3 months or more from the time of diagnosis to first systemic therapy, in 31 of 97 patients with newly diagnosed MCL.[14] There were no predefined criteria for initial observation although lymphoma-related symptoms, significant cytopenias or organ involvement, high tumor burden, and rapidly progressive disease were reasons for initiating treatment. All patients with stage I and II were observed, and the seven patients with blastoid histology were in the early treatment group. Median OS of the observation group was statistically longer than that of the early treatment group (not reached vs 64 months; $P = .004$). The median time to treatment (TTT) was 12 months and did not predict OS in multivariate analysis, suggesting that the longer OS is not attributable to greater treatment sensitivity and likely reflects more favorable clinical presentation and disease biology. Likewise, a short TTT (<14 days) seems to be associated with aggressive disease features and inferior OS despite an increased likelihood of treatment with intensive induction regimens.[15]

Subsequent studies of deferred therapy in MCL are summarized in **Table 1**.[16–22] In a large national cohort analysis using the National Cancer Database, 492 (6%) of 8029 patients were expectantly monitored for more than 90 days with a median TTT of 121 days (91–1152 days).[18] The investigators found that deferred therapy was an independent predictor of improved OS (hazard ratio, 0.79; 95% confidence interval [CI], 0.7–0.9; $P = .005$). Of note, observed patients were more likely to be managed at a high-volume academic institution and reside in the Northeast or West regions, which may be in part caused by referral selection bias but also highlights likely differences in practice patterns.

The British Columbia Cancer Agency (BCCA) published on 440 newly diagnosed patients, including 75 (17%) patients who were observed for 3 months or more.[19] The median TTT was 35 months (range, 5–79), including 60 patients (80%) who

Table 1
Reported studies of deferred initial therapy in patients with newly diagnosed mantle cell lymphoma

Study	Patient Selection	Observation (>3 mo)	Median TTT (Range)	Survival Outcomes (OBS vs Early Treatment)	Predictors of Deferred Therapy
Martin et al,[14] 2009	97 patients diagnosed 1997–2007 at single US academic center	31 patients (32%)	12 mo (4–128 mo)	Median OS not reached vs 64 mo (P = .004)	ECOG PS 0, stage I-II, lower-risk IPI score
Eve et al,[16] 2009	49 patients diagnosed 1994–2008 at single UK academic center	16 patients (33%)	11.1 mo (3.7–131.1 mo)	Median OS 34.7 mo vs 39.2 mo (not significant)	Median age <60, ECOG PS 0–1, lymphocytosis
Abrahamsson et al,[17] 2014	1389 patients diagnosed 2000–2011 from the Swedish Cancer Registry and Danish Lymphoma Registry	29 patients (2%, defined as ≥2 y)	Not reported	3-y OS of 79.8% (favorable)	ECOG PS 0–1, normal LDH
Cohen et al,[18] 2016	8209 patients diagnosed 2004–2011 from the National Cancer Database	492 patients (6%)	121 d (91–1152 d)	Median OS improved (HR, 0.79; 95% CI, 0.7–0.9; P = .005)	Stage I-II, extranodal, no B symptoms, treatment at academic center, residence in the Northeast or West
Abrisqueta et al,[19] 2017	440 patients diagnosed 1998–2014 from the British Columbia Cancer Agency Lymphoid Cancer Database	75 patients (17%)	35 mo (5–79 mo)	Median OS 72 mo vs 52.5 mo (P = .041)	ECOG PS 0–1, no B symptoms, normal LDH, nonbulky, nonnodal, nonblastoid, Ki67 <30%
Calzada et al,[20] 2018	395 patients diagnosed 1993–2015 at 5 US academic centers	72 patients (18%)	233 d (90–3651 d)	Median OS 11.8 y vs 11.6 y (P = .352)	ECOG PS 0, no B symptoms, normal LDH

(continued on next page)

Table 1
(continued)

Study	Patient Selection	Observation (>3 mo)	Median TTT (Range)	Survival Outcomes (OBS vs Early Treatment)	Predictors of Deferred Therapy
Kumar et al,[21] 2019	404 patients diagnosed 2000–2014 at single US academic center	90 patients (22%)	23 mo	Median OS 11.4 y vs 9.4 y (P = .043)	No B symptoms, normal LDH, extranodal sites <2, leukemic, nonblastoid, Ki67 <30%, lower-risk IPI score
McCulloch et al,[22] 2019	315 patients diagnosed 2015–2018 at 58 centers in the United Kingdom (ongoing)	87 patients (27.6%)	Not reported	Not reported	Female sex, no measurable disease on imaging, Ki67 <30%, normal LDH

Abbreviations: CI, confidence interval; HR, hazard ratio; IPI, International Prognostic Index; OBS, observation.
Data from Refs.[14,16–22]

were observed for at least 12 months. The only variable that was significantly associated with TTT was clinical presentation: nodal (median TTT, 25 months), nonnodal (median TTT, not reached), and gastrointestinal (median TTT, 59 months) ($P = .012$). Median OS was significantly longer in the observation group (72 vs 52.5 months; $P = .041$) and was not compromised by deferring therapy. In another population-based series using the Swedish and Danish Lymphoma Registries, 29 patients (2.4%) were observed for 2 years or longer and demonstrated a favorable 3-year OS of 79.8%.[17]

More recently, Calzada and colleagues[20] reported outcomes for 395 patients diagnosed with MCL at five academic sites in the United States. The median TTT was 3.2 years (range, 2.1–10.0 years), and the median OS was 5.2 years from diagnosis and 3.0 years from the time of initial therapy. There was no difference between the 72 (18%) patients who were initially observed compared with those who received immediate therapy, with a median OS of 11.8 versus 11.6 years, respectively ($P = .352$). In their multicenter cohort analysis, the 14 cases of deferred therapy for more than 2 years were characterized by normal LDH level (100%), no bulky adenopathy greater than 5 cm (85%), lack of B symptoms (85%), simple karyotype (80%), ECOG PS less than or equal to one (75%), and no splenomegaly (69%).

Survival rates were similarly high in the Memorial Sloan Kettering (MSK) cohort of 404 patients diagnosed with MCL between 2000 and 2014.[21] In the 90 (22%) patients with deferred treatment, there was a significant survival advantage of 11.4 years compared with 9.4 years in those who received immediate therapy ($P = .043$). Also concordant with our initial study, the OS difference between the groups disappeared when comparing time from start of treatment to death ($P = .99$). The median duration of observation was 23 months (95% CI, 17–28 months) and only the presence of lymphadenopathy greater than 1.5 cm was significantly associated with a shorter TTT. The investigators reviewed the baseline characteristics of the 30 patients who were observed for 2 years or longer and identified three dominant clinical categories of indolent MCL: (1) leukemic phase disease with minimal nodal disease (n = 9), (2) low tumor-burden disease without leukemic phase disease (n = 17), and (3) gastrointestinal tract–only disease (n = 4).[21]

The prospective MCL Biobank Observational Study in the United Kingdom presented interim results of 87 of 315 patients (27.6%) who were observed 90 days beyond diagnosis, and one-half remain on watch and wait at 2 years.[22] Most observed cases had measurable lymphadenopathy and were not the leukemic nonnodal subtype, and 40% of females were managed with initial observation. Other ongoing studies include the Lymphoma Epidemiology Outcomes study (NCT02736357) and A Disease Registry of Patients With Mantle Cell Lymphoma (NCT03816683).

Collectively, these studies support that a subgroup of patients with MCL can be safely observed at initial diagnosis without adversely impacting their outcomes. Although leukemic nonnodal MCL was associated with deferred therapy, a significant portion of observed patients had nodal disease, albeit low-volume and nonbulky. Criteria correlating with asymptomatic and lower disease burden, including lower ECOG PS, lack of B symptoms, and normal LDH levels, consistently predicted the use of expectant management at diagnosis. Other key clinical and biologic criteria are reviewed next.

MCL International Prognostic Index

The MIPI is an important and widely used clinical tool in MCL, but its prognostic significance in the modern era of novel targeted therapies is unclear, with varying findings across different trials.[23–28] Furthermore, the MIPI has not been prospectively studied to guide clinical management. In the Cornell and MSK cohorts and BCCA series, the MIPI was not predictive for either observation versus immediate treatment or the length of observation.[14,19,21] In contrast, the International Prognostic Index did correlate with treatment group in the Cornell and MSK cohorts. This was perhaps caused by age, LDH, and white blood cell count being continuous variables in the MIPI, which can drive up the score without reflecting the underlying indolent presentation.

Ki67 Proliferation Index

In MCL, the Ki67 proliferation index is a well-established prognostic marker independent of MIPI. In the Cornell cohort, Ki67 did not associate significantly with treatment group, although limited data were available. In the BCCA series, patients with a Ki67 less than 30% were more likely to be observed; however, within the observed group there was no significant difference in median TTT for patients with Ki67 less than 30% or Ki67 of 30% or greater (29 vs 20 months; $P = .447$).[19] As with the BCCA study, patients in the MSK cohort with a Ki67 of 30% or higher were more likely to receive immediate therapy; however, this may be caused by the providers being uncomfortable with expectant monitoring because of perceived high-risk disease behavior. Note that 15 patients with a Ki67 of 30% or higher were observed for a median of 22 months (95% CI, 7–33 months).[21] The Ki67 absolute value was also not significantly associated with length of observation.

TP53 Mutation

As with other malignancies, *TP53* mutation and protein overexpression in MCL are associated with a poor prognosis. In two small series published in 1996, *TP53*-mutated MCL cases had a median OS of 1.3 and 1.5 years.[10,29] Similarly, in the more recent study of 183 younger patients treated on the Nordic MCL2 and MCL3 trials, *TP53*-mutated cases had a median OS of 1.8 years compared with 12.7 years for *TP53*-unmutated cases ($P<.0001$) with inferior responses to induction- and high-dose chemoimmunotherapy and ASCT.[30] A study described patients with leukemic nonnodal MCL and *TP53* mutations who had stable disease for 6 to 38 months without need for therapy.[31] In the BCCA series, there was no significant difference between the observation periods for *TP53*-positive and *TP53*-negative patients: median TTT was 18 months and 24 months, respectively.[19] The MSK cohort also had three patients with a *TP53* mutation and they were observed for 4, 18, and 20 months.[21]

Complex Karyotype

Complex karyotype (CK), defined as the presence of three or more unrelated cytogenetic abnormalities, is an independent predictor of inferior outcomes in MCL. In a series of 483 patients, where a CK was found to be associated with a shorter progression-free survival (PFS; 1.9 vs 4.4 years; $P<.01$) and OS (4.5 vs 11.6 years; $P<.01$) independent of MIPI and Ki67 and regardless of the intensity of induction therapy or consolidation with ASCT.[9] Furthermore, patients with *TP53* mutation combined with a CK have a worse PFS and OS compared with the presence of either risk factor alone.[11] Intriguingly, Calzada and colleagues[20] found that among the 12 patients with a CK in their multicenter cohort, the median PFS was improved for those who deferred therapy ($P = .047$), raising the possibility of chemotherapy-induced resistance in cases with more genetic instability.

ADVANTAGES AND DISADVANTAGES OF WATCH AND WAIT

As with other indolent and incurable lymphomas, there has been no evidence of any detrimental effect with the watch and wait approach at initial diagnosis of MCL for a subset of patients. One benefit of expectant monitoring is the avoidance of treatment-related toxicities for a potentially prolonged period of time. Although this is evident when considering the adverse effects of intensive chemoimmunotherapy induction regimens and consolidation with ASCT, the risk-benefit analysis is not as straightforward with less aggressive yet effective therapies, such as the novel agents.

Another possible advantage of deferring therapy is giving the patient time to come to terms with the diagnosis and to seek out a consensus of other opinions. However, we realize this approach may be anxiety-inducing for some patients. In a phase 3 trial of rituximab compared with watch and wait in patients with asymptomatic follicular lymphoma (FL), the maintenance rituximab group had significant improvements in two quality-of-life assessments, the Mental Adjustment to Cancer and Illness Coping Style, from baseline to month 7 compared with the watchful waiting group.[32] The investigators attributed this finding to patients feeling more empowered and better adjusted to their diagnosis, possibly because something active was being done. Of note, the negative effect of a diagnosis of lymphoma decreased over time for the all treatment groups, as was also reported in the RESORT study randomizing patients with FL to maintenance rituximab versus surveillance and rituximab retreatment.[33]

One proposed argument against deferring treatment is that it allows time for the development of mutations that may confer chemotherapy resistance. It is also plausible that immediate treatment may improve survival in this subset of patients with indolent MCL presentations and likely more favorable disease biology. However, there are currently no data supporting these hypotheses from reported studies in MCL that have either shown superior survival or no impact with watch and wait. Although prospective data in MCL are lacking, several randomized trials of observation versus immediate treatment of early stage, indolent lymphomas, such as FL and chronic lymphocytic leukemia (CLL), have shown no survival advantage with early treatment using chemotherapy or a monoclonal antibody.[32,34-36] More recently, in the phase 3 randomized trial of the BTK inhibitor ibrutinib versus placebo in patients with asymptomatic, treatment-naive, early stage CLL, ibrutinib significantly improved PFS but also did not show an OS benefit.[37]

It would be helpful to have an objective method using a biomarker to prospectively and more definitively identify patients who are most likely to benefit and least likely to be harmed by observation without therapy. The Lymphoma/Leukemia Molecular Profiling Project recently proposed a gene expression-based assay (MCL35) using NanoString technology for formalin-fixed paraffin-embedded biopsies that contains a 17-gene proliferation signature to define groups of patients with significantly different OS independent of the MIPI.[38] Additionally, the L-MCL16 assay distinguishes between classical MCL and leukemic nonnodal MCL in leukemic samples.[31] The latter subgroup had a better OS (3-year OS 92% vs 69%; $P = .006$) and longer time to first treatment. Both assays require further validation and prospective study but have the potential for guiding therapy. Until such a predictive biomarker exists, the advantages and disadvantages of observation and early treatment should be discussed with patients who do not have a clear indication for therapy at the time of diagnosis.

FUTURE DIRECTIONS

MCL outcomes seem to be improving overall, likely because of the introduction of rituximab, new therapeutic regimens, and novel agents.[39-41] Unfortunately, current treatment strategies are not curative in most cases, and a risk-stratified approach is crucial to avoid unnecessary toxicities while maximizing survival and quality of life. Clinical trials that prospectively stratify patients on the basis of MCL biology and disease risk will be especially informative regarding the true heterogeneity of MCL presentations and the evolving patterns of care. An example is the phase 2 trial of time-limited ibrutinib and rituximab as frontline treatment of patients with indolent MCL, defined by asymptomatic presentation, ECOG PS 0 to 1, stable disease without therapy need for at least 3 months, nonblastoid histology, Ki67 less than 30%, and largest tumor diameter less than or equal to 3 cm.[42] Preliminary results were promising, with an overall response rate of 82%, a complete response rate of 75%, and 87% of complete response patients with undetectable minimal residual disease testing. Another strong consideration should be for phase 3 studies of watch and wait compared with early treatment in indolent MCL using predefined criteria, similar to those performed in FL and CLL, particularly in patients with high-risk features, such as *TP53* mutations and CK.

SUMMARY

It is now recognized that "watch and wait" is safe and appropriate in a subset of patients with MCL, potentially for an extended period of time without compromising long-term outcomes. This approach seems to be increasingly adopted, highlighting a fundamental shift in the management of newly diagnosed MCL.[22] Diagnostic criteria to prospectively identify this group of patients with "indolent MCL," however, remains to be clearly defined. Currently, the recommendation for initial observation relies primarily on clinical criteria rather than the underlying disease biology. Data from observational studies indicate that lack of lymphoma-related symptoms, good PS, and normal LDH level are strongly associated with deferred therapy. The MIPI is evidently not predictive, and the usefulness of Ki67 is uncertain. Additionally, the presence of negative prognosticators including diffuse adenopathy, high-risk MIPI score, *TP53* mutation, and CK alone should not exclude an asymptomatic patient from a period of initial observation. Improved understanding of the biologic differences driving the heterogeneity of MCL will likely help to develop better targets, personalize therapy, and ultimately improve patient outcomes.

DISCLOSURE

The authors have nothing to disclose.

REFERENCES

1. Swerdlow SH, Campo E, Pileri SA, et al. The 2016 revision of the World Health Organization classification of lymphoid neoplasms. Blood 2016;127(20): 2375–90.
2. Jares P, Colomer D, Campo E. Molecular pathogenesis of mantle cell lymphoma. J Clin Invest 2012;122(10):3416–23.
3. Orchard J, Garand R, Davis Z, et al. A subset of t(11;14) lymphoma with mantle cell features displays mutated IgVH genes and includes patients with good prognosis, nonnodal disease. Blood 2003;101(12):4975–81.
4. Ondrejka SL, Lai R, Smith SD, et al. Indolent mantle cell leukemia: a clinicopathological variant characterized by isolated lymphocytosis, interstitial bone marrow involvement, kappa light chain restriction, and good prognosis. Haematologica 2011;96(8):1121–7.

5. Carvajal-Cuenca A, Sua LF, Silva NM, et al. In situ mantle cell lymphoma: clinical implications of an incidental finding with indolent clinical behavior. Haematologica 2012;97(2):270–8.

6. Ambinder AJ, Shenoy PJ, Nastoupil LJ, et al. Using primary site as a predictor of survival in mantle cell lymphoma. Cancer 2013;119(8):1570–7.

7. Hoster E, Dreyling M, Klapper W, et al. A new prognostic index (MIPI) for patients with advanced-stage mantle cell lymphoma. Blood 2008;111(2):558–65.

8. Hoster E, Rosenwald A, Berger F, et al. Prognostic value of Ki-67 index, cytology, and growth pattern in mantle-cell lymphoma: results from randomized trials of the European Mantle Cell Lymphoma Network. J Clin Oncol 2016;34(12):1386–94.

9. Greenwell IB, Staton AD, Lee MJ, et al. Complex karyotype in patients with mantle cell lymphoma predicts inferior survival and poor response to intensive induction therapy. Cancer 2018;124(11):2306–15.

10. Greiner TC, Moynihan MJ, Chan WC, et al. p53 mutations in mantle cell lymphoma are associated with variant cytology and predict a poor prognosis. Blood 1996;87(10):4302–10.

11. Obr A, Prochazka V, Jirkuvova A, et al. TP53 mutation and complex karyotype portends a dismal prognosis in patients with mantle cell lymphoma. Clin Lymphoma Myeloma Leuk 2018;18(11):762–8.

12. Pinyol M, Hernandez L, Cazorla M, et al. Deletions and loss of expression of p16INK4a and p21Waf1 genes are associated with aggressive variants of mantle cell lymphomas. Blood 1997;89(1):272–80.

13. Maddocks K. Update on mantle cell lymphoma. Blood 2018;132(16):1647–56.

14. Martin P, Chadburn A, Christos P, et al. Outcome of deferred initial therapy in mantle-cell lymphoma. J Clin Oncol 2009;27(8):1209–13.

15. Epperla N, Switchenko JM, Shanmugasundaram K, et al. Short time to treatment is associated with inferior survival in newly diagnosed patients with mantle cell lymphoma. Blood 2019;134(Supplement_1):3997.

16. Eve HE, Furtado MV, Hamon MD, et al. Time to treatment does not influence overall survival in newly diagnosed mantle-cell lymphoma. J Clin Oncol 2009;27(32):e189–90 [author reply: e191].

17. Abrahamsson A, Albertsson-Lindblad A, Brown PN, et al. Real world data on primary treatment for mantle cell lymphoma: a Nordic Lymphoma Group observational study. Blood 2014;124(8):1288–95.

18. Cohen JB, Han X, Jemal A, et al. Deferred therapy is associated with improved overall survival in patients with newly diagnosed mantle cell lymphoma. Cancer 2016;122(15):2356–63.

19. Abrisqueta P, Scott DW, Slack GW, et al. Observation as the initial management strategy in patients with mantle cell lymphoma. Ann Oncol 2017;28(10):2489–95.

20. Calzada O, Switchenko JM, Maly JJ, et al. Deferred treatment is a safe and viable option for selected patients with mantle cell lymphoma. Leuk Lymphoma 2018;59(12):2862–70.

21. Kumar A, Ying Z, Alperovich A, et al. Clinical presentation determines selection of patients for initial observation in mantle cell lymphoma. Haematologica 2019;104(4):e163–6.

22. McCulloch R, Smith A, Wainman B, et al. 40% of females with mantle cell lymphoma are managed with initial observation: results from the MCL biobank observational study. Blood 2019;134(Supplement_1):2821.

23. Ruan J, Martin P, Shah B, et al. Lenalidomide plus rituximab as initial treatment for mantle-cell lymphoma. N Engl J Med 2015;373(19):1835–44.

24. Martin P, Maddocks K, Leonard JP, et al. Postibrutinib outcomes in patients with mantle cell lymphoma. Blood 2016;127(12):1559–63.
25. Rule S, Dreyling M, Goy A, et al. Outcomes in 370 patients with mantle cell lymphoma treated with ibrutinib: a pooled analysis from three open-label studies. Br J Haematol 2017;179(3):430–8.
26. Jerkeman M, Eskelund CW, Hutchings M, et al. Ibrutinib, lenalidomide, and rituximab in relapsed or refractory mantle cell lymphoma (PHILEMON): a multicentre, open-label, single-arm, phase 2 trial. Lancet Haematol 2018;5(3):e109–16.
27. Tam CS, Anderson MA, Pott C, et al. Ibrutinib plus venetoclax for the treatment of mantle-cell lymphoma. N Engl J Med 2018;378(13):1211–23.
28. Martin P, Bartlett NL, Blum KA, et al. A phase 1 trial of ibrutinib plus palbociclib in previously treated mantle cell lymphoma. Blood 2019;133(11):1201–4.
29. Hernandez L, Fest T, Cazorla M, et al. p53 gene mutations and protein overexpression are associated with aggressive variants of mantle cell lymphomas. Blood 1996;87(8):3351–9.
30. Eskelund CW, Dahl C, Hansen JW, et al. TP53 mutations identify younger mantle cell lymphoma patients who do not benefit from intensive chemoimmunotherapy. Blood 2017;130(17):1903–10.
31. Clot G, Jares P, Gine E, et al. A gene signature that distinguishes conventional and leukemic nonnodal mantle cell lymphoma helps predict outcome. Blood 2018;132(4):413–22.
32. Ardeshna KM, Qian W, Smith P, et al. Rituximab versus a watch-and-wait approach in patients with advanced-stage, asymptomatic, non-bulky follicular lymphoma: an open-label randomised phase 3 trial. Lancet Oncol 2014;15(4):424–35.
33. Wagner LI, Zhao F, Hong F, et al. Anxiety and health-related quality of life among patients with low-tumor burden non-Hodgkin lymphoma randomly assigned to two different rituximab dosing regimens: results from ECOG trial E4402 (RESORT). J Clin Oncol 2015;33(7):740–8.
34. Shustik C, Mick R, Silver R, et al. Treatment of early chronic lymphocytic leukemia: intermittent chlorambucil versus observation. Hematol Oncol 1988;6(1):7–12.
35. Dighiero G, Maloum K, Desablens B, et al. Chlorambucil in indolent chronic lymphocytic leukemia. French Cooperative Group on Chronic Lymphocytic Leukemia. N Engl J Med 1998;338(21):1506–14.
36. Ardeshna KM, Smith P, Norton A, et al. Long-term effect of a watch and wait policy versus immediate systemic treatment for asymptomatic advanced-stage non-Hodgkin lymphoma: a randomised controlled trial. Lancet 2003;362(9383):516–22.
37. Langerbeins P, Bahlo J, Rhein C, et al. Ibrutinib versus placebo in patients with asymptomatic, treatment-naïve early stage CLL: primary endpoint results of the phase 3 double-blind randomized CLL12 trial. Hematol Oncol 2019;37(S2):38–40.
38. Scott DW, Abrisqueta P, Wright GW, et al. New molecular assay for the proliferation signature in mantle cell lymphoma applicable to formalin-fixed paraffin-embedded biopsies. J Clin Oncol 2017;35(15):1668–77.
39. Smith A, Roman E, Appleton S, et al. Impact of novel therapies for mantle cell lymphoma in the real world setting: a report from the UK's Haematological Malignancy Research Network (HMRN). Br J Haematol 2018;181(2):215–28.
40. Fu S, Wang M, Li R, et al. Increase in survival for patients with mantle cell lymphoma in the era of novel agents in 1995-2013: findings from Texas and national SEER areas. Cancer Epidemiol 2019;58:89–97.

41. Kumar A, Sha F, Toure A, et al. Patterns of survival in patients with recurrent mantle cell lymphoma in the modern era: progressive shortening in response duration and survival after each relapse. Blood Cancer J 2019;9(6):50.
42. Gine E, De La Cruz MDF, Grande C, et al. Efficacy and safety of ibrutinib in combination with rituximab as frontline treatment for indolent clinical forms of mantle cell lymphoma (MCL): preliminary results of Geltamo IMCL-2015 phase II trial. Blood 2019;134(Supplement_1):752.

Is Limited-Stage Mantle Cell Lymphoma Curable and How Is It Best Managed?

Jason T. Romancik, MD, Jonathon B. Cohen, MD, MS*

KEYWORDS

- Mantle cell lymphoma • Non-Hodgkin lymphoma • Limited-stage • Early-stage
- Radiation therapy

KEY POINTS

- Limited-stage (stage I–II) mantle cell lymphoma (MCL) is encountered in only 5% to 15% of newly diagnosed cases, and there are limited data to guide management of these patients.
- Gastrointestinal and bone marrow evaluation are essential in suspected cases of limited-stage MCL because these are common sites of disseminated disease that may not be apparent on positron emission tomography/computed tomography.
- Radiation therapy can be considered for patients with local symptoms. There are limited data to support the use of combined chemoradiation.
- Watchful waiting is a reasonable approach for asymptomatic patients with limited-stage MCL.

INTRODUCTION

Mantle cell lymphoma (MCL) accounts for 3% to 10% of all cases of non-Hodgkin lymphoma (NHL) and is characterized by the chromosomal translocation t(11;14) leading to overexpression of cyclin D1.[1] MCL is more common in older adults with a median age at diagnosis of 67 years.[2] A majority of patients present with advanced-stage disease (Ann Arbor stage III–IV), which is incurable and characterized by a pattern of continued relapses, although outcomes have improved substantially with therapeutic advances in recent years. Limited-stage (Ann Arbor stage I–II) disease is present in approximately 5% to 15% of patients with newly diagnosed MCL, but the prognosis and best approach to treatment of these patients remains undefined. Intensive induction chemotherapy in younger, fit patients with advanced-stage disease, often followed by consolidation with an autologous stem cell transplant (ASCT), can lead to

Department of Hematology and Medical Oncology, Emory University – Winship Cancer Institute, 1365C Clifton Road, Northeast, Suite B4000D, Atlanta, GA 30322, USA
* Corresponding author.
E-mail address: Jonathon.cohen@emory.edu

Hematol Oncol Clin N Am 34 (2020) 849–859
https://doi.org/10.1016/j.hoc.2020.06.003
0889-8588/20/© 2020 Elsevier Inc. All rights reserved.

hemonc.theclinics.com

prolonged remissions and a median overall survival (OS) in excess of 10 years.[3,4] Novel agents, such as bortezomib, lenalidomide, and the Bruton tyrosine kinase inhibitors, are active in MCL and their use also has led to improved outcomes in patients with advanced disease.[5–8] The role of these treatment approaches, however, in patients with limited-stage MCL is unclear because these patients often are excluded from prospective clinical trials. Radiation therapy (RT) is effective and potentially curative for patients with certain subtypes of indolent NHL presenting with early-stage/localized disease, but there are no prospective data to support this approach for patients with limited-stage MCL. Due to the rarity of limited-stage MCL, the available data used to inform treatment decisions is composed mainly of retrospective studies. This article reviews the available evidence pertaining to the management of patients with limited-stage MCL and describe the authors' approach to treating these patients.

EPIDEMIOLOGY OF LIMITED-STAGE MANTLE CELL LYMPHOMA

The overall incidence of MCL has increased over the past 2 decades, yet the proportion of patients presenting with localized disease has declined substantially over this same time period.[9–11] An analysis of the Surveillance, Epidemiology, and End Results (SEER) database showed that the proportion of patients diagnosed with limited-stage disease had decreased from 30.5% during the time period between 1992 and 1999 to just 5.8% between 2004 and 2007.[12] An increased understanding of disease biology and patterns of spread along with more-sensitive staging techniques likely contribute to this trend. MCL is a fluorodeoxyglucose-avid disease, so the use of positron emission tomography (PET)/computed tomography (CT) as part of the initial staging workup likely has resulted in upstaging for at least some patients, although PET/CT is not sensitive enough to reliably detect extranodal involvement of the bone marrow or GI tract.[13–15] The bone marrow is involved in 50% to 80% of MCL patients, so a bone marrow biopsy is required as part of the initial staging even if it appears negative on PET scan. The gastrointestinal (GI) tract also is a common site of extranodal disease, and, although GI symptoms are present in only 15% to 25% of cases, disease involvement at the microscopic level can be detected in up to 88% of patients based on the results of 2 prospective studies where upper and lower endoscopies with random biopsies were performed on patients with newly diagnosed MCL.[16,17] As a result, the incidence of truly limited-stage disease is likely quite low.

IN SITU MANTLE CELL NEOPLASIA

In situ mantle cell neoplasia (ISMCN) is a rare incidental finding in reactive lymph nodes that merits brief discussion given the similar appearance to MCL. ISMCN is characterized by the proliferation of cyclin D1–positive B cells in the mantle zone without disruption of the normal lymph node architecture.[18–20] When ISMCN is encountered, a thorough work-up, including biopsy of any other suspicious lymph nodes or masses along with peripheral blood flow cytometry, is recommended because the lesion may coexist with overt MCL or other B-cell lymphomas, in which case treatment should be initiated based on the stage and histologic subtype of the lymphoma that is identified.[20] Consultation with an experienced hematopathologist is critical when considering a diagnosis of ISMCN and adequate tissue—preferably an excisional lymph node biopsy—must be available for review to ensure that there is no concurrent lymphoma. In the absence of overt lymphoma, no treatment is indicated, and the patient can be observed. The lesion appears to have indolent behavior, but the true incidence and overall malignant potential of isolated ISCM are not known. One series retrospectively evaluated 1292 reactive lymph nodes from unselected surgical cases of 131 patients without a lymphoma diagnosis and found no cases of ISMCN, highlighting the rarity of this entity.[21] Another series identified only 23 cases from 11 international sites over an 8-year period, and only 1 of 8 patients with isolated ISMCN managed with watchful waiting went on to develop overt lymphoma 4 years later.[22]

RATIONALE FOR RADIATION THERAPY IN THE TREATMENT OF LIMITED-STAGE MANTLE CELL LYMPHOMA

RT is a potentially curative treatment modality for patients with other forms of indolent NHL that present with localized disease.[23–28] It also is utilized in combination with shorter courses of chemotherapy for patients with limited-stage diffuse large B-cell lymphoma who are being treated with curative intent, although this strategy recently has been challenged by the results of the FLYER and SWOG1001 trials, which reported that RT can be omitted after an abbreviated course of chemotherapy without compromising outcomes in favorable-risk patients or those treated with a PET-adapted approach.[29–31] The data supporting the use of RT in MCL all are retrospective, but current treatment guidelines and expert opinion support the use of RT with or without chemotherapy as part of the initial treatment strategy for patients with confirmed limited-stage disease.[32–35]

In vitro experiments demonstrated the radiosensitivity of MCL cell lines as a result of several distinct molecular mechanisms, including mutations of the p53 and ATM genes, abnormalities of DNA repair proteins, and an abnormal telomerase status.[36] Early retrospective studies published in the 1990s provided the initial clinical evidence that favorable outcomes can be achieved when RT is used to treat limited-stage MCL. Vandenberghe and colleagues[37] reported the clinical outcomes for 69 patients with MCL who were treated prior to 1995 and, therefore, staged without PET/CT. Sixteen of these patients were reported to have limited-stage disease. A bone marrow biopsy was performed in the majority (91%) of patients in this series and extranodal disease involving the GI tract was reported in 12 patients, although it was not specified if these evaluations were performed in all patients with limited-stage disease. Fifteen of the 16 patients with limited-stage disease were treated with RT alone, which resulted in 12 complete responses. A majority of these patients eventually relapsed but 3 of them remained in complete response at 156 months, 190 months, and 192 months. Similarly, Meusers and Hense[38] found that 8 of 13 patients treated with RT alone for limited-stage disease remained in remission for up to 60 months. A more recent retrospective analysis of 657 patients with stage I–II MCL in the SEER database and found that the 178 (27%) patients who received RT as part of the initial treatment strategy had a significant improvement in median OS compared with those who did not receive RT (103 vs 66 months, respectively; $P = .002$), although the investigators did not specify if any patients received chemotherapy in addition to RT as part of the initial treatment approach, which limits the interpretation of these results.[39]

Further evidence to support the efficacy of RT for treatment of MCL was obtained when Rosenbluth and Yahalom[40] demonstrated that involved field RT (IFRT) leads to high local response rates when used for palliation in a cohort composed mainly of patients with advanced-stage or relapsed disease. The patients included in this analysis were treated with IFRT with a mean dose of 30 Gy and had a local response rate of 100% (complete response 64%), with 94% of patients experiencing an improvement in local symptoms. Local progression occurred at 34% of the disease sites, with a median duration of local response of 9 months. The toxicity generally was mild, and no grade III adverse effects were observed. The median follow-up was relatively short, at 13 months (range 1–59 months), so the durability of response remains a question. Together, these results demonstrate the feasibility of using RT for the management of limited-stage MCL.

DEFERRED THERAPY FOR LIMITED-STAGE MANTLE CELL LYMPHOMA

A subset of patients with MCL have an indolent disease course and can be observed safely after diagnosis. Martin and colleagues[41] provided the first description of a group of patients with MCL who were managed with deferred therapy and reported that patients can be monitored safely for a median of 12 months (range 4–128 months) with no detrimental impact on OS. Five of 20 patients with staging information available had limited-stage disease in this series. Similar findings were reported by Abrisqueta and colleagues[42] in a cohort that included 8 patients with stage I–II disease of a total of 74 patients. The median time to treatment and median OS were not reached in the patients with limited-stage disease. A national cohort analysis from the National Cancer Database included 8029 patients, 15% of whom had stage I–II disease.[43] The presence of stage I–II disease did not significantly influence the OS of patients who initially received deferred therapy. Finally, in a retrospective analysis of 179 patients with limited-stage MCL, Dabaja and colleagues[44] reported favorable outcomes (5-year OS rate of 92%) for the 12 patients who were managed with initial observation. Consistent clinical predictors of initial management with deferred therapy include a good performance status, lack of B symptoms, and normal lactate dehydrogenase. These factors often are present in patients with limited-stage MCL and as a result deferred therapy can be considered in this patient population.

SUMMARY OF RETROSPECTIVE STUDIES FOR THE TREATMENT OF LIMITED-STAGE MANTLE CELL LYMPHOMA

Table 1 summarizes the retrospective series, addressing the treatment of limited-stage MCL. There was no standard approach to treatment of the patients included in these reports; some received combined modality therapy whereas others were treated with chemotherapy or RT alone; 5-year OS rates in these series range from 60% to 80%, and younger patients and those with stage I disease consistently had superior outcomes. It is clear that RT is effective in achieving local control and its use can lead to prolonged remissions in some patients, although distant relapse remains a significant problem. Interpreting the results of these series is challenging, however, due to the inherit limitations of retrospective studies, the small numbers of patients included in some studies, and the lack of baseline characteristics reported in others. This is complicated further by the use of outdated chemotherapy regimens—often without rituximab—in the earlier studies. The added value of combining chemotherapy with RT is unclear and there is little guidance for selecting a treatment regimen and number of cycles of therapy. Also, details pertaining to the management of patients at time of relapse were not reported in these studies, so it is unclear how the initial treatment approach influences the response to second-line therapy. As a result, no clear treatment paradigm for patients with limited-stage MCL has emerged from the literature.

Leitch and colleagues[45] provided the first detailed description of the clinical characteristics and outcomes for patients who were treated for limited-stage MCL. In this study, records from patients treated at the British Columbia Cancer Agency were reviewed retrospectively, and 26 patients with stage I–II, nonbulky (<10 cm) MCL were identified. Twelve (46%) patients had stage I disease, and 11 (42%) patients had disease localized to the head and neck region. Of the 22 patients who received

Table 1
Summary of retrospective studies for limited-stage mantle cell lymphoma

Publication (Ref.)	Patients (n)	Chemotherapy Alone	Radiation Therapy Alone	Combined Modality Therapy	Progression-Free Survival	Overall Survival	Comment
Leitch et al,[45] 2003	26	CHOP (n = 2) Clb (n = 2)	IFRT 25–35 Gy (n = 11)	Multiagent chemotherapy + IFRT n = 4) Single-agent chemotherapy + IFRT (n = 2)	RT vs no RT; 5-y PFS, 68%, vs 11%, respectively (P = .002)	RT vs no RT; 6-y OS, 71% vs 25%, respectively (P = .13)	No patients treated with rituximab
Bernard et al,[46] 2013	26	CHOP - > ASCT (n = 1), R-CHOP (n = 1)	EFRT, 35 Gy (n = 1) IFRT, 30 Gy (n = 1)	CHOP (n = 12), R-CHOP (n = 4), CVP (n = 1), Plus IFRT (median dose, 35 Gy)	5-y PFS, 43.8%	5-y OS, 62%	No comparison made between treatment modalities
Dabaja et al,[44] 2017	179	N = 44 (72% received rituximab)	IFRT (n = 24) Median dose, 36 Gy	N = 99 (55% received rituximab)	5-y FFP, 65%	5-y OS, 76%	No significant change in FFP, OS based on treatment modality
Jo et al,[47] 2020	41	R-CHOP (n = 17), CHOP (n = 8), HyperCVAD (n = 5), BR (n = 5), CVP (n = 2)	N = 2	None	42-mo RFS, 59.1%	5-y OS, 80.4%	
Gill et al,[48] 2015	2539	70%	11%	19%	Not reported	3-y OS; 79.8% CMT vs 72.4% chemotherapy only vs 68.2% RT only (P = .018)	No details regarding chemotherapy regimen reported

Abbreviations: BR, bendamustine plus rituximab; CHOP, cyclophosphamide, doxorubicin, vincristine, and prednisone; Clb, chlorambucil; CMT, combined modality therapy; CVP, cyclophosphamide, vincristine, and prednisone; EFRT, extended-field RT; HyperCVAD, hyperfractionated cyclophosphamide, vincristine, doxorubicine, and dexamethasone.
Data from Refs.[44–48]

treatment, 11 received RT alone. Six patients received combined chemotherapy plus RT and 4 received chemotherapy alone. No patients received rituximab as part of the treatment regimen. The median follow-up time was 59 months (range 5–85 months). The 17 patients who received RT as part of the initial treatment strategy had significantly improved 5-year progression-free survival (PFS) compared with those who did not (73% vs 13%, respectively; $P = .02$) as well as improved 5-year OS, although these results were not statistically significant due to the small sample size (71% vs 25%, respectively; $P = .13$). Patients less than 60 year old also had an improved 5-year PFS (83% vs 39%, respectively; $P = .04$) and there was a trend toward improved PFS in patients with stage I disease. Four patients who were treated with RT relapsed outside of the radiation field, and all 4 patients who received chemotherapy alone relapsed, three of these relapses occurred at the original site of disease.

More recently, Bernard and colleagues[46] retrospectively analyzed the outcomes of 26 patients who were treated for stage I–II MCL between 1990 and 2007 at the Princess Margaret Hospital in Toronto. Ten (38%) patients presented with stage I disease. Bulky disease (>5 cm) was present in 5 (19%) patients. Similar to Leitch and colleagues' report,[45] the head and neck region was a common site of involvement, with 19 (73%) patients presenting with disease localized to this area. Five patients in this cohort were managed with palliative intent and were not included in the survival analysis. Of the remaining 21 patients who received aggressive therapy, 17 were treated with a combination of chemotherapy and RT. Two patients were treated with RT alone. Two patients were treated with chemotherapy alone and 1 went on to receive an ASCT. Only 5 patients received rituximab as part of the treatment regimen. For the 21 patients who were treated with aggressive therapy, the median PFS and OS were 3.2 and 6.4 years, respectively. No comparison between the different treatment modalities was provided. Patients with stage I disease had improved outcomes compared with those with stage II, with estimated median PFSs of 10.8 years and 2.8 years, respectively. Distant relapse occurred in 2 of 8 patients with stage I disease and in 7 of 13 patients with stage II disease site, and 3 of these relapses occurred in the GI tract. None of these patients had an upper endoscopy or colonoscopy at the time of diagnosis.

Dabaja and colleagues[44] expanded on this series by conducting a retrospective analysis that combined the data from 13 institutions from the International Lymphoma Radiation Oncology Group, including the 26 patients from Bernard and colleagues' study[46]; 179 patients who were treated for stage I–II MCL between 1990 and 2013 were included in the analysis. Ninety-six (54%) patients presented with stage I disease and 27 (17%) had bulky disease. Disease was localized to the head and neck region in 135 (75%) patients. A bone marrow analysis was conducted in all but 22 (12%) patients and a GI work-up was conducted in 59 (33%) patients as part of the initial staging. Ninety-nine (55%) patients were treated with chemotherapy followed by RT. Chemotherapy alone was given to 44 (25%) patients, RT alone was 24 (13%) patients, and 12 (7%) were observed. Rituximab plus cyclophosphamide, doxorubicin, vincristine, and prednisone (R-CHOP) was the most common chemotherapy regimen and was used in 57% of patients. The median follow-up was 60 months, and the 5-year and 10-year OS rates for the entire cohort were 76% and 64%, respectively. The 5-year and 10- year freedom from progression (FFP) rates were 65% and 42%, respectively. In contrast to the prior studies, the treatment modality used (combined modality vs chemotherapy alone vs RT alone) did not significantly influence the FFP or OS, although the use of RT was associated with a decreased risk of local failure. Age greater than 60 years old and the presence of bulky disease (defined as a mass >5 cm) were found to be adverse prognostic factors and there was a trend toward inferior FFP in patients with stage II disease; 68 of the 179 (38%) patients experienced treatment failure with a median time to relapse of 38 months (range 1–186 months). Relapse at the initial site of disease was predominant in those who received chemotherapy alone (10/14) compared with those who received combined modality therapy (7/34) or those who received RT alone (0/10).

Jo and colleagues[47] recently reported the outcomes of patients with limited-stage MCL who, in contrast to the prior studies, were treated mostly with chemotherapy alone as the initial treatment strategy. The study included 41 patients with stage I–II MCL who were treated between 2000 and 2016. Thirty-seven patients were treated with chemotherapy alone as their first therapeutic strategy, and 23 received a rituximab-containing regimen. Only 2 patients were treated with RT. With a median follow-up duration of 40.6 months, the 42-month relapse-free survival (RFS) rate was 59.1% and the median OS was not reached for the entire group. The estimated 5-year PFS and OS rates were 37.6% and 80.4%, respectively. Overall, 16 patients experienced relapse, which occurred locally in 5 patients, at a distant site in 7 patients, and both locally and distant in 4 patients. Because only 2 patients received RT on this study, no meaningful comparison can be made between the 2 treatment modalities.

In the largest series of limited-stage MCL to date, Gill and colleagues[48] retrospectively analyzed the trends in practice patterns and outcomes for 2539 patients with limited-stage MCL who were included in the National Cancer Database; 54.1% of patients had stage I disease and 27.8% of patients presented with extranodal disease, with the head and neck region and GI tract the most common sites involved. A majority of patients were treated with chemotherapy alone (69.8%) and the remaining patients received either RT alone (11.5%) or combined modality therapy (18.7%). No description of the chemotherapy regimens used was provided. With a median follow-up of 42.8 months, the median survival was 77.0 months, resulting in 3-year and 5-year OS estimates of 70.7% and 57.4%, respectively. The combined modality approach was associated with significantly greater 3-year estimated OS compared with chemotherapy or RT alone (79.8% vs 72.4% vs 67.8%, respectively; $P<.001$). Patients with stage I disease had greater survival than those with stage II disease (3-year OS 73.1% vs 68.2%, respectively; $P = .018$).

IS LIMITED-STAGE MANTLE CELL LYMPHOMA CURABLE?

The curability of limited stage MCL remains uncertain based on the available data. Incorporating RT into the treatment of limited-stage MCL is an effective strategy to achieve local disease control and can achieve prolonged remissions in some patients (up to 192 months in Vandenberghe and colleagues' report[37]), but MCL is a disease characterized by late relapses, as demonstrated by a patient in Dabaja and colleagues' series,[44] who relapsed after 186 months of remission. An analysis of patients with stage I NHL from the SEER database included 944 patients with MCL and, despite a 5-year disease-specific survival of 77%, there was no plateau on the survival curve, suggesting that late relapse and death from MCL continue to occur over time.[49] Similarly, patients with advanced-stage MCL who receive intensive induction therapy followed by ASCT can enjoy prolonged remissions, but a continued pattern of relapse is again seen with ongoing disease-related mortality and no plateau on the survival curves even after 12 years of follow-up. Much longer follow-up is needed with more patients achieving lasting remissions before RT can be confidently declared a curative treatment modality. MCL is largely a systemic disease, which further complicates the use of RT with curative intent. MCL is not curable with chemotherapy alone, so the addition of chemotherapy to RT is unlikely to increase the likelihood of cure significantly. Distant relapses remain a significant problem for patients treated with RT and suggest that disseminated disease often is present at the time of initial diagnosis but is not identified on initial staging. A recent study of patients with localized follicular lymphoma reported that only 40% achieved MRD negativity after treatment with RT, which further emphasizes the fact that current methods of disease detection in NHL are inadequate to truly rule out disseminated disease.[50] Further development of more-sensitive staging techniques may help better identify patients with the highest potential for cure with the use of RT.

RECOMMENDED APPROACH TO LIMITED-STAGE MANTLE CELL LYMPHOMA

Fig. 1 summarizes the authors' recommended approach for the management of patients with limited-stage MCL. If a patient presents with suspected limited-stage MCL, it is critical to perform a thorough staging evaluation, including a PET scan and bone marrow biopsy. Given the high frequency of GI involvement, an upper endoscopy and colonoscopy also should be strongly considered, even in asymptomatic patients, especially if local therapy with RT is planned. The presence of gross GI involvement leads to upstaging of the disease, although the clinical implications of occult GI involvement on a random mucosal biopsy are not known. For patients who appear to have truly limited-stage disease, especially those who are experiencing local symptoms, IFRT (30–36 Gy) should be considered because this approach is effective in achieving local control and can lead to prolonged remissions even though it is unlikely curative. If RT is not given, then an initial strategy of watchful waiting is appropriate because this approach has been shown to have no adverse effect on OS. The data supporting the use of combined chemotherapy and RT are lacking, so the authors do not recommend this treatment approach. The evidence to support the use of attenuated or abbreviated courses of chemotherapy also is lacking, so this strategy should be avoided. Patients with systemic symptoms thought to be related to MCL and those with bulky stage II disease should be treated with a full course of systemic therapy. Once a decision is made to treat systemically, a contemporary treatment regimen can be selected based on patient age, comorbidities, and disease biology just as for patients with advanced-stage disease.

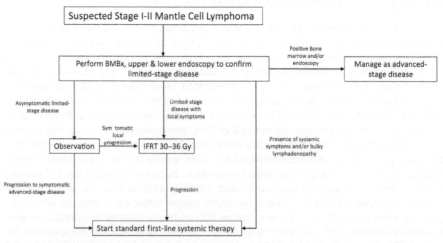

Fig. 1. Recommended initial approach to patients with suspected limited-stage MCL. BMBx, bone marrow biopsy.

DISCLOSURE

The authors have nothing to disclose.

REFERENCES

1. Teras LR, DeSantis CE, Cerhan JR, et al. 2016 US lymphoid malignancy statistics by World Health Organization subtypes. CA Cancer J Clin 2016;66(6):443–59.
2. Epperla N, Hamadani M, Fenske TS, et al. Incidence and survival trends in mantle cell lymphoma. Br J Haematol 2018;181(5):703–6.
3. Eskelund CW, Kolstad A, Jerkeman M, et al. 15-year follow-up of the Second Nordic Mantle Cell Lymphoma trial (MCL2): prolonged remissions without survival plateau. Br J Haematol 2016;175(3):410–8.
4. Chihara D, Cheah CY, Westin JR, et al. Rituximab plus hyper-CVAD alternating with MTX/Ara-C in patients with newly diagnosed mantle cell lymphoma: 15-year follow-up of a phase II study from the MD Anderson Cancer Center. Br J Haematol 2016;172(1):80–8.
5. Robak T, Huang H, Jin J, et al. Bortezomib-based therapy for newly diagnosed mantle-cell lymphoma. N Engl J Med 2015;372(10):944–53.
6. Ruan J, Martin P, Shah B, et al. Lenalidomide plus Rituximab as Initial Treatment for Mantle-Cell Lymphoma. N Engl J Med 2015;373(19):1835–44.
7. Wang ML, Rule S, Martin P, et al. Targeting BTK with ibrutinib in relapsed or refractory mantle-cell lymphoma. N Engl J Med 2013;369(6):507–16.
8. Wang M, Rule S, Zinzani PL, et al. Acalabrutinib in relapsed or refractory mantle cell lymphoma (ACE-LY-004): a single-arm, multicentre, phase 2 trial. Lancet 2018;391(10121):659–67.
9. Zhou Y, Wang H, Fang W, et al. Incidence trends of mantle cell lymphoma in the United States between 1992 and 2004. Cancer 2008;113(4):791–8.
10. Fu S, Wang M, Lairson DR, et al. Trends and variations in mantle cell lymphoma incidence from 1995 to 2013: A comparative study between Texas and National SEER areas. Oncotarget 2017;8(68):112516–29.
11. Aschebrook-Kilfoy B, Caces DB, Ollberding NJ, et al. An upward trend in the age-specific incidence patterns for mantle cell lymphoma in the USA. Leuk Lymphoma 2013;54(8):1677–83.
12. Chandran R, Gardiner SK, Simon M, et al. Survival trends in mantle cell lymphoma in the United States over 16 years 1992-2007. Leuk Lymphoma 2012;53(8):1488–93.
13. Elstrom R, Guan L, Baker G, et al. Utility of FDG-PET scanning in lymphoma by WHO classification. Blood 2003;101(10):3875–6.
14. Tsukamoto N, Kojima M, Hasegawa M, et al. The usefulness of (18)F-fluorodeoxyglucose positron emission tomography ((18)F-FDG-PET) and a comparison of (18)F-FDG-pet with (67)gallium scintigraphy in the evaluation of lymphoma: relation to histologic subtypes based on the World Health Organization classification. Cancer 2007;110(3):652–9.
15. Hosein PJ, Pastorini VH, Paes FM, et al. Utility of positron emission tomography scans in mantle cell lymphoma. Am J Hematol 2011;86(10):841–5.
16. Romaguera JE, Medeiros LJ, Hagemeister FB, et al. Frequency of gastrointestinal involvement and its clinical significance in mantle cell lymphoma. Cancer 2003;97(3):586–91.
17. Salar A, Juanpere N, Bellosillo B, et al. Gastrointestinal involvement in mantle cell lymphoma: a prospective clinic, endoscopic, and pathologic study. Am J Surg Pathol 2006;30(10):1274–80.

18. Richard P, Vassallo J, Valmary S, et al. In situ-like" mantle cell lymphoma: a report of two cases. J Clin Pathol 2006;59(9):995–6.

19. Koletsa T, Markou K, Ouzounidou S, et al. In situ mantle cell lymphoma in the nasopharynx. Head Neck 2013;35(11):E333–7.

20. Carbone A, Santoro A. How I treat: diagnosing and managing "in situ" lymphoma. Blood 2011;117(15):3954–60.

21. Adam P, Schiefer AI, Prill S, et al. Incidence of preclinical manifestations of mantle cell lymphoma and mantle cell lymphoma in situ in reactive lymphoid tissues. Mod Pathol 2012;25(12):1629–36.

22. Carvajal-Cuenca A, Sua LF, Silva NM, et al. In situ mantle cell lymphoma: clinical implications of an incidental finding with indolent clinical behavior. Haematologica 2012;97(2):270–8.

23. Brady JL, Binkley MS, Hajj C, et al. Definitive radiotherapy for localized follicular lymphoma staged by (18)F-FDG PET-CT: a collaborative study by ILROG. Blood 2019;133(3):237–45.

24. Goda JS, Gospodarowicz M, Pintilie M, et al. Long-term outcome in localized extranodal mucosa-associated lymphoid tissue lymphomas treated with radiotherapy. Cancer 2010;116(16):3815–24.

25. Vaughan Hudson B, Vaughan Hudson G, MacLennan KA, et al. Clinical stage 1 non-Hodgkin's lymphoma: long-term follow-up of patients treated by the British National Lymphoma Investigation with radiotherapy alone as initial therapy. Br J Cancer 1994;69(6):1088–93.

26. Kamath SS, Marcus RB Jr, Lynch JW, et al. The impact of radiotherapy dose and other treatment-related and clinical factors on in-field control in stage I and II non-Hodgkin's lymphoma. Int J Radiat Oncol Biol Phys 1999;44(3):563–8.

27. Wilder RB, Jones D, Tucker SL, et al. Long-term results with radiotherapy for Stage I-II follicular lymphomas. Int J Radiat Oncol Biol Phys 2001;51(5):1219–27.

28. Campbell BA, Voss N, Woods R, et al. Long-term outcomes for patients with limited stage follicular lymphoma: involved regional radiotherapy versus involved node radiotherapy. Cancer 2010;116(16):3797–806.

29. Persky DO, Unger JM, Spier CM, et al. Phase II study of rituximab plus three cycles of CHOP and involved-field radiotherapy for patients with limited-stage aggressive B-cell lymphoma: Southwest Oncology Group study 0014. J Clin Oncol 2008;26(14):2258–63.

30. Poeschel V, Held G, Ziepert M, et al. Four versus six cycles of CHOP chemotherapy in combination with six applications of rituximab in patients with aggressive B-cell lymphoma with favourable prognosis (FLYER): a randomised, phase 3, non-inferiority trial. Lancet 2019;394(10216):2271–81.

31. Persky DO, Li H, Stephens DM, et al. PET-Directed Therapy for Patients with Limited-Stage Diffuse Large B-Cell Lymphoma - Results of Intergroup Nctn Study S1001. Blood 2019;134(Supplement_1):349.

32. Ghielmini M, Zucca E. How I treat mantle cell lymphoma. Blood 2009;114(8):1469–76.

33. Straus DJ. How I treat mantle cell lymphoma. J Oncol Pract 2007;3(5):281–2.

34. Zelenetz AD, Gordon LI, Wierda WG, et al. Non-Hodgkin's lymphomas, version 4.2014. J Natl Compr Cancer Netw 2014;12(9):1282–303.

35. Sandoval-Sus JD, Sotomayor EM, Shah BD. Mantle cell lymphoma: contemporary diagnostic and treatment perspectives in the age of personalized medicine. Hematol Oncol Stem Cell Ther 2017;10(3):99–115.

36. M'Kacher R, Bennaceur A, Farace F, et al. Multiple molecular mechanisms contribute to radiation sensitivity in mantle cell lymphoma. Oncogene 2003; 22(39):7905–12.
37. Vandenberghe E, De Wolf-Peeters C, Vaughan Hudson G, et al. The clinical outcome of 65 cases of mantle cell lymphoma initially treated with non-intensive therapy by the British National Lymphoma Investigation Group. Br J Haematol 1997;99(4):842–7.
38. Meusers P, Hense J. Management of mantle cell lymphoma. Ann Hematol 1999; 78(11):485–94.
39. Guru Murthy GS, Venkitachalam R, Mehta P. Effect of radiotherapy on the survival of patients with stage I and stage II mantle cell lymphoma: analysis of the Surveillance, Epidemiology and End Results database. Clin Lymphoma Myeloma Leuk 2014;14(Suppl):S90–5.
40. Rosenbluth BD, Yahalom J. Highly effective local control and palliation of mantle cell lymphoma with involved-field radiation therapy (IFRT). Int J Radiat Oncol Biol Phys 2006;65(4):1185–91.
41. Martin P, Chadburn A, Christos P, et al. Outcome of deferred initial therapy in mantle-cell lymphoma. J Clin Oncol 2009;27(8):1209–13.
42. Abrisqueta P, Scott DW, Slack GW, et al. Observation as the initial management strategy in patients with mantle cell lymphoma. Ann Oncol 2017;28(10):2489–95.
43. Cohen JB, Han X, Jemal A, et al. Deferred therapy is associated with improved overall survival in patients with newly diagnosed mantle cell lymphoma. Cancer 2016;122:2356–63.
44. Dabaja BS, Zelenetz AD, Ng AK, et al. Early-stage mantle cell lymphoma: a retrospective analysis from the International Lymphoma Radiation Oncology Group (ILROG). Ann Oncol 2017;28(9):2185–90.
45. Leitch HA, Gascoyne RD, Chhanabhai M, et al. Limited-stage mantle-cell lymphoma. Ann Oncol 2003;14(10):1555–61.
46. Bernard M, Tsang RW, Le LW, et al. Limited-stage mantle cell lymphoma: treatment outcomes at the Princess Margaret Hospital. Leuk Lymphoma 2013;54(2): 261–7.
47. Jo JC, Kim SJ, Lee HS, et al. Clinical features and treatment outcomes of limited-stage mantle cell lymphoma: consortium for improving survival of lymphoma report. Ann Hematol 2020;99(2):223–8.
48. Gill BS, Vargo JA, Pai SS, et al. Management trends and outcomes for stage I to II mantle cell lymphoma using the national cancer data base: ascertaining the ideal treatment paradigm. Int J Radiat Oncol Biol Phys 2015;93(3):668–76.
49. Chihara D, Oki Y, Fanale MA, et al. Stage I non-Hodgkin lymphoma: no plateau in disease-specific survival ? Ann Hematol 2019;98(5):1169–76.
50. Pulsoni A, Tosti ME, Ferrero S, et al. EARLY STAGE Follicular Lymphoma: First Results of the FIL "Miro" Study, a Multicenter Phase II Trial Combining Local Radiotherapy and MRD-driven immunotherapy. Blood 2019;134(Supplement_1):124.

Initial and Consolidation Therapy for Younger Patients with Mantle Cell Lymphoma

Daniel Guy, MD, Brad S. Kahl, MD*

KEYWORDS

- Mantle cell lymphoma • Autologous stem cell transplantation • Novel therapeutics
- Clinical trials

KEY POINTS

- For young, fit mantle cell lymphoma (MCL) patients, remission duration is improved by the inclusion of high-dose cytarabine.
- Consolidation with high-dose chemotherapy followed by autologous stem cell transplantation provides a significant benefit in progression-free survival. An overall survival benefit is not proven at this time.
- Maintenance therapy with rituximab following autologous stem-cell transplantation increases both progression-free survival and overall survival.
- Novel agents, such as Bruton tyrosine kinase inhibitors, immunomodulatory drugs, and BCL2 inhibitors, have promising activity in the relapsed and refractory setting and are now being investigated in the front-line setting.
- Patients who harbor a TP53 mutation have markedly worse prognosis and may not benefit from standard intensive therapy. Treatment of these patients in a clinical trial setting is highly recommended.

Mantle cell lymphoma (MCL) is an incurable cancer that behaves aggressively in most patients. Advanced stage presentation is the general rule, and most patients require treatment at the time of diagnosis. Despite advances in the field, the treatment of young fit patients varies widely among centers, and to date, there is no standard induction treatment regimen that has shown superiority to others.

Generally, the current treatment paradigm for younger fit patients consists of immunochemotherapy followed by consolidation with high-dose chemotherapy and autologous stem-cell transplantation.

Division of Medical Oncology, Department of Medicine, Washington University School of Medicine, 660 South Euclid Avenue, Campus Box 8056-29, St Louis, MO 63108, USA
* Corresponding author.
E-mail address: bkahl@wustl.edu

Hematol Oncol Clin N Am 34 (2020) 861–870
https://doi.org/10.1016/j.hoc.2020.06.004
0889-8588/20/© 2020 Elsevier Inc. All rights reserved.

hemonc.theclinics.com

The use of intensive induction regimens for fit patients provides high response rates.

The MD Anderson Cancer Center pioneered the use of alternating cycles of hyper-fractionated cyclophosphamide, vincristine, doxorubicin, and dexamethasone (hyper-CVAD) with high-dose cytarabine and methotrexate followed by consolidation with high-dose chemotherapy and autologous or allogeneic stem-cell transplantation.[1] Forty-five patients, of which 25 were treatment naïve, began the treatment protocol. Thirty-four patients proceeded to transplant and had an impressive response with all patients achieving a complete remission (CR). Event-free survival (EFS) and overall survival (OS) for previously untreated patients were 72% (95% confidence interval [CI], 45%–98%) and 92% (95% CI, 80%–100%), respectively. Despite these results, the treatment was associated with significant toxicity, which precluded stem cell mobilization and autologous stem cell transplantation (ASCT) in a significant proportion of patients.[1] A follow-up phase 2 study of 97 treatment-naïve patients with MCL added rituximab (R) to the same chemotherapy backbone and eliminated the use of ASCT as consolidation.[2] Patients were treated with alternating cycles of R-hyperCVAD and R-Methotrexate/Cytarabine. The overall response rate (ORR) was high with 87% of the patients achieving a complete response or unconfirmed CR. At a median follow-up of 40 months, the 3-year failure-free survival (FFS) and OS were 64 and 82%, respectively.[2] Unfortunately, this regimen was associated with significant morbidity with 29% of patients discontinuing treatment because of treatment-related toxicity. In addition, 8 cases of treatment-related mortality occurred.[2] Follow-up reports showed that the 5-, 10-, and 15-year FFS rates were 49% (95% CI, 38%–58%), 26% (95% CI, 17%–35%), and 22% (95% CI 15%–31%), respectively. The 5-, 10-, and 15-year OS rates were 67% (95% CI, 57%–75%), 52% (95% CI, 42%–62%), and 33% (95% CI, 22%–43%), respectively.[3,4] The median FFS and OS were 4.8 and 10.7 years, respectively. At a median follow-up of 13.4 years, 6 patients developed treatment-related myelodysplastic syndrome or acute myeloid leukemia.[3] Interestingly, the FFS appeared to plateau after 10 years with an FFS of 30% in the young patients.

Further experience with the hyperCVAD/cytarabine/methotrexate regimen was obtained from 2 other large cohorts. A multicenter trial from the Gruppo Italiano Studio Linfomi enrolled 60 patients with newly diagnosed previously untreated MCL. CR and ORR were 72% and 83%, respectively. Sixty-three percent of the patients discontinued therapy because of treatment-related toxicity, and 3 treatment-related deaths occurred. After a median follow-up of 46 months, the estimated 5-year OS and progression-free survival (PFS) were 73% (95% CI, 59%–83%) and 61% (95% CI 45%–73%), respectively.[5] In the phase 2 SWOG 0213 study, 49 patients with previously untreated MCL were treated with R-hyperCVAD/cytarabine/MTX. CR/Complete remission unconfirmed (CRu) was achieved in 58% of the patients. The median PFS and OS were 4.8 and 6.8 years, respectively. Treatment-related toxicity led to discontinuation of therapy in 39% of the patients.[6] Although the R-hyperCVAD/cytarabine/methotrexate regimen achieves good responses and relatively long remissions, significant toxicity and difficulties in stem-cell mobilization before ASCT limited its widespread use.

The Cancer and Leukemia Group B (CALGB) designed the phase 2 CALGB 59909 trial incorporating 2 cycles of R-M-CHOP (rituximab, methotrexate, and augmented cyclophosphamide, hydroxydaunorubicin-vincristine [oncovin], and prednisone [CHOP]) with a cycle of EAR (high-dose etoposide and cytarabine with rituximab) followed by high-dose chemotherapy and ASCT.[7] The complete response rate was 69%. With a median follow-up of 4.7 years, the 5-year PFS and OS were 56% (95% CI, 43%–68%) and 64% (95% CI, 50%–75%), respectively.[7]

Several other European groups have developed treatment approaches that incorporated consolidation with high-dose chemotherapy and ASCT in the upfront setting.

In the phase 2 Nordic MCL2 trial, 160 patients younger than 66 years with newly diagnosed MCL were treated with dose-intensified induction therapy with rituximab, cyclophosphamide, doxorubicin, and prednisone (R-maxi-CHOP) alternating with rituximab and high-dose cytarabine.[8] Overall response and complete response rates were 96% and 54%, respectively. The responding patients continued treatment with high-dose chemotherapy and ASCT. The 6-year PFS and OS were 66% and 70%, respectively.[8] Long-term results with a median follow-up of 14 years showed median PFS of 8.5 years with a median OS of 12.7 years.[9,10] Despite improved and long response durations, late relapses were common, and survival curves never plateaued.

The role of high-dose cytarabine was illustrated in a few additional trials. In a French phase 2 study, the addition of dexamethasone, cisplatin, and high-dose cytarabine (DHAP) sequentially to CHOP chemotherapy increased the CR rate from 7% to 82%. The responding patients underwent high-dose chemotherapy followed by ASCT. The median EFS and OS were 51 months (95% CI, 43- upper limit not reached) and 81 months (95% CI, 66- upper limit not reached), respectively.[11,12] In a follow-up phase 2 study (n = 60) by the French cooperative group (GELA), rituximab was added to sequential therapy with CHOP and DHAP, followed by ASCT. The ORR was 95% with 57% achieving complete response. After a median follow-up of 67 months, the median PFS was 84 months, and the median OS has not been reached.[13] The European MCL network was the first to show the importance of high-dose cytarabine in a randomized controlled trial.[14] In this phase 3 study, investigators compared induction with 6 cycles of R-CHOP chemotherapy followed by ASCT to 6 cycles of alternating R-CHOP and R-DHAP followed by ASCT. Patients who received R-DHAP containing induction achieved higher complete response rates before ASCT compared with R-CHOP alone (55% vs 39%; $P = .0005$). After a median follow-up of 6.1 years, patients who received high-dose cytarabine had a significantly longer PFS (9.1 vs 4.3 years; $P < .0001$). OS, however, was not significantly different between the groups. The Lymphoma Study Association (LYSA) also evaluated the use of R-DHAP induction regimen in a phase 3 study that evaluated the role of rituximab maintenance after ASCT.[15] Patients were treated with 4 consecutive cycles of R-DHAP followed by high-dose chemotherapy and ASCT. R-DHAP was chosen in order to eliminate the exposure to anthracyclines or alkylating agents. The exact platinum compound was physician's choice: 184 patients were treated with cisplatin; 76 patients with carboplatin; and 38 patients with oxaliplatin.[16] The ORR to R-DHAP was 93%, including a complete response in 77% of the patients.[15] In a subsequent subgroup analysis, there was a trend toward improved PFS and OS in the oxaliplatin-treated patients that did not reach statistical significance.[16] A summary of trial outcomes using different intensive therapy strategies is shown in **Table 1**.

CONSOLIDATION WITH AUTOLOGOUS STEM CELL TRANSPLANTATION

The use of high-dose chemotherapy and ASCT as consolidation in young transplant-eligible patients is a widely accepted approach. The European MCL Network was the only one to date to show the benefit of ASCT in a randomized controlled trial.[17] They randomized 122 patients aged less than 65 with newly diagnosed advanced stage MCL to either high-dose chemotherapy followed by ASCT or to interferon-alpha maintenance. All patients were treated with CHOP-like induction therapies. Patients who underwent ASCT had a significantly longer median PFS compared with interferon-alpha maintenance (39 vs 17 months; $P = .0108$). No survival benefit was observed in this trial.[17] Multiple other trials incorporated high-dose chemotherapy and showed an increase in PFS in comparison to historical controls, but no OS benefit was proven.

Table 1
Summary of outcomes using different intensive strategies in mantle cell lymphoma

Regimen	Author/ Study	Median Age	Number of Patients	Median PFS	OS
R-hyperCVAD/ R-MTX-AraC	Romaguera et al,[2] 2005; Chihara et al,[3] 2016	56	65	5.5 y	Median OS 13.4 y 5-y PFS: 75%
R-hyperCVAD/ R-MTX-AraC	Merli et al,[5] 2012	57	60	Estimated 5-y PFS: 61%	ES 5-y: 73%
R-hyperCVAD/ R-MTX-AraC	Bernstein et al,[6] 2013	57	49	4.8 y	Median OS: 6.8
R-M-CHOP, EAR, ASCT	Damon et al,[7] 2009	57	78	5-y PFS: 56%	5-y OS: 64%
R-maxi-CHOP/ HiDAC, ASCT	Eskelund et al,[9] 2016	56	160	8.5 y	Median: 12.7 y
CHOP, DHAP, ASCT	Lefrere et al,[11,12] 2002, 2004	56	28	Median EFS 4.25 y	6.75 y
R-CHOP/R-DHAP, ASCT	Delarue et al,[13] 2013	57	60	5-y EFS: 64%	5- y OS: 75%
R-CHOP + ASCT vs R-CHOP/R-DHAP + ASCT	Hermine et al,[14] 2016	55	234 vs 232	4.3 vs 9.1 y	Median not reached vs 12.7 y
R-DHAP + ASCT	Le Gouill et al,[15] 2017	57	299	4-y PFS 68%	4-y OS 78%

There is currently no other randomized prospective data about the benefit of consolidation with ASCT. Retrospective analyses, however, reached conflicting conclusions. A small retrospective analysis of 42 patients treated at the University Hospital Zurich compared the outcomes of patients treated with R-hyperCVAD or R-CHOP/ASCT.[18] With a mean follow-up of 5.7 years, the 10-year PFS for all patients was 32% and OS was 76% with no difference between the 2 treatment groups.[18] Analysis of 127 cases from the non-Hodgkin lymphoma (NHL) outcomes database of the National Comprehensive Cancer Network showed no difference in PFS between aggressive induction regimens (R-hyperCVAD, R-CHOP + ASCT, or R-hyperCVAD + ASCT), but they all demonstrated superior PFS compared with R-CHOP induction ($P<.004$). Despite the benefit in PFS, no survival benefit was attributed to intensive upfront treatment.[19] On the other hand, analysis of data pertaining to 10,290 patients from the National Cancer Data Base did find an association between ASCT and improved OS (hazard ratio [HR] 0.46, 95% CI 0.41–0.52; $P<.001$).[20] The OS benefit remained statistically significant following propensity score matched analysis. Conflicting results were obtained in a recently published large retrospective analysis. Investigators pooled data from 25 medical centers for 1254 transplant-eligible patients under the age of 65. On *unadjusted* analysis, ASCT was associated with improved PFS (75 vs 44 months; $P<.01$) as well as OS (147 vs 115 months; $P<.05$) when compared with chemotherapy alone. This survival benefit lost its statistical significance on multivariate regression analysis (HR 0.77, 95% CI 0.98–1.01; $P = .06$). Refinement of these results with propensity-score weighted analysis (using inverse probability of treatment weighting) further decreased the difference in OS (147 vs 138 months; $P = .24$).[21]

The intergroup trial EA4151 (NCT03267433) is a randomized phase 3 trial that attempts to shed light on the role of ASCT. Patients who achieve CR with a negative minimal residual disease (MRD) state are randomized into either rituximab maintenance or to autologous stem-cell transplantation followed by rituximab maintenance. This trial may help future tailoring of the correct consolidation therapy for patients based on biological markers (MRD status).

Despite the conflicting evidence regarding the effect of consolidation with high-dose chemotherapy and ASCT on OS, it has become common practice because patients have the benefit of long remissions. An additional consideration supporting intensive strategies upfront is that many patients with MCL are diagnosed in the seventh decade of life and may lose their "window of opportunity" to receive more intensive approaches as they age or develop other comorbid conditions.

It is particularly important to recognize the young patient who may not benefit from an intensive upfront therapy. Analysis of samples from the Nordic MCL trials found patients who harbor TP53 mutations to represent a unique subset of MCL patients who have markedly shorter remissions as well as decreased survival. The CR rate after induction and ASCT in TP53 mutated cases was 45% compared with 90% in unmutated cases ($P<.0001$). The median OS and PFS of TP53 mutated cases versus unmutated cases were 1.8 years versus OS not reached and 0.9 versus 10.2 years, respectively.[22] The optimal approach to TP53 mutated cases is currently unknown, and treatment in a clinical trial setting using novel agents is highly recommended.

The role of maintenance therapy with rituximab was clarified in a phase 3 randomized control trial by the LYSA Group.[15] Eligible patients received 4 cycles of R-DHAP chemotherapy followed by autologous stem-cell transplantation with R-BEAM (rituximab, BCNU, etoposide, cytarabine, melphalan) conditioning. Two hundred forty transplanted patients were then randomized to receive rituximab maintenance therapy (at a dose of 375 mg/m² every 2 months for 3 years) or to undergo observation. At a median follow-up of 50.2 months from randomization, the median PFS and OS were not reached in either group. Albeit, the 4-year rates of EFS, PFS, and OS were significantly higher in the rituximab maintenance group. The 4-year EFS from randomization was 79% (95% CI, 70%–86%) in the rituximab group versus 61% (95% CI, 51%–70%) in the observation group ($P = .001$). The 4-year PFS was 83% (95% CI, 73%–88%) versus 64% (95% CI, 55%–73%; $P<.001$), and the 4-year OS was 89% (95% CI, 81%–94%) in the rituximab group versus 80% (95% 72%–88%) in the observation group ($P = .004$). The added benefit in terms of PFS and OS led to widespread adoption of maintenance rituximab therapy following ASCT.

FUTURE DIRECTIONS

The lack of a plateau in survival curves of patients with MCL led investigators to try to improve on current treatments. Although less intensive induction regimens are mostly used in the elderly MCL population, recent studies provided important information for future therapy.

The proteasome inhibitor bortezomib has shown promising activity against MCL. It was initially approved as monotherapy for treatment of relapsed MCL in 2006.[23] It then showed benefit in the upfront setting for patients who were ineligible for intensive regimens.[24]

Bendamustine and rituximab (BR) is a less intensive regimen that has shown high activity in indolent NHL and in MCL. The STIL trial was a phase 3 randomized controlled study that showed a PFS benefit to BR over R-CHOP in transplant-ineligible patients (35.4 vs 22.1 months, HR 0.49, 95% CI 0.28–0.79; P = .00044).[25] The BRIGHT trial confirmed these results in the subset of patients with MCL yielding a 5-year PFS rate of 39.7% in the BR arm versus 14.2% in the R-CHOP arm (95% CI, 0.21–0.75; P = .0035).[26,27] The SWOG study S1106 compared BR to R-hyperCVAD as an induction regimen before ASCT in fit young patients with MCL.[28] The study was prematurely closed after accruing 53 out of planned 160 patients because of unacceptably high mobilization failure rate on the R-hyperCVAD arm (29%). Although limited by small numbers, BR was associated with an ORR of 82.9% versus 94.1% in the R-hyper-CVAD arm and CR rate of 40% versus 35%.[28] A phase 2 study at the Dana-Farber Cancer Institute combined BR with high-dose cytarabine. Twenty-three transplant-eligible patients received 3 cycles of BR, followed by 3 cycles of high-dose cytarabine. The CR rate was 96% with a PFS of 96% at a median follow-up of 13 months.[29] A single-institution study at Washington University in St. Louis evaluated alternating cycles of BR with rituximab plus high-dose cytarabine in transplant-eligible patients (NCT02728531). A pooled analysis of these 2 trials as well as a cohort of patients treated off-trial demonstrated an ORR of 98% with a CR rate of 92%.[30] The same regimen is currently being tested in the phase 2 intergroup trial EA4181 (NCT04115631).

Multiple targeted agents have been investigated either as monotherapy or in combination in patients with relapsed and refractory MCL. There are now attempts to move these agents to the front-line setting in order to try to achieve deeper remissions and better clinical outcomes.

The Bruton tyrosine kinase (BTK) inhibitors, ibrutinib, acalabrutinib, and zanubrutinib, are highly active in B-cell malignancies and have been approved as monotherapies for relapsed/refractory MCL.[31–33] Several clinical trials are currently testing the role of BTK inhibitors in newly diagnosed patients with MCL. MD Anderson Cancer Center is testing an induction regimen with ibrutinib and rituximab followed by consolidation with hyperCVAD chemotherapy (Window-1 trial, NCT02427620). The European MCL Network is conducting a multicenter phase 3 trial looking at the role of ibrutinib in induction therapy for young fit patients (TRIANGLE trial). Patients are randomized to either alternating cycles of R-CHOP/R-DHAP followed by myeloablative ASCT, R-CHOP + ibrutinib alternating with R-DHAP followed by ibrutinib maintenance for 2 years, or R-CHOP + ibrutinib alternating with R-DHAP and followed by myeloablative ASCT and ibrutinib maintenance for 2 years (NCT02858258). Washington University in St. Louis has piloted a combined regimen of acalabrutinib with consecutive cycles of bendamustine/rituximab followed by cytarabine/rituximab (NCT03623373). The same regimen is now part of the phase 2 intergroup trial EA1418 comparing 3 induction therapies in young fit patients: bendamustine/rituximab followed by cytarabine/rituximab, acalabrutinib with bendamustine/rituximab followed by acalabrutinib with cytarabine/rituximab, and acalabrutinib with bendamustine/rituximab (NCT04115631). The immunomodulating drug lenalidomide was approved as monotherapy for patients with relapsed MCL after bortezomib treatment.[34] It is now being tested in combination with acalabrutinib and rituximab in patients with untreated MCL, including ones who are eligible for high-dose chemotherapy and ASCT (NCT03863184). Other targets have shown promising results in treatment of MCL in the relapsed setting. The BCL2 inhibitor venetoclax combined with ibrutinib showed improved outcomes in patients with relapsed disease.[35] MD Anderson Cancer Center is currently studying an induction regimen of ibrutinib and rituximab followed by consolidation with venetoclax and hyperCVAD in young fit patients (Window II trial, NCT03710772). Venetoclax is also being evaluated in the front-line setting in both

Table 2
Ongoing clinical trials in mantle cell lymphoma

ClinicalTrials.gov Identifier	Study Name	Regimen	Phase of Study	Study Start	Estimated Completion	Estimated Enrollment	Status
NCT04115631	EA4181	1. BR + CR 2. BR + CR + Acalabrutinib 3. BR + Acalabrutinib	2	Mar 2019	Mar 2025	369 patients	Recruiting
NCT03623373	FIT MCL 2.0	BR + CR + Acalabrutinib	Pilot	Nov 2018	Nov 2025	15 patients	
NCT02427620	WINDOW-1	Induction: Ibrutinib + Rituximab Consolidation: hyperCVAD	2	Jun 2015	Jun 2022	131 patients	Recruiting
NCT03710772	WINDOW-2	Induction: Ibrutinib + Rituximab Consolidation: hyperCVAD + Venetoclax	2	May 2019	May 2021	50 patients	Recruiting
NCT02858258	TRIANGLE	1. R-CHOP/R-DHAP ASCT consolidation 2. R-CHOP + Ibrutinib/R-DHAP ASCT consolidation Ibrutinib maintenance 3. R-CHOP + Ibrutinib/R-DHAP Ibrutinib maintenance	3	Jul 2016	May 2026	870 patients	Recruiting
NCT03863184		Acalabrutinib + Lenalidomide + Rituximab	2	Oct 2019	Nov 2024	24 patients	Recruiting
NCT03523975		Lenalidomide + Rituximab + Venetoclax	1	Dec 2018	Jul 2022	28 patients	Recruiting
NCT03872180		Bendamustine + Obinutuzumab + Venetoclax	2	Apr 2019	Apr 2026	27 patients	Recruiting
NCT03267433	EA4151	Patients with MRD(−) after induction: 1. ASCT, then Rituximab maintenance 2. No ASCT; Rituximab maintenance only	3	Aug 2017	Jan 2032	689 patients	Recruiting

transplant-eligible and transplant-ineligible patients in combination with lenalidomide and rituximab (NCT03523975) or with bendamustine and obinutuzumab (NCT03872180). A summary of ongoing clinical trials is shown in **Table 2**.

Novel cellular therapies and immunotherapies are currently evaluated in the relapsed/refractory setting. Allogeneic stem cell transplantation has the potential for long remissions, but the risk of nonrelapse morbidity and mortality is significant.[36] Chimeric antigen receptor (CAR) T-cell therapies as well as T-cell engagers are being evaluated in the relapsed setting and may provide another opportunity for long-term remissions.

SUMMARY

Most young fit patients achieve long remissions with an intensive upfront approach that includes a combination of immunochemotherapy containing rituximab and high-dose cytarabine, followed by high-dose chemotherapy and autologous stem-cell transplantation. The addition of maintenance therapy with rituximab following autologous stem-cell transplantation prolongs the time to relapse and increases OS. Despite an intensive approach, late relapses are common and are usually treated with novel agents. Current research is focused on testing novel agents such as BTK inhibitors and BCL2 inhibitors in the frontline setting.

DISCLOSURE

D. Guy: Nothing to disclose; B.S. Kahl: Genentech, Roche, Celgene, Pharmacyclics, AstraZeneca, BeiGene.

REFERENCES

1. Khouri IF, Romaguera J, Kantarjian H, et al. Hyper-CVAD and high-dose methotrexate/cytarabine followed by stem-cell transplantation: an active regimen for aggressive mantle-cell lymphoma. J Clin Oncol 1998;16(12):3803–9.

2. Romaguera JE, Fayad L, Rodriguez MA, et al. High rate of durable remissions after treatment of newly diagnosed aggressive mantle-cell lymphoma with rituximab plus hyper-CVAD alternating with rituximab plus high-dose methotrexate and cytarabine. J Clin Oncol 2005;23(28):7013–23.

3. Chihara D, Cheah CY, Westin JR, et al. Rituximab plus hyper-CVAD alternating with MTX/Ara-C in patients with newly diagnosed mantle cell lymphoma: 15-year follow-up of a phase II study from the MD Anderson Cancer Center. Br J Haematol 2016;172(1):80–8.

4. Romaguera JE, Fayad LE, Feng L, et al. Ten-year follow-up after intense chemoimmunotherapy with Rituximab-HyperCVAD alternating with Rituximab-high dose methotrexate/cytarabine (R-MA) and without stem cell transplantation in patients with untreated aggressive mantle cell lymphoma. Br J Haematol 2010;150(2):200–8.

5. Merli F, Luminari S, Ilariucci F, et al. Rituximab plus HyperCVAD alternating with high dose cytarabine and methotrexate for the initial treatment of patients with mantle cell lymphoma, a multicentre trial from Gruppo Italiano Studio Linfomi. Br J Haematol 2012;156(3):346–53.

6. Bernstein SH, Epner E, Unger JM, et al. A phase II multicenter trial of hyperCVAD MTX/Ara-C and rituximab in patients with previously untreated mantle cell lymphoma; SWOG 0213. Ann Oncol 2013;24(6):1587–93.

7. Damon LE, Johnson JL, Niedzwiecki D, et al. Immunochemotherapy and autologous stem-cell transplantation for untreated patients with mantle-cell lymphoma: CALGB 59909. J Clin Oncol 2009;27(36):6101–8.
8. Geisler CH, Kolstad A, Laurell A, et al. Long-term progression-free survival of mantle cell lymphoma after intensive front-line immunochemotherapy with in vivo-purged stem cell rescue: a nonrandomized phase 2 multicenter study by the Nordic Lymphoma Group. Blood 2008;112(7):2687–93.
9. Eskelund CW, Kolstad A, Jerkeman M, et al. 15-year follow-up of the Second Nordic Mantle Cell Lymphoma trial (MCL2): prolonged remissions without survival plateau. Br J Haematol 2016;175(3):410–8.
10. Geisler CH, Kolstad A, Laurell A, et al. Nordic MCL2 trial update: six-year follow-up after intensive immunochemotherapy for untreated mantle cell lymphoma followed by BEAM or BEAC + autologous stem-cell support: still very long survival but late relapses do occur. Br J Haematol 2012;158(3):355–62.
11. Lefrere F, Delmer A, Levy V, et al. Sequential chemotherapy regimens followed by high-dose therapy with stem cell transplantation in mantle cell lymphoma: an update of a prospective study. Haematologica 2004;89(10):1275–6.
12. Lefrere F, Delmer A, Suzan F, et al. Sequential chemotherapy by CHOP and DHAP regimens followed by high-dose therapy with stem cell transplantation induces a high rate of complete response and improves event-free survival in mantle cell lymphoma: a prospective study. Leukemia 2002;16(4):587–93.
13. Delarue R, Haioun C, Ribrag V, et al. CHOP and DHAP plus rituximab followed by autologous stem cell transplantation in mantle cell lymphoma: a phase 2 study from the Groupe d'Etude des Lymphomes de l'Adulte. Blood 2013;121(1):48–53.
14. Hermine O, Hoster E, Walewski J, et al. Addition of high-dose cytarabine to immunochemotherapy before autologous stem-cell transplantation in patients aged 65 years or younger with mantle cell lymphoma (MCL Younger): a randomised, open-label, phase 3 trial of the European Mantle Cell Lymphoma Network. Lancet 2016;388(10044):565–75.
15. Le Gouill S, Thieblemont C, Oberic L, et al. Rituximab after autologous stem-cell transplantation in mantle-cell lymphoma. N Engl J Med 2017;377(13):1250–60.
16. Le Gouill S, Thieblemont C, Oberic L, et al. R-DHA-oxaliplatin before autologous stem cell transplantation prolongs PFS and OS as compared to R-DHA-carboplatin and R-DHA-cisplatin in patients with mantle cell lymphoma, a subgroup analysis of the LyMa trial. Blood 2017;130(S1):1496.
17. Dreyling M, Lenz G, Hoster E, et al. Early consolidation by myeloablative radiochemotherapy followed by autologous stem cell transplantation in first remission significantly prolongs progression-free survival in mantle-cell lymphoma: results of a prospective randomized trial of the European MCL Network. Blood 2005;105(7):2677–84.
18. Widmer F, Balabanov S, Soldini D, et al. R-hyper-CVAD versus R-CHOP/cytarabine with high-dose therapy and autologous haematopoietic stem cell support in fit patients with mantle cell lymphoma: 20 years of single-center experience. Ann Hematol 2018;97(2):277–87.
19. LaCasce AS, Vandergrift JL, Rodriguez MA, et al. Comparative outcome of initial therapy for younger patients with mantle cell lymphoma: an analysis from the NCCN NHL Database. Blood 2012;119(9):2093–9.
20. Sawalha Y, Radivoyevitch T, Tullio K, et al. The role of upfront autologous hematopoietic cell transplantation in the treatment of mantle cell lymphoma, a population based study using the national cancer data base (NCDB). Blood 2017;130(S1):2009.

21. Gerson JN, Handorf E, Villa D, et al. Survival outcomes of younger patients with mantle cell lymphoma treated in the rituximab era. J Clin Oncol 2019;37(6): 471–80.

22. Eskelund CW, Dahl C, Hansen JW, et al. TP53 mutations identify younger mantle cell lymphoma patients who do not benefit from intensive chemoimmunotherapy. Blood 2017;130(17):1903–10.

23. Fisher RI, Bernstein SH, Kahl BS, et al. Multicenter phase II study of bortezomib in patients with relapsed or refractory mantle cell lymphoma. J Clin Oncol 2006; 24(30):4867–74.

24. Robak T, Huang H, Jin J, et al. Bortezomib-based therapy for newly diagnosed mantle-cell lymphoma. N Engl J Med 2015;372(10):944–53.

25. Rummel MJ, Niederle N, Maschmeyer G, et al. Bendamustine plus rituximab versus CHOP plus rituximab as first-line treatment for patients with indolent and mantle-cell lymphomas: an open-label, multicentre, randomised, phase 3 non-inferiority trial. Lancet 2013;381(9873):1203–10.

26. Flinn IW, van der Jagt R, Kahl B, et al. First-line treatment of patients with indolent non-Hodgkin lymphoma or mantle-cell lymphoma with bendamustine plus rituximab versus R-CHOP or R-CVP: results of the BRIGHT 5-year follow-up study. J Clin Oncol 2019;37(12):984–91.

27. Flinn IW, van der Jagt R, Kahl BS, et al. Randomized trial of bendamustine-rituximab or R-CHOP/R-CVP in first-line treatment of indolent NHL or MCL: the BRIGHT study. Blood 2014;123(19):2944–52.

28. Chen RW, Li H, Bernstein SH, et al. RB but not R-HCVAD is a feasible induction regimen prior to auto-HCT in frontline MCL: results of SWOG Study S1106. Br J Haematol 2017;176(5):759–69.

29. Armand P, Redd R, Bsat J, et al. A phase 2 study of Rituximab-Bendamustine and Rituximab-Cytarabine for transplant-eligible patients with mantle cell lymphoma. Br J Haematol 2016;173(1):89–95.

30. Merryman RD, Natasha B, Redd RA, et al. Rituximab/bendamustine and rituximab/cytarabine (RB/RC) induction chemotherapy for transplant-eligible patients with mantle cell lymphoma: a pooled analysis of two phase 2 clinical trials and off-trial experience. Blood 2018;132(S1):858–67.

31. Wang M, Rule S, Zinzani PL, et al. Acalabrutinib in relapsed or refractory mantle cell lymphoma (ACE-LY-004): a single-arm, multicentre, phase 2 trial. Lancet 2018;391(10121):659–67.

32. Wang ML, Blum KA, Martin P, et al. Long-term follow-up of MCL patients treated with single-agent ibrutinib: updated safety and efficacy results. Blood 2015; 126(6):739–45.

33. Wang ML, Rule S, Martin P, et al. Targeting BTK with ibrutinib in relapsed or refractory mantle-cell lymphoma. N Engl J Med 2013;369(6):507–16.

34. Goy A, Sinha R, Williams ME, et al. Single-agent lenalidomide in patients with mantle-cell lymphoma who relapsed or progressed after or were refractory to bortezomib: phase II MCL-001 (EMERGE) study. J Clin Oncol 2013;31(29):3688–95.

35. Tam CS, Anderson MA, Pott C, et al. Ibrutinib plus Venetoclax for the treatment of mantle-cell lymphoma. N Engl J Med 2018;378(13):1211–23.

36. Fenske TS, Zhang MJ, Carreras J, et al. Autologous or reduced-intensity conditioning allogeneic hematopoietic cell transplantation for chemotherapy-sensitive mantle-cell lymphoma: analysis of transplantation timing and modality. J Clin Oncol 2014;32(4):273–81.

Approach to the Initial Treatment of Older Patients with Mantle Cell Lymphoma

Jia Ruan, MD, PhD

KEYWORDS

- MCL • Older patients • Induction • Maintenance • Novel agents

KEY POINTS

- Chemoimmunotherapies, such as bendamustine and rituximab (BR) induction and rituximab plus cyclophosphamide, doxorubicin, vincristine, and prednisone (R-CHOP) induction followed by rituximab maintenance, are common initial therapies for older mantle cell lymphoma patients who are physically fit. BR induction is noninferior to R-CHOP.
- BR forms the induction backbone for multiple ongoing phase 3 studies evaluating the efficacy of adding novel agents, including bortezomib and Bruton tyrosine kinase (BTK) inhibitors.
- Maintenance rituximab prolongs progression-free survival and overall survival after R-CHOP induction. The role of rituximab maintenance after BR induction remains unclear.
- Chemotherapy-free combinations have the potential as induction and maintenance options.
- Minimal residual disease correlates with response duration and is being explored as an experimental endpoint for response-adapted treatment strategy.

INTRODUCTION

Mantle cell lymphoma (MCL) is a distinct subtype of non-Hodgkin lymphoma characterized by t(11;14) (q13;q32) translocation leading to cyclin D1 overexpression and cell-cycle dysregulation.[1] With a median age of 65 years, MCL affects predominantly older patients with comorbidities. Initial treatment is not standardized but usually builds on chemotherapy backbones that are not curative. Although the introduction of high-dose cytarabine to rituximab-based chemoimmunotherapy followed by consolidative autologous stem cell transplant has significantly improved the outcome of young and fit patients, the intensity and toxicity associated with such approach generally were prohibitive for older MCL patients. Instead, clinical development with less-intensive treatment regimens incorporating rituximab, maintenance therapy, and novel

Division of Hematology and Medical Oncology, Meyer Cancer Center, Weill Cornell Medicine, 1305 York Avenue, New York, NY 10065, USA
E-mail address: jruan@med.cornell.edu

Hematol Oncol Clin N Am 34 (2020) 871–885
https://doi.org/10.1016/j.hoc.2020.06.005
hemonc.theclinics.com

agents has steadily improved treatment options and outcomes for older MCL patients.[2]

There is no clear definition of elderly in MCL therapy. Clinical trials often use a cutoff of 65 years or older as an empirical threshold to gauge tolerance to treatment intensity, with the threshold ranging from 60 years to 70 years in various studies. Exception and limitation to such definition, however, are well recognized in real-world clinical practice. For example, patients younger than 65 with comorbidities often are considered for less-intensive treatment, whereas some patients well into their 70s do quite well with high-dose therapy with stem cell transplant.[3] Ultimately, making effective treatment tailored to individual risk profiles and broadly applicable to all patients will make treatment decisions less reliant on age factor, while delivering the promise of improving quality of life and prolonging survival.

This review summarizes current initial management approach for older MCL patients who require treatment, focusing on data from chemoimmunotherapy studies, with additional discussion on emerging novel agents and combinations.

INITIAL TREATMENT WITH CHEMOIMMUNOTHERAPY

Conventional outpatient-based chemoimmunotherapy is the primary treatment modality for older and fit patients (**Table 1**; see **Table 3**). Rituximab plus cyclophosphamide, doxorubicin, vincristine, and prednisone (R-CHOP)–based or rituximab-bendamustine (BR)–based regimens provide median progression-free survival (PFS) of 3 years to 5 years, with median overall survival (OS) exceeding 7 years.

Rituximab-CHOP–Based Strategies

Randomized phase 3 studies have established that building on the R-CHOP backbone, either by adding the biologic agent bortezomib during induction (VR-CAP) or with rituximab maintenance (MR) after R-CHOP induction (European MCL Network Elderly trial), significantly improves PFS and OS compared with R-CHOP alone.[4–7]

Based on phases II studies in MCL patients, which demonstrated feasibility and efficacy combining bortezomib with R-CHOP–based induction,[8–10] the LYM-3002 randomized phase 3 trial compared VR-CAP (replacing vincristine with bortezomib at 1.3 mg/m^2 given on days 1, 4, 8, and 11) with standard-dose R-CHOP in 483 patients ineligible for stem cell transplant, including 73% patients over the age of 60 years and 50% over the age of 65 years.[4] VR-CAP was superior in terms of complete response (CR) rate (53% vs 42%, respectively) and primary endpoint of median PFS (24.7 months vs 14.4 months, respectively; P<.001). In the final data analyses, at a median follow-up of 82 months, median OS remained significantly longer in the VR-CAP group (90.7 months vs 55.7 months, respectively; P = .001).[5] Hematologic toxicities, including neutropenia and thrombocytopenia, were higher in VR-CAP arm and manageable. The LYM-3002 study is the first to show long-term survival benefit of bortezomib-based chemoimmunotherapy induction compared with R-CHOP in transplant-ineligible patients, including older MCL patients. Maintenance strategy, however, was not explored.

In the European MCL Network Elderly trial, 560 older MCL patients at the median age of 70 were first randomized to induction regimens of either R-CHOP or R-fludarabine and cyclophosphamide, followed by a second randomization to maintenance of either with rituximab or interferon alfa.[6] After a median follow-up of 7.6 years, patients treated with R-CHOP induction followed by MR had superior median PFS and OS times of 5.4 years and 9.8 years, respectively, compared with 1.9 years (P<.001) and 7.1 years (P = .0026), respectively, to patients assigned to interferon alfa. MR was ongoing 2 years and 5 years from start of maintenance in 58% and 32%,

Table 1
Chemotherapy-based initial therapy for older mantle cell lymphoma patients

	Regimen	Phase	N	Age (Year) (Range)	Overall Response Rate (Complete Response/ Unconfirmed Complete Response)	Progression-Free Survival	Overall Survival	Notable Adverse Effect Profiles Greater Than or Equal to Grade 3
R-CHOP based	MCL Elderly: R-CHOP/MR	III	267	70 (60–87)	86% (34%)	mPFS, 5.4 y	mOS, 9.8 y	Thrombocytopenia, 57%; Neutropenia, 15%; Febrile neutropenia, 15%
	LYM-2003: VR-CAP	III	243	65 (26–88)	92% (53%)	mPFS, 25 mo	mOS, 90.7 mo	Thrombocytopenia, 1%; Febrile neutropenia, 1%; Neuropathy, 8%
BR based	StiL: BR	III	46	64 (34–83)	93% (40%)	mPFS, 35 mo	N/R	Thrombocytopenia, 6%; Neutropenia, 29%; Skin rash (all grades), 15%
	BRIGHT: BR	III	36	60 (28–84)	94% (50%)	5-y PFS, @ 40%	5y-OS, @ 59%	Thrombocytopenia, 10%; Neutropenia, 39%; Skin rash (all grades) 20%
	FIL: R-BAC	II	57	71 (67–75)	91% (91%)	3-y PFS, @ 76%	N/R	Thrombocytopenia, 52%; Neutropenia, 49%; Febrile neutropenia, 8%
	LYSA: RiBVD	II	74	73 (64–83)	84% (75.5%)	4-y PFS, @ 58%	4-y OS, @71%	Thrombocytopenia, 35%; Febrile neutropenia, 15%; Neuropathy, 15%
	NLG/MCL4: LBR	I/II	51	71 (62–84)	80% (64%)	mPFS, 42 mo	3-y OS, @73%	Thrombocytopenia, 20%; Neutropenia, 75%; Infections, 42%

Abbreviations: LBR, lenalidomide, bendamustine, rituximab; mOS, median overall survival; mPFS, median progression free survival; N/R, not reported; @, at.
Data from Refs.[4–7,12–17]

respectively, of patients treated with R-CHOP.[7] These long-term data support that R-CHOP induction followed by MR is an effective and safe initial treatment option for older MCL patients and that prolonged rituximab beyond 2 years is feasible.

As a follow-up to the European MCL Network Elderly trial, the MCL-R2 Elderly trial (NCT01865110) is an ongoing phase 3 study of the European MCL Network comparing 8 cycles of R-CHOP versus an experimental induction with 3 cycles of R-CHOP and 3 cycles of R-HAD (rituximab, cytarabine, and dexamethasone) in older MCL patients (≥60 years old) followed by maintenance. The primary endpoint is PFS at 2.5 years after maintenance randomization.[11]

Bendamustine-Rituximab–Based Strategies

Induction with bendamustine and rituximab

The combination BR, which has been increasingly adapted as induction therapy in outpatient practice, has demonstrated noninferiority in efficacy compared with R-CHOP in the randomized phase 3 Study Group Indolent Lymphoma (StiL) and BRIGHT studies, albeit with a different toxicity profile.[12–14] The German StiL study, which enrolled 64% patients over the age of 60, randomly assigned 46 MCL patients to BR (bendamustine given at 90 mg/m^2 on days 1–2 of a 4-week cycle) and 48 MCL patients to R-CHOP. The international BRIGHT study, which compared BR with a standard rituximab-chemotherapy regimen of either R-CHOP or R-CVP, included 74 treatment-naive MCL patients at the median age of 60 years and randomized 36 patients to the BR arm. BR treatment was associated with significantly improved median PFS of 35.4 months compared with 22.1 months with R-CHOP ($P = .0044$) in the StiL study.[12] BR showed improved CR rate (50% vs 27%, respectively), 5-year PFS rate (65.5% vs 55.8%, respectively; $P = .0025$) in the BRIGHT study.[13,14] No significant difference in OS, however, was observed. BR treatment was associated with more incidences of drug hypersensitivity skin reactions, whereas R-CHOP had more cytopenias, peripheral neuropathy/paresthesia, and alopecia.

Induction with bendamustine and rituximab plus

Approaches to augment BR backbone, such as adding (1) low-dose cytarabine (FIL [Fondazione Italiana Linfomi]: rituximab, bendamustine, and cytarabine [R-BAC]),[15] (2) bortezomib (LYSA [The Lymphoma Study Association]: RiBVD [rituximab, bendamustine, bortezomib, dexamethasone]),[16] and (3) lenalidomide (NLG/MCL4 [Nordic Lymphoma Group/MCL4]: Lena-Berit [lenalidomide, bendamustine and rituximab]),[17] were explored in phase 2 trials, which demonstrated improvement in CR at the expense of increased toxicities. In particular, the combination of Lena-Berit was associated with a high degree of severe infections and SPMs, limiting further clinical application.[17]

FIL: rituximab, bendamustine, and cytarabine R-BAC was evaluated in a multicenter phase 2 trial, including 57 treatment-naive patients (median age 71 years) who were ineligible for transplant.[15] Patients received RBAC500 regimen (rituximab, 375 mg/m^2 on day 1; bendamustine 70 mg/m^2 on days 2 and 3; and cytarabine 500 mg/m^2 on days 2–4) every 4 weeks for up to 6 cycles, without maintenance. The overall response rate (ORR) and CR rates were 91%. The most frequent grade 3 to 4 hematological toxicities were neutropenia (49%) and thrombocytopenia (52%), which were manageable with supportive care and dose reductions. The 2-year OS was 86%, and 2-year PFS was 81%. In multivariate analysis, elevated Ki-67 and blastoid variant were independent predictors of worse PFS. The FIL high-risk elderly MCL study (NCT03567876) is a follow-up phase 2 study currently under way, which adds venetoclax (VEN) as consolidation and maintenance after R-BAC for patients with high-risk features, such as elevated Ki-67, blastoid cytology, and TP53 mutation.

LYSA: RiBVD In the LYSA phase 2 RiBVD study for older MCL patients, bortezomib given subcutaneous, 1.3 mg/m^2 on days 1, 4, 8, and 11, and dexamethasone, 40 mg intravenously (IV) on day 2, was combined with BR in 76 patients aged 65 years or older (median age 73), without maintenance.[16] CR/unconfirmed CR rate was 76% at the end of treatment; 2-year PFS was 70%. The main grade 3/4 toxicities included neutropenia (51%), thrombocytopenia (35%), and neuropathy (15%). The peripheral blood (PB) minimal residual disease (MRD) rate was 87% in responding patients after 6 cycles of treatment. Four-year OS rate was 87% in patients who achieved MRD negativity compared with 29% in those with detectable MRD at end of treatment ($P<.0001$). Conventional prognostic index, such as MCL International Prognostic Index or Ki-67, did not differentiate survival.

NLG/MCL4: Lena-Berit The phase 1/2 Nordic MCL4 Lena-Berit trial evaluated the addition of lenalidomide to BR, given at 10 mg days 1 to 14 of a 28-day cycle during induction, followed by lenalidomide maintenance (days 1–21) for a maximum 52-week treatment, in 51 treatment-naive elderly MCL patients greater than 65 years.[17] The Lena-Berit regimen demonstrated improved CR rate at 64% after 6 cycles of induction, including 36% MRD-negative CR. Treatment was associated, however, with significant grade 3/4 neutropenia (38%), opportunistic infections (42%), and secondary malignancies (16%), which limited further clinical application.

Ongoing clinical trials with bendamustine and rituximab plus novel agent induction
Phase 2 US intergroup study: Eastern Cooperative Oncology Group *E1411* E1411 is an ongoing randomized phase 2 US intergroup study examining the effect of addition of bortezomib to BR induction therapy, followed by a second randomization with either rituximab alone or lenalidomide and rituximab (LR) as maintenance therapy (NCT01415752) in patients over the age of 60. In addition to routine image-based response assessment, the study measures MRD after cycle 3 (I3), end of induction, and after 4 cycles of consolidation.[18] Efficacy analysis by treatment groups to differentiate the impact of novel agents during induction (bortezomib) and maintenance (rituximab alone, or LR) on PFS is eagerly awaited.

Phase 3 studies of bendamustine and rituximab with BTK inhibitors In transplant-ineligible patients, an ongoing randomized, double-blind, placebo-controlled phase III global study is comparing the effect of addition of ibrutinib to BR induction and MR with BR and MR on PFS in patients 65 years of age or older with newly diagnosed MCL (the SHINE study [NCT01776840]). Study subjects responding to induction therapy will receive 12 doses of MR given every other cycle, in addition to continuous therapy with blinded study drug (ibrutinib or placebo). A similarly designed global phase 3 study, ACE-LY-308, is examining the efficacy outcome of randomized study drug (acalabrutinib or placebo) to BR (NCT02972840).

Phase 2 Eastern Cooperative Oncology Group PrE0405 study ECOG is leading a phase 2 study evaluating the combination of BR plus BCL-2 inhibitor VEN as induction therapy for treatment-naive MCL patients over 60 years of age (NCT03834688).[19] The study induction treatment is planned for up to 6 cycles, and maintenance rituximab is allowed per physician discretion.

Maintenance Strategies After Chemoimmunotherapy

Rituximab given every 2 months until progression after R-CHOP induction was associated with superior PFS and OS in the European MCL Network Elderly trial, with MR ongoing beyond 5 years in one-third of patients.[7] In contrast, MR for either 2 years or

4 years after BR induction did not demonstrate survival advantage to date in the randomized MAINTAIN study after a median follow-up time of 4.5 years,[20] suggesting that quality of induction may influence MR outcome.

Given the efficacy of immunomodulatory agent lenalidomide in MCL, the synergy of antibody-dependent cell-mediated cytotoxicity when combined with rituximab,[21] and the feasibility of chronic LR maintenance as demonstrated in the chemotherapy-free LR frontline regimen,[22] LR doublet is being compared with rituximab alone as maintenance strategy in several ongoing phase 2/3 trials for older MCL patients. This includes the randomized phase 2 E1411 study and the randomized phase 3 MCL-R2 study, as discussed previously, in older patients ($\geq$60 years old) with MCL. The primary endpoint analysis of PFS differentiating LR versus rituximab alone maintenance awaits accrual maturation.

BCL-2 inhibitor VEN is being evaluated as a consolidation and maintenance strategy after R-BAC in the FIL high-risk elderly MCL study (NCT03567876). Consolidation study treatment consists of single-agent VEN, at 800 mg daily for 4 cycles (with initial ramp-up), which is followed by maintenance with VEN, 400 mg daily for a total of 2 years.

Alternative Anti-CD20 Antibody for Chemoimmunotherapy Backbone

Obinutuzumab is a type II, glyco-engineered, humanized anti-CD20 monoclonal antibody, which was superior to rituximab in MCL xenograft models. In the phase 2 GAUGUIN study, single-agent obinutuzumab demonstrated clinical activity in patients with relapsed/refractory (R/R) MCL, including those with rituximab-refractory disease.[23] Several frontline phase 2 trials, which recruit older MCL patients, are assessing the efficacy of bendamustine plus obinutuzumab (instead of rituximab) combinations. For example, investigators at University of Wisconsin is leading a phase II single-arm multicenter study (NCT03311126) evaluating the efficacy and safety of induction chemoimmunotherapy with bendamustine and obinutuzumab followed by consolidation therapy and maintenance therapy with obinutuzumab. Investigators at Emory University are leading a phase 2 trial studying how well bendamustine, obinutuzumab, and VEN work as induction therapy (NCT03872180). Patients receive VEN, orally on days 1 to 28 of course 1 and days 1 to 10 of subsequent courses; bendamustine, IV on days 1 and 2; and obinutuzumab IV on days 1, 8, and 15 of course 1 and day 1 of subsequent courses. Treatment repeats every 28 days for up to 6 courses.

THE POTENTIAL OF CHEMOTHERAPY-FREE INITIAL THERAPY

Over the past decade, 5 nonchemotherapy biologic agents, namely bortezomib, lenalidomide, ibrutinib, acalabrutinib, and zanubrutinib, have received regulatory approval from US Food and Drug Administration for treatment of R/R MCL. Although other agents, such as BCL-2 inhibitor VEN and PI3K inhibitors, also have demonstrated significant clinical activities, the introduction of novel agents, in particular oral drugs, has fundamentally changed the care, for older MCL patients, in particular, by providing community-based outpatient treatment that is accessible, convenient, and effective. Compared with conventional intensive chemotherapy regimens, which often are prescribed in the inpatient hospital setting, novel agents deliver disease control without the typical dose-limiting adverse events (AEs) of cytotoxic chemotherapy, making chronic treatment feasible. Furthermore, rational combinations of novel agents have shown preliminary potential as an effective alternative to chemotherapy in high-risk MCL harboring chemotherapy-resistance genes, such as TP53 mutations. Several exploratory phase 1/2 studies have demonstrated feasibility and preliminary efficacy of chemotherapy-free combinations as initial therapy (**Tables 2** and **3**), paving the way for large studies with comparators, including conventional chemoimmunotherapy.

Lenalidomide Plus Rituximab as Initial Induction and Maintenance

Single-agent lenalidomide, given at 25 mg on days 1 to 21 every 28 days, has moderate activity in R/R MCL (ORR 28%–40%, including CR 5%–8%).[24,25] Addition of rituximab to lenalidomide improved response rates (ORR 57% with CR 36%).[26] The combination LR doublet given as induction and maintenance therapy was the first chemotherapy-free novel combination evaluated in the initial therapy setting in a multicenter phase 2 study with 38 treatment-naive MCL patients. A majority of patients were elderly at study entry with the median age of 65 years, including 24 (63%) patients over the age of 60, 10 (26%) over age 70, and 5 (13%) over age 80. Lenalidomide was given at 20 mg daily on days 1 to 21 of every 28-day cycle for 12 cycles as induction therapy, followed by maintenance at 15 mg daily on days 1 to 21 of every 28-day cycle. Rituximab was given weekly for the first 4 weeks and then once every other cycle. Treatment was continuous until disease progression or unacceptable toxicity.

Initial therapy with LR combination is the first chemotherapy-free study with long-term follow-up to show that rational combination of biologic agents is feasible, safe, and effective as induction and maintenance strategy in MCL. The study treatment generally is well tolerated with expected side effects, while delivering high response rates and durable remissions, with ORR of 92%, CR of 64%, and 5-year PFS and OS of 64% and 77%, respectively, in long-term follow-up.[22,27] MRD-negative remissions in PB were achieved in 8 of 10 subjects with available samples. Hematologic AEs included asymptomatic grades 3 to 4 cytopenias, and mostly grades 1 to 2 infections managed in outpatient setting. Nonhematologic AEs, such as constitutional and inflammatory symptoms, occurred in reduced frequency and intensity during maintenance compared with induction.

Building on LR regimen for additional synergy, triple combination with BCL-2 inhibitor VEN (NCT03523975) currently is in phase 1 dose escalation and expansion trial, whereas a triple-combination , which combines second-generation BTK inhibitor acalabrutinib with LR (ALR) as induction and maintenance treatment, is under way in phase 2 study (NCT03863184). The ALR study has incorporated next-generation sequence–based real-time MRD analysis as biomarker to assess response and to guide responses-adaptive maintenance strategy.[28]

Ibrutinib-Based Combinations

BTK inhibitors are the most effective class of novel agent to date for MCL in R/R setting, providing ORR in the range of 65% to 84%, CR 21% to 59%, and median PFS 13 months to 20 months, based on single-arm phase II studies.[29–31] Earlier access to ibrutinib after 1 prior line of therapy was shown to be associated with improved PFS.[32] Adding rituximab to ibrutinib further improved response rates in R/R disease, with ORR at 88% and CR at 44%.[33] The second-generation BTK inhibitors acalabrutinib and zanubrutinib are highly selective inhibitors of BTK with minimal off-target activity. Class-specific AEs specific to BTK inhibitors, such as hypertension, bleeding/bruising, and atrial arrhythmia, appear to differ between first-generation and second-generation agents. For example, compared with ibrutinib, acalabrutinib is associated with less atrial fibrillation and fewer cutaneous toxicities, making it potentially more appealing for combination strategy.

Table 2
Chemotherapy-free initial therapy for older mantle cell lymphoma patients

Regimen	Regimen	Phase	N	Age (Range)	Overall Response Rate (Complete Response/ Unconfirmed Complete Response)	Progression-Free Survival/ Event-Free Survival/Time-to-Failure	Overall Survival	Adverse Effect Profiles	Ref.
Lenalidomide combination	Len (L) + R	II	38	65 (42–86)	92% (64%)	5y-PFS @64%	5-y OS @77%	Neutropenia (induction), 42% Neutropenia (maintenance), 32% Rash (induction), 29%	
Ibrutinib combinations	MDACC MCL Older: I + R	II	50	71 (65–84)	98% (60%)	mDOR, 19 mo	Not reported	Fatigue, neutropenia, atrial fibrillation, myalgia	
	GELTAMO IMCL-2015: I + R	II	40	66	82% (75%)	15-mo PFS @ 96%	Not reported	Cytopenias, atrial fibrillation, rash, asthenia	
	OAsIS step C: I + VEN	I	15	65 (51–77)	100% (47%)	Not reported	Not reported	Neutropenia, lymphocytosis, rash, hepatobiliary abnormality	

Abbreviations: I, ibrutinib; Len (L), lenalidomide; MDACC, MD Anderson Cancer Center; mDOR, median duration of response; R, rituximab.
Data from Refs. [22,27,28,34,39]

Table 3
Ongoing frontline studies under evaluation for older mantle cell lymphoma patients

Strategy	Regimen	Phase	N	Treatment	Outcomes	ClinicalTrials.gov
Chemotherapy based	E1411	II	332	BR- > MR BR- > MRL BRV- > MR BRV- > MRL	First: PFS	NCT01415752
	SHINE BR ± ibrutinib	III	523	BR- > MR BRI- > MRI	First: PFS	NCT01776840
	BR ± acalabrutinib	III	546	BR- > MR BRA- > MRA	First: PFS	NCT02972840
	MCL-R2 Elderly	III	633	First: R-CHOP vs R-CHOP/R-HAD Second: MR vs MRL	First: PFS	NCT01865110
	ENRICH	II/III	400	R-chemotherapy with MR vs IR with MR	FirstFirst: PFS	N/A
	PrE0405	II	56	BR + VEN	First: CR	NCT03834688
	FIL Elderly MCL	II	130	VEN maintenance after R-BAC	First: PFS	NCT03567876
	Emory U.	II	27	BO + VEN	First: CR	NCT03872180
	U. Wisconsin	II	32	BO- > MO	First: PFS	NCT03311126
Chemotherapy-free	WINDOW II: VIR	II	50	Group 3: VIR	First: CR	NCT03710772
	ALR	II	24	Induction: ALR cycles 1–12 Maintenance: cycles 13-POD	First: MRD-neg CR	NCT03863184
	VLR	I	28	VLR cycles 1–12	First: MTD	NCT03523975
Chemotherapy vs novel agents	ENRICH	II/III	400	R-chemotherapy with MR vs IR with MR	First: PFS	N/A
	Beigene	III	500	BR vs zanbrutinib + R	First: PFS	NCT04002297

WINDOW II study contains chemotherapy-free treatment of VEN, ibrutinib, and rituximab in group 3. ENRICH study has chemotherapy-free arm with IR.

Abbreviations: ->, followed by; BO, bendamustine and obinutuzumab; IR, ibrutinib and rituximab; MI, ibrutinib maintenance; MO, obinutuzumab maintenance; MRA, rituximab and acalabrutinib maintenance; MRI, rituximab and ibrutinib maintenance; MRL, rituximab and lenalidomide maintenance; R-HAD, rituximab, high-dose cytarabine, and dexamethasone; VIR, VEN, ibrutinib, and rituximab; VLR, VEN, lenalidomide, and rituximab.

Ibrutinib plus rituximab

The IR combination is under evaluation as initial therapy for transplant ineligible patients in several studies, notably the MD Anderson MCL older patients study (NCT01880567), the Spanish GELTAMO IMCL-2015 trial (NCT02682641), and the UK ENRICH (chemotherapy-free arm) study. The accrual for the UK randomized ENRICH trial (2015-000832-13) currently is under way, which compares chemotherapy-free ibrutinib and rituximab combination with standard rituximab and chemotherapy, either R-CHOP or BR, in MCL patients 60 years and older.

In the phase 2 MD Anderson older MCL study, which enrolled patients over 65 years of age, the ORR was 98% with 60% CR, whereas the MRD-negative CR by flow cytometry was 81% among the evaluable patients. At a median follow-up of 28 months, the median PFS and OS were not reached, and the median duration on study was 19 months. Notable grade 3/4 AEs included 14% myalgias, 14% fatigue, 10% shortness of breath, 8% neutropenia, and 8% new-onset atrial fibrillation; 39% of patients discontinued treatment due to either disease progression (including transformation) or treatment-related toxicities, and 53% of patients required dose reduction.[34]

Forty patients with indolent MCL received treatment in the phase 2 GELTAMO IR study with ibrutinib, 560 mg daily, and a total of 8 doses of rituximab 375 mg/m2. The study stipulated that ibrutinib could be discontinued after 2 years of treatment provided that patients stayed in negative MRD for at least 6 months.[28] High response rates, including ORR 82% with 75% CR and MRD-negative rate of 87% in evaluable patients were observed. AE profile was predictable, including hematological toxicity, rash, gastrointestinal intolerance, arthralgias, atrial fibrillation, and asthenia. Remissions appeared to be durable, including in patients in MRD-negative CR who discontinued treatment, although longer follow-up is needed.

Ibrutinib plus venetoclax combinations

VEN is a BH3-mimetic that inhibits BCL2, which has marked single-agent efficacy in MCL.[35,36] The combination of VEN and ibrutinib has demonstrated synergy as shown in the Australian AIM study. The treatment consisted of monotherapy of ibrutinib (560 mg) for first 4 weeks followed by addition of VEN in week 5, with weekly ramp-up to 400-mg to 800-mg dose level. The CR rate at 16 weeks was 42%, MRD clearance was 67% in bone marrow by flow cytometry, and 38% in PB by allele-specific oligonucleotide–polymerase chain reaction, suggesting high efficacy with the dual targeting of BTK and BCL2, compared with historical data with ibrutinib monotherapy.[37] The responses appeared to be durable, including in 4 patients who remained in MRD-negative CR after electively interrupted treatment after a median 18.5 months of therapy.[38]

In the frontline setting, the dual inhibition by ibrutinib plus VEN has been evaluated in an ongoing phase 1/2 study (OAsIs, NCT02558816) with anti-CD20 obinutuzumab, given at 1000 mg IV, C1D1, 8, 15, C2–6 D1 (cycle 1 day 1, 8, 15, cycle 2-6 day 1) and every 2 months for 2 years. The study consists of a stepwise enrollment: step A with obinutuzumab plus ibrutinib combination in R/R MCL, step B with triple combination in R/R MCL, and step C with the triplet in treatment-naive patients.[39] Patients in step C were treated with obinutuzumab, at 1000 mg IV on C1D1, 8, 15, C2–6 D1 and every 2 months for up to 2 years. VEN was given at 400 mg daily for up to 2 years, whereas ibrutinib was given as a standard dose, at 560 mg daily, until progression. Preliminary data on 15 treatment-naive patients showed ORR of 100% when assessed at end of cycle 2 treatment. MRD, CR rate, and survival analyses are ongoing. The phase 2 WINDOW II (NCT03710772) study has a chemotherapy-free arm to assess the efficacy of the combination of VEN plus ibrutinib and rituximab (VIR) as induction and maintenance therapy in treatment-naive MCL patients.

Phase 3 Studies Comparing Chemotherapy-Free Combination with Chemoimmunotherapy

The UK randomized ENRICH trial (2015-000832-13) is under way for accrual and study maturation, which compares chemotherapy-free ibrutinib and rituximab combination with standard rituximab and chemotherapy, either R-CHOP or BR, in MCL patients 60 years and older to assess PFS benefit. MR is permitted in both arms. A global phase 3 study is enrolling patients with treatment-naive MCL to compare safety and efficacy of chemotherapy-free combination of zanubrutinib plus rituximab with the combination of BR chemoimmunotherapy (NCT04002297).

MINIMAL RESIDUAL DISEASE AND RESPONSE-ADAPTED STRATEGIES

Remission duration and survival outcome in MCL have been shown to correlate to MRD status in chemotherapy-based clinical trials, including intensive treatment protocols incorporating high-dose cytarabine and consolidative autologous stem cell transplant as well as less-intensive strategies.[40] As consistently demonstrated in the Nordic MCL 2 and MCL 3 studies,[41] the European MCL Network Younger and Elderly trials,[42] as well as the US CALGB 59909 and S1106 studies,[43,44] molecular remission after induction treatment was highly predictive of response duration and disease progression. In older MCL patients, sustained molecular remission was predictive of outcome during maintenance.[42] MRD assays increasingly are incorporated into prospective clinical trials as correlative biomarkers for response quality measurement as well as in some cases as an experimental endpoint to guide MRD-adjusted treatment strategy. For example, as discussed previously, the Spanish GELTAMO IMCL-2015 phase 2 trial with ibrutinib plus rituximab combination allows for ibrutinib discontinuation based on MRD-negative status after 2 years of treatment.

SUMMARY

MCL remains a clinical challenge due to its heterogeneous clinical course and general incurability despite therapeutic advancement. Most MCL patients are elderly and less able to tolerate or wish to avoid aggressive treatment. The main therapeutic goal is to deliver the most effective therapy tailored to patient and disease factors in order to extend survival while preserving quality of life whenever possible. The incorporation of novel agents in clinical practice has significantly improved treatment options and outcome for nearly all patients, especially for older MCL patients who are not candidates for intensive regimens and stem cell transplant due to age and/or comorbidities.

A majority of older MCL patients who are physically fit are candidates for initial treatment with chemoimmunotherapy. Based on randomized phase 3 studies, the induction therapy with R-CHOP followed by MR, or induction regimens of either VR-CAP or BR, are commonly employed frontline strategies that deliver median PFS of 3 years to 5 years, and median OS in the range of 6 years to 10 years. BR is noninferior in efficacy and has a different toxicity profile compared with R-CHOP. Fortifying BR induction with additional chemotherapy ingredients or novel agents generally is associated with more toxicity, but careful application of dose adjustment, as in the case of R-BAC, can be done safely and effectively for older MCL patients.

For older MCL patients who are frail, rituximab and nonchemotherapy-based novel agents either in sequence or combination are possible options. Data from exploratory phase 2 studies have shown feasibility and efficacy of chemotherapy-free combinations as initial treatment options, including the doublet of LR and the combinations of BTK inhibitor ibrutinib with either rituximab or VEN. With the exception of LR doublet, longitudinal follow-up is needed to understand the full spectrum of clinical activity and treatment-associated side effects with the ibrutinib combinations. Ultimately, larger studies, including randomized comparison between novel agents and chemotherapy, are warranted to compare efficacy and toxicity.

Chronic therapy with maintenance appears to be an important management strategy associated with less intensive induction regimens in older MCL patients. The optimal duration and intensity of maintenance therapy, however, are not well defined for specific agents or combinations. Given the potential side effects and financial ramification associated with long-term treatment, exploration of response-adaptive strategy is warranted. MRD has emerged as an important biomarker/surrogate PFS endpoint for clinical trials to assess response quality, providing a cross-sectional comparison of efficacy of various regimens. In addition, it provides an experimental endpoint for MRD-adjusted strategy to guide treatment intensity/duration.

ACKNOWLEDGMENTS

The author would like to thank ongoing collaboration and support from Drs Peter Martin and John Leonard of the lymphoma program at Weill Cornell Medicine and grant support from a Mantle Cell Lymphoma Research Initiative Award from the Leukemia & Lymphoma Society (PI: Dr. Chen-Kiang).

REFERENCES

1. Swerdlow SH, Campo E, Pileri SA, et al. The 2016 revision of the World Health Organization classification of lymphoid neoplasms. Blood 2016;127:2375–90.
2. Ruan J. Molecular profiling and management of mantle cell lymphoma. Hematology 2019;2019:30–40.
3. Abrahamsson A, Albertsson-Lindblad A, Brown PN, et al. Real world data on primary treatment for mantle cell lymphoma: a Nordic Lymphoma Group observational study. Blood 2014;124:1288–95.
4. Robak T, Huang H, Jin J, et al. Bortezomib-based therapy for newly diagnosed mantle-cell lymphoma. N Engl J Med 2015;372:944–53.
5. Robak T, Jin J, Pylypenko H, et al. Frontline bortezomib, rituximab, cyclophosphamide, doxorubicin, and prednisone (VR-CAP) versus rituximab, cyclophosphamide, doxorubicin, vincristine, and prednisone (R-CHOP) in transplantation-ineligible patients with newly diagnosed mantle cell lymphoma: final overall survival results of a randomised, open-label, phase 3 study. Lancet Oncol 2018; 19:1449–58.
6. Kluin-Nelemans HC, Hoster E, Hermine O, et al. Treatment of Older Patients with Mantle-Cell Lymphoma. N Engl J Med 2012;367:520–31.
7. Kluin-Nelemans HC, Hoster E, Hermine O, et al. Treatment of older patients with mantle cell lymphoma (MCL): long-term follow-up of the Randomized European MCL elderly trial. J Clin Oncol 2020;38:248–56.
8. Ruan J, Martin P, Furman RR, et al. Bortezomib Plus CHOP-rituximab for previously untreated diffuse large B-cell lymphoma and mantle cell lymphoma. J Clin Oncol 2011;29:690–7.
9. Till BG, Li H, Bernstein SH, et al. Phase II trial of R-CHOP plus bortezomib induction therapy followed by bortezomib maintenance for newly diagnosed mantle cell lymphoma: SWOG S0601. Br J Haematol 2016;172:208–18.

10. Chang JE, Li H, Smith MR, et al. Phase 2 study of VcR-CVAD with maintenance rituximab for untreated mantle cell lymphoma: an Eastern Cooperative Oncology Group study (E1405). Blood 2014;123:1665–73.
11. Ribrag V, Feugier P, Doorduijn J, et al. MCL-R2 elderly: a phase III study of the European MCL network assessing efficacy of alternating immunochemotherapy (R-CHOP/R-HAD) and a rituximab-lenalidomide maintenance. Hematological Oncol 2017;35:421.
12. Rummel MJ, Niederle N, Maschmeyer G, et al. Bendamustine plus rituximab versus CHOP plus rituximab as first-line treatment for patients with indolent and mantle-cell lymphomas: an open-label, multicentre, randomised, phase 3 non-inferiority trial. Lancet 2013;381:1203–10.
13. Flinn IW, van der Jagt R, Kahl BS, et al. Randomized trial of bendamustine-rituximab or R-CHOP/R-CVP in first-line treatment of indolent NHL or MCL: the BRIGHT study. Blood 2014;123(19):2944–52.
14. Flinn IW, van det Jagt R, Kahl B, et al. First-line treatment of patients with indolent non-hodgkin lymphoma or mantle-cell lymphoma with bendamustine plus rituximab versus R-CHOP or R-CVP: results of the BRIGHT 5-year follow-up study. J Clin Oncol 2019;37:984–91.
15. Visco C, Chiappella A, Nassi L, et al. Rituximab, bendamustine, and low-dose cytarabine as induction therapy in elderly patients with mantle cell lymphoma: a multicentre, phase 2 trial from Fondazione Italiana Linfomi. Lancet Haematol 2017;4:e15–23.
16. Gressin R, Daguindau N, Tempescul A, et al. A phase 2 study of rituximab, bendamustine, bortezomib and dexamethasone for first-line treatment of older patients with mantle cell lymphoma. Haematologica 2019;104:138–46.
17. Albertsson-Lindblad A, Kolstad A, Laurell A, et al. Lenalidomide-bendamustine-rituximab in patients older than 65 years with untreated mantle cell lymphoma. Blood 2016;128:1814–20.
18. Smith M, Jegede O, Parekh S, et al. Minimal residual disease (MRD) assessment in the ECOG1411 randomized phase 2 trial of front-line bendamustine-rituximab (BR)-based induction followed by rituximab (R) ± lenalidomide (L) consolidation for mantle cell lymphoma (MCL). Blood 2019;134:751.
19. Portell CA, Bennani NN, Jegede O, et al. Bendamustine and rituximab plus venetoclax in untreated mantle cell lymphoma over 60 years of age (PrE0405): a phase II study. Blood 2019;134:5243.
20. Rummel M, Buske C, Hertenstein B, et al. Four versus two years of rituximab maintenance (R-maintenance) following bendamustine plus rituximab (B-R): results of a prospective, randomized multicenter phase 3 study in first-line follicular lymphoma (the StiL NHL7-2008 MAINTAIN Study). Clin Lymphoma Myeloma Leuk 2018;18:S101–3.
21. Gribben JG, Fowler N, Morschhauser F. Mechanisms of action of lenalidomide in B-cell non-hodgkin lymphoma. J Clin Oncol 2015;33:2803–11.
22. Ruan J, Martin P, Christos P, et al. Five-year follow-up of lenalidomide plus rituximab as initial treatment of mantle cell lymphoma. Blood 2018;132:2016–25.
23. Morschhauser FA, Cartron G, Thieblemont C, et al. Obinutuzumab (GA101) Monotherapy in Relapsed/Refractory Diffuse Large B-Cell Lymphoma or Mantle-Cell Lymphoma: Results From the Phase II GAUGUIN Study. J Clin Oncol 2013;31:2912–9.
24. Goy A, Sinha R, Williams ME, et al. Single-agent lenalidomide in patients with mantle-cell lymphoma who relapsed or progressed after or were refractory to bortezomib: phase II MCL-001 (EMERGE) Study. J Clin Oncol 2013;31:3688–95.

25. Trněný M, Lamy T, Walewski J, et al. Lenalidomide versus investigator's choice in relapsed or refractory mantle cell lymphoma (MCL-002; SPRINT): a phase 2, randomised, multicentre trial. Lancet Oncol 2016;17:319–31.

26. Wang M, Fayad L, Wagner-Bartak N, et al. Lenalidomide in combination with rituximab for patients with relapsed or refractory mantle-cell lymphoma: a phase 1/2 clinical trial. Lancet Oncol 2012;13:716–23.

27. Ruan J, Martin P, Shah B, et al. Lenalidomide plus Rituximab as Initial Treatment for Mantle-Cell Lymphoma. N Engl J Med 2015;373:1835–44.

28. Gine E, De La Cruz MdF, Grande C, et al. Efficacy and safety of ibrutinib in combination with rituximab as frontline treatment for indolent clinical forms of mantle cell lymphoma (MCL): preliminary results of geltamo IMCL-2015 phase II trial. Blood 2019;134:752.

29. Wang ML, Rule S, Martin P, et al. Targeting BTK with ibrutinib in relapsed or refractory mantle-cell lymphoma. N Engl J Med 2013;369:507–16.

30. Wang M, Rule S, Zinzani PL, et al. Acalabrutinib in relapsed or refractory mantle cell lymphoma (ACE-LY-004): a single-arm, multicentre, phase 2 trial. Lancet 2018;391:659–67.

31. Song Y, Zhou K, Zou D, et al. Safety and activity of the investigational bruton tyrosine kinase inhibitor zanubrutinib (BGB-3111) in patients with mantle cell lymphoma from a phase 2 trial. Blood 2018;132:148.

32. Rule S, Dreyling M, Goy A, et al. Outcomes in 370 patients with mantle cell lymphoma treated with ibrutinib: a pooled analysis from three open-label studies. Br J Haematol 2017;179:430–8.

33. Wang ML, Lee H, Chuang H, et al. Ibrutinib in combination with rituximab in relapsed or refractory mantle cell lymphoma: a single-centre, open-label, phase 2 trial. Lancet Oncol 2016;17:48–56.

34. Jain P, Lee HJ, Steiner RE, et al. Frontline Treatment with Ibrutinib with Rituximab (IR) combination is highly effective in elderly (≥65 years) patients with mantle cell lymphoma (MCL) - results from a phase II trial. Blood 2019;134:3988.

35. Davids MS, Roberts AW, Seymour JF, et al. Phase I first-in-human study of venetoclax in patients with relapsed or refractory non-hodgkin lymphoma. J Clin Oncol 2017;35:826–33.

36. Eyre TA, Walter HS, Iyengar S, et al. Efficacy of venetoclax monotherapy in patients with relapsed, refractory mantle cell lymphoma after Bruton tyrosine kinase inhibitor therapy. Haematologica 2019;104:e68–71.

37. Tam CS, Anderson MA, Pott C, et al. Ibrutinib plus Venetoclax for the Treatment of Mantle-Cell Lymphoma. N Engl J Med 2018;378:1211–23.

38. Handunnetti SM, Anderson MA, Burbury K, et al. Three year update of the phase II ABT-199 (venetoclax) and ibrutinib in mantle cell lymphoma (AIM) study. Blood 2019;134:756.

39. Le Gouill S, Morschhauser F, Bouabdallah K, et al. Ibrutinib, venetoclax plus obinutuzumab in newly diagnosed mantle cell lymphoma patients. Blood 2019;134:1530.

40. Hoster E, Pott C. Minimal residual disease in mantle cell lymphoma: insights into biology and impact on treatment. Hematology Am Soc Hematol Educ Program 2016;2016:437–45.

41. Kolstad A, Pedersen LB, Eskelund CW, et al. Molecular monitoring after autologous stem cell transplantation and preemptive rituximab treatment of molecular relapse; results from the nordic mantle cell lymphoma studies (MCL2 and MCL3) with median follow-up of 8.5 years. Biol Blood Marrow Transplant 2017;23:428–35.

42. Pott C, Hoster E, Delfau-Larue M-H, et al. Molecular remission is an independent predictor of clinical outcome in patients with mantle cell lymphoma after combined immunochemotherapy: a European MCL intergroup study. Blood 2010; 115:3215–23.
43. Liu H, Johnson JL, Koval G, et al. Detection of minimal residual disease following induction immunochemotherapy predicts progression free survival in mantle cell lymphoma: final results of CALGB 59909. Haematologica 2012;97:579–85.
44. Kamdar M, Li H, Chen RW, et al. Five-year outcomes of the S1106 study of R-hyper-CVAD vs R-bendamustine in transplant-eligible patients with mantle cell lymphoma. Blood Adv 2019;3:3132–5.

Minimal Residual Disease in Mantle Cell Lymphoma
Methods and Clinical Significance

Marco Ladetto, MD[a,*], Rita Tavarozzi, MD[a],
Christiane Pott, MD, PhD[b]

KEYWORDS

- Polymerase chain • Reaction • Next-generation sequencing • Molecular response
- Molecular relapse

KEY POINTS

- Mantle cell lymphoma (MCL) has considerable biological and clinical heterogeneity; several baseline clinical histologic and biological predictors have been identified, including Mantle Cell Lymphoma International Prognostic Index, proliferation index, blastoid histology, and genetic mutations.
- In recent years, minimal residual disease (MRD) detection has been established as a critical posttreatment outcome predictor and a considerable amount of data has been generated.
- MRD has been most often assessed through polymerase chain reaction–based molecular tools, but considerable interest is now placed on next-generation sequencing–based tools.
- MRD evaluation has clearly underlined the progress observed in the clinical management of MCL.
- Clinical studies exploiting MRD-tailored treatment have been conducted and are ongoing.

INTRODUCTION

Mantle cell lymphoma (MCL) is an uncommon subtype of non-Hodgkin lymphoma occurring in adults and elderly people with a peculiar male predominance. Genetically, it is characterized by the t(11;14) translocation to overexpression of cyclin D1. MCL is recognized as incurable; recurrences are frequent and, despite recent improvements, survival is lower compared with other non-Hodgkin lymphoma subtypes.[1] Most significant improvements in the outcome of patients with MCL have been achieved over the

[a] Struttura Complessa di Ematologia, Azienda Ospedaliera SS Antonio e Biagio e Cesare Arrigo, via Venezia 16, Alessandria 15121, Italy; [b] Second Medical Department, University Hospital Schleswig-Holstein, Campus Kiel, Arnold-Heller-Straße 3, Kiel 24105, Germany
* Corresponding author.
E-mail addresses: marco.ladetto@ospedale.al.it; marco.ladetto@unito.it

Hematol Oncol Clin N Am 34 (2020) 887–901
https://doi.org/10.1016/j.hoc.2020.06.006
0889-8588/20/© 2020 Elsevier Inc. All rights reserved.

hemonc.theclinics.com

last 2 decades thanks to the addition of rituximab to conventional chemotherapy,[1,2] and chemotherapeutic intensification, including the use of high doses of arabinosylcy-tosine (Ara-C) (HA),[3,4] and consolidation with high-dose chemotherapy and autolo-gous stem cell transplant (ASCT).[5,6] Moreover, the use of rituximab maintenance has provided further benefit with improvement of progression-free survival (PFS) and overall survival.[7,8] In addition, several novel agents, including targeted drugs such as ibrutinib and venetoclax, novel monoclonal antibodies, and cellular therapies, proved effective in the treatment of relapsed/refractory MCL and hold promise for a substantial impact on the management of these patients.[8,9]

Several baseline prognosticators have been identified in MCL, including Mantle Cell Lymphoma International Prognostic Index (MIPI), proliferation index (and their combi-nation [c-MIPI]), and blastoid histology genetic landscape (particularly tp53 and KMT2D mutations).[10-12] In recent years, growing evidence has shown that presence of minimal residual disease (MRD) detectable in peripheral blood (PB) or bone marrow (BM) may be a strong prognostic and predictive factor potentially suitable for treat-ment guiding in the near future.[13,14] The success of MRD monitoring was mostly caused by remarkable development of laboratory techniques. This progress has been achieved thanks to both intrinsic technical progress and collaborative efforts for standardization.[13-15]

MRD diagnostics is not a recent introduction because the first reports were gener-ated in the last decade of the previous millennium.[16,17] Nevertheless, substantial improvement has occurred in diagnostic techniques with increased robustness, accu-racy, applicability, and standardization.[13,17,18] This article describes methods suitable for MRD monitoring in MCL, outlining advantages and disadvantages. It describes the contribution of MRD diagnostics to the development of effective treatment of MCL and summarizes current standards on the clinical application of MRD in the treatment of MCL.

TECHNIQUES FOR MINIMAL RESIDUAL DISEASE ANALYSIS

Several methods have been used for MRD monitoring in the context of MCL and other lymphoid tumors in BM or PB. At present, there is no single technique that could be considered superior to others in any disease and any clinical context.[16,17] However, real-time quantitative (RQ) polymerase chain reaction (PCR) remains the gold standard for MCL,[18] although next-generation sequencing (NGS) is gaining considerable inter-est also in this entity.

Available approaches have different sensitivity, specificity, and accuracy of target quantification. Moreover, potential technical biases are different, as is the level of stan-dardization between different laboratories.[17-19] In addition some approaches are easily available worldwide, whereas others can be performed only at highly specialized sites.

It should also be noted that timing for sampling has not been uniform across studies, resulting in a lack of clear indication on which treatment phase should be considered optimal for MRD monitoring as opposed to other neoplasms, such as acute lympho-blastic leukemia.

For the methodological point of view, with the exception of the earliest generation of studies, MRD reports on MCL have used RQ-PCR, which still is the most extensively validated method. However, methodological progress has been relevant in the last 5 to 7 years, and comparative studies have been performed and are currently in prog-ress. These studies could promote a progressive change in the methodological approach, with progressive broader adoption of novel next-generation PCR methods, and improved flow cytometry (FC) and NGS tools.[17,19,20]

Flow Cytometry–Based Methods for Minimal Residual Disease Detection

FC is a commonly used tool in laboratory diagnostics for hematological cancers, including lymphomas. It is performed by the identification of immunophenotypic abnormalities and the identification of the light-chain restriction of immunoglobulins, which is a critical clonality marker in B-cell tumors. It is a fast and easily available tool compared with molecular methods, capable of providing a clinically useful output in just a few hours. Consequently, it is an interesting method for the detection of MRD.[21,22] On the other hand, MCL is immunophenotypically very heterogeneous, requiring widespread marker combinations for effective and sensitive MRD detection. Moreover, there are no antibody panels validated for MRD evaluation.

In MCL, the sensitivity of the conventional 4-color flow MRD is in the range of less than 10^{-4}, which is lower than that of molecular biology techniques such as allele-specific oligonucleotide real-time quantitative PCR and NGS (10^{-4} to 10^{-5}).[23] A comparative study showed that a single 8-color multiparametric flow cytometry (MFC) tube provides specific MRD evaluation with a solid sensitivity of 0.01% in all patients[21]; nevertheless, using the 0.01% cutoff level, MFC identified MRD in only 80% of patients who were MRD positive by RQ-PCR.[24]

The Euro Flow consortium of the European Scientific Foundation for the Haematooncology Laboratory (ESLHO) has elaborated guidelines for instrument setup, panel composition, and data interpretation.[25,26] Moreover, it carries on a quality control program for the MRD collection of MFC-based methods in most hematological tumors.[27,28] In order to achieve sensitivity levels suitable for MRD monitoring, both carefully optimized MFC strategies based on highly effective antibody panels as well as well-designed and adapted bioinformatics tools are needed to achieve sensitivity comparable with RQ-PCR. In addition, these assays need to be validated in the context of clinical trials with regard to applicability and prognostic impact to show their value as new MRD instruments for patients with MCL. Given that it is more complex to centralize FC-based MRD detection, this has still not been fully achieved in MCL, as opposed to other fields such as multiple myeloma.[29]

Polymerase Chain Reaction–Based Methods for Minimal Residual Disease Detection

PCR-based MRD methods investigate the persistence of residual tumor burden through amplification of the lymphoma's genotype, reaching a high degree of sensitivity. PCR methods are by far the most extensively used tool for MRD detection in MCL. RQ-PCR is considered the gold standard for the MRD because it is sensitive, standardized, and validated in large multicenter studies.[17,18,22]

Two different genetic targets are suitable for MRD detection in mature B-cell lymphomas and specifically in MCL: tumor-specific translocations and antigen receptor rearrangements.

The most widely applicable MRD marker in malignant B-cell lymphomas relies on a physiologic rearrangement typical of B-cell differentiation: the rearrangement of the immunoglobulin heavy chain gene (IGHV). A marker based on the IGHV rearrangement can be obtained in most B-cell tumors and is more easily detected in neoplasms with modest or no somatic hypermutation load. Clonal sequences of the complementarity determining regions are amplified using consensus PCR primers derived from the VH and JH region and then sequenced to identify tumor-specific variable (VH), diversity (DH) and joining (JH) genes (VH-DH-JH) rearrangement. This method allows the construction of an allele-specific oligonucleotide (ASO) suitable for quantitative approach measurement of tumor load by RQ-PCR. Because of a very low somatic hypermutation load, in MCL, IGHV clonal rearrangements are detectable in more than 90% of patients[19] and are the most frequently used MRD target.

Other markers that can be used for MRD detection in lymphoma are structural chromosome translocations typical for histologic subtypes of mature lymphoid neoplasms, such as t(14;18) in FL and t(11;14) in MCL. In MCL, the t(11;14) involves a 360-kb 5′ region of the cyclin D1 gene (CCND1); in almost half of these cases, the breaking points on the chromosome cluster 11 in an 85-bp region called the major translocation cluster region (BCL1-MTC). Chromosome translocations are ideal PCR targets because of high stability and lack of somatic mutations.[30] Even if present in most patients with MCL and detectable by fluorescence in situ hybridization, breakpoints in the BCL1-MTC region scatter up to 2 kb downstream of the MTC region, resulting in only 35% of t(11;14) translocations being detectable by PCR. Target locus amplification methodology has recently been shown to be able to identify a suitable MRD target derived from t(11;14) in almost 80% of patients, holding promise for a wider application of this target in patients with MCL.[31,32]

As opposed to acute lymphoblastic leukemia, in many patients with MCL, a substantial tumor infiltration may be lacking in samples used for target identification. This lack can limit the identification of a tumor marker in a proportion of patients and can hamper the generation of a suitable quantitative serial dilution. This problem represents one of the most important limitations of RQ-PCR, as discussed later.

The first approaches to PCR-based detection of MRD were based on qualitative end-point amplification approaches and particularly on nested PCR, consisting of a double amplification step with internal primers during the second round of amplification (**Fig. 1**A).[33–35] These approaches provided useful information but were strictly qualitative and had several technical biases, including high risk of contamination.

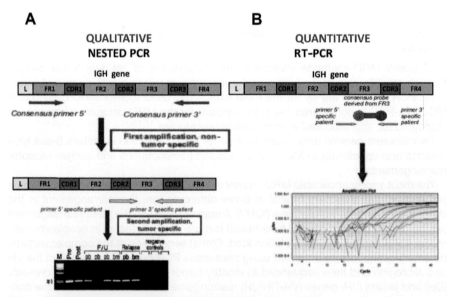

Fig. 1. Standard molecular MRD techniques. Comparison between qualitative method, nested PCR (A), and quantitative method, RQ-PCR (B).

Compared heat to head with RQ-PCR, qualitative PCR was less predictive than RQ-PCR.[35] Both qualitative nested PCR and RQ-PCR using ASO primers for IGHV rearrangement or translocation (11;14) achieve reproducible detection limits of 1 MCL cell in a background of 100,000 white blood cells (10^{-5}), with a slightly superior sensitivity of nested PCR because of the larger amounts of DNA used.

The development and standardization of RQ-PCR[36,37] represented a major technical advance in the detection of MRD in lymphoid malignancies (**Fig. 1B**). RQ-PCR is robust, accurate, and reproducible, and substantially minimizes the risk of contamination caused by closed-tube output analysis, lack of reamplification, and target-specific amplification. In addition, development of multilaboratory standardization efforts has substantially increased the value and applicability of RQ-PCR and allowed a very high level of reproducibility to be achieved between different MRD laboratories. The standardization of MRD assessment and the conduction of interlaboratory quality controls is essential to guarantee a high comparability of MRD data, which could be the basis for MRD-driven treatment. The feasibility of such an approach is shown by at least 1 major international phase III multicenter randomized trial currently being conducted in Europe in patients aged 18 to 65 years, which includes standardized MRD evaluation performed in several laboratories affiliated to the Euro-MRD consortium (EudraCT [European Union Drug Regulating Authorities Clinical Trials Database] number: 2014-001363-12).

Despite its advantages, RQ-PCR also has several limitations. It is not an absolute quantification tool, and requires a standard curve obtained from samples with known amounts of target diagnostic DNA, which might not be available in adequate amounts and requires a laborious setup procedure. Moreover, because of discrepancies between sensitivity and quantitative range, there are numerous samples that cannot be fully quantified and are usually defined as nonquantifiable positives (PNQs).[38] In addition, RQ-PCR is also sensitive to chemical inhibitors that can severely affect results if not taken in proper consideration.

In recent years, digital droplet PCR (ddPCR) allowed some of these limitations to be overcome.[18] ddPCR is an absolute quantification method based on Poisson statistics and, being an end-point quantification tool, it is much more tolerant of PCR inhibitors (**Fig. 2**). ddPCR and RQ-PCR have comparable sensitivity but ddPCR is able to quantify a large proportion of cases classified as PNQ by RQ-PCR.[39] Despite these technical merits, ddPCR has yet to prove to be as predictive as RQ-PCR in a controlled clinical setting.[18] This work is currently being undertaken by the Euro-MRD consortium in cooperation with the EU-MCL network in large multicenter clinical trials.

Minimal Residual Disease Detection by Next-Generation Sequencing

New molecular biology technologies are based on high-performance sequencing of IGHV clonal rearrangement. These technologies could allow some of the disadvantages of classic ASO–RQ-PCR–based MRD approaches to be overcome.[17] In particular NGS can ensure higher specificity and spare the time-consuming and potentially subjective laboratory design of patient-specific tests (**Fig. 3**). Compared head to head, the 2 methods have shown similar sensitivity, but NGS has the potential to further increase sensitivity and specificity.[17]

For MRD detection by NGS, the first step is multiplex PCR for amplification of V-D-J rearrangements of Immunoglobulin gene (IG) or T cell receptor (TR) genes followed by a second PCR round with barcoded primers that allows library preparation and subsequent high-throughput sequencing.

For MRD analysis, it is essential to identify the correct index sequence specific for the tumor IG/TR rearrangement that is followed in follow-up samples. The whole

MRD detection by digital droplet PCR (ddPCR)

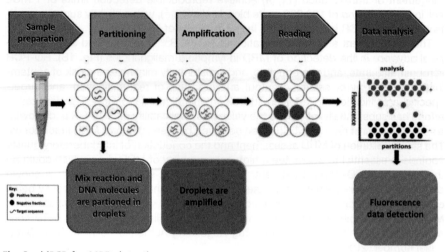

Fig. 2. ddPCR for MRD detection.

NGS of clonal IGHV rearrangements

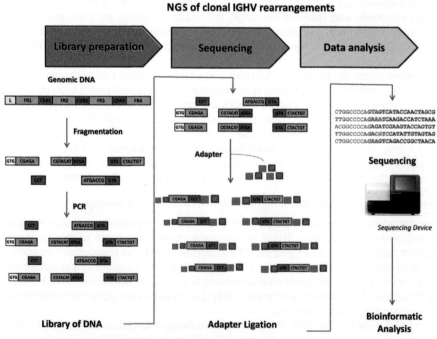

Fig. 3. Workflow for MRD evaluation by high-throughput sequencing methods. The immunoglobulin heavy chain (IGH) sample is fragmented and amplified, resulting in a library of DNA. Amplified fragments, known as amplicons, are immobilized on a solid support in order to sequence all DNA fragments in a parallel high-throughput process. This technique is only 1 possible approach to NGS. Alternative methods are also available.

analysis requires a well-established bioinformatics approach. The first studies on NGS-based MRD were conducted on acute lymphoid leukemia, showing that the 5% frequency cutoff is correctly used to allocate a clone as coming from cancer.[17,40] This threshold may be difficult to reach in BM or PB samples from patients with lymphoma because of decreased infiltration and unrelated B-cell and T-cell clones. Therefore, NGS has some applicability limitations in cases of low-level lymphoma cell infiltration. A further problem in amplicon-based sequencing approaches is somatic mutations at the primer binding sites that impair correct primer binding. This problem is particularly important in hypermutated B-cell neoplasms such as multiple myeloma.[40]

Another aspect that has not been adequately covered in recent publications is the correct quantification of MRD, particularly if the polyclonal background of B cells is low. The measurement of MRD by quantifying the number of index sequences and dividing them by the total number of IG reads is susceptible to error, because multiplex IG/TR PCR amplifies only the rearranged IG/TR genes, so cells with the respective gene in the germline configuration are not targeted. This omission could lead to false results, particularly in situations with a low number of polyclonal background B cells, because preferential sequencing of rearranged immunoglobulin heavy chain (IGH) B cells could lead to a considerable overestimation of the residual tumor load. Therefore, standardized internal controls should be included in each PCR reaction for correct MRD determination.

The EuroClonality-NGS consortium (www.EuroClonality.org) was formed in the context of ESLHO with the main objective of developing, standardizing, and validating the entire IG/TR NGS test workflow. Recently, articles have been published focusing on an amplicon-based NGS approach for the identification of MRD markers and the identification of clonality in lymphoid neoplasms.[20,40,41] In summary, robust validated procedures, standardized processing, regular quality controls, and guidelines for the interpretation of results are critical requirements for tailored MRD treatment in lymphoid neoplasms. The ultimate goal of any MRD assessment approach will to provide a fast, predictable, and reproducible tool that is sensitive enough to detect the disease before clinical relapse; NGS holds considerable promise in this regard but still requires extensive standardization and clinical validation.

HOW MINIMAL RESIDUAL DISEASE DATA HAVE AFFECTED THERAPEUTIC PARADIGMS IN MANTLE CELL LYMPHOMA

MRD has been extensively investigated in several large multicenter studies in MCL and proved to be a reliable and effective method to predict the clinical outcome of patients with MCL, particularly in terms of risk of recurrence. Early studies were based on the use of nested PCR, whereas more recent studies have primarily used RQ-PCR.[42–46] When systematically compared, RQ-PCR showed a better predictive value at most time points.[33]

Both PB and BM have been investigated in order to identify which source could be more predictive. In different trials, both tissues have shown typically informative but contrasting results on which source was superior from different experiences.[4,33,45] Given the lack of consensus on which source is the most informative, most ongoing trials include testing of both sources at least at some points. Both early and late time points proved to be informative in most settings, although later time points have been associated with a more rapid relapse pattern, indicating that persistent MRD positivity is usually not compatible with a prolonged disease remission.[33,45,47–49]

A criticism of MRD detection in lymphoma has been the supposed localized nature of most lymphomas, which could hamper a successful detection of residual tumors in liquid tissues such as PB and/or BM. This hypothesis is not justified in MCL because this neoplasm substantially invades PB or BM in greater than 90% of cases.[21] Moreover, a large bulk of data have shown that even apparently localized relapses are often heralded by signals of disease activity in PB or BM. Integration of imaging tools such as PET and MRD tools is a major field of interest that could allow an even more complete characterization of these complex entities.

Experience to date has shown that MRD is a strong and independent predictor of results and could provide a reliable tool to tailor treatment to the presence of residual tumor burden and the kinetics of the disease. The main experiences available can be summarized as follows:

- The use of CHOP (cyclophosphamide, hydroxydaunorubicin, oncovin, prednisone)-like chemotherapy alone, without the addition of rituximab, does not provide an effective clearance of molecularly detectable disease, including patients achieving clinical remission, as reported in the Nordic MCL5 study.[5] This finding underlines the inadequacy of CHOP-like regimens in MCL.[50] Immunochemotherapy with rituximab plus CHOP (R-CHOP) in the MCL Younger and MCL Elderly trials showed modest rates of molecular remission (MRD negativity) of 40%, with 21% of patients with MRD negative at midterm induction.[4,51,52]
- The use of rituximab in combination with intensive high-dose Ara-C chemotherapy is a very successful induction strategy inducing deeper remissions compared with previously used regimens. This result was originally observed using the High Dose Sequential Chemotherapy with Rituximab (R-HDS) regimen and then confirmed in the MCL Younger trial.[42,53,54] Intensification of induction treatment with HA in the arm that used alternating R-CHOP and Rituximab, dexamethasone, cytarabine, cisplatin (R-DHAP) was associated with 66% molecular remissions.[54] Others studies provided similar evidence in the context of the EU-MCL network studies.[4]
- Fludarabine-based regimens induced a profound clearance of MRD in patients with MCL.[55] However, these approaches are no longer used in MCL, because of their toxicity.
- Limited MRD data are available for bendamustine-based immunochemotherapy.[43,56,57] In the Nordic MCL4 study, after 6 cycles of rituximab, bendamustine, and lenalidomide, the percentage of 32 evaluable patients who were MRD positive by qualitative nested PCR was 56% in BM and 61% in PB.[43,56] The R-BAC combination also seems to induce a very high rate of molecular remission.[58]
- The use of ASCT enhances the outcome of patients with MCL. The effect of high-dose chemotherapy and subsequent ASCT has increased clinical response and long-term survival.[6] In European MCL trials, ASCT increases molecular remission rates after R-CHOP from 47% to 68% in PB and from 26% to 59% in BM.[4] In the Nordic MCL3 study, ASCT increased the proportion of MRD-negative patients in PB and/or BM from 53% after alternating R-CHOP/R-HA to 83%.[53] In an intermediate analysis of the LYSA-sponsored LYMA study, ASCT increased MRD negativity among patients in clinical remission after 4 cycles of R-DHAP from 80% to 95% in PB and from 66% to 82% in BM.[49]
- Several studies have shown the high prognostic value of MRD status at the end of induction after ASCT and during subsequent follow-up on PFS.[49,59–61] In the MCL Younger study, MRD positivity before ASCT was highly predictive for shorter PFS (hazard ratio in PB, 2.7; in BM, 1.8), independently of the induction treatment arm.[4] Similar results were observed in the French LYMA study.[49]

- Long-term monitoring of MRD in the follow-up of patients in disease remission is of substantial clinical relevance. Data from the MCL European network show that the reappearance of MRD in clinical remission is associated with clinical relapse.[3,4,33,55,61,62] Post-ASCT MRD status is highly prognostic for PFS, with PFS at 4 years of about 38% (median PFS about 3 years)[4] and is independent of MIPI score, Ki-67 index, and clinical response. In the MCL0208 study, MRD positivity was linked to an increased risk of recurrence at multiple follow-up time points, whereas the presence of at least 2 consecutive MRD-negative results indicated a significantly reduced risk of recurrence.[33] Similar results have been observed in studies focusing on elderly patients.[55,62,63]
- Posttreatment maintenance has a well-defined role in MCL.[64] However, the impact of maintenance on MRD kinetics is not well characterized yet. Results from the LYMA trial suggest that MRD-positive patients have a meaningful benefit when receiving maintenance.[49] The LYMA-101 study investigating obinutuzumab maintenance after Obinutuzumab, dexamethasone, cytarabine, cisplatin (O-DHAP) and ASCT gave excellent results in terms of MRD response and is actively exploring the role of MRD-tailored maintenance in this population.[8]
- Because MRD positivity anticipates an imminent relapse, this may lead to the personalization of the treatment, with the aim of preventing or delaying a clinical relapse. In several prospective and retrospective reports, preventive treatment with rituximab of MRD-positive patients was able to convert them to MRD negativity, with the possibility of prolonging their PFS.[34,61,65] Another alternative could be the use of MRD in order to identify patients that could benefit from treatment reduction, based on an excellent molecular response. However, patients achieving molecular response are not necessarily ideal candidates for treatment reduction, as shown in a large study in follicular lymphoma.[66]
- Allogeneic BM transplant can induce MRD negativity in patients who have failed other therapies.[67,68]
- The emergence of new drugs in MCL therapy has enhanced patient outcomes. Data on MRD evaluation are still scarce. At present, the TRIANGLE trial, a randomized, 3-arm, parallel-group, phase 3 trial with open-phase international targets, is investigating whether the addition of ibrutinib to the current standard treatment could improve results (EudraCT number: 2014-001363-12). This study will include standardized multi–time-point MRD detection across the entire test population and will therefore allow the impact of Bruton tyrosine kinase inhibitors on MRD kinetics in MCL to be established.

In summary, the data available prove that MRD is a major predictor in MCL. Most of the current generation of MCL clinical studies include MRD negativity as a secondary end point, and some studies, such as LYMA-101, are prospectively exploring the value of tailor-made treatment of MRD in this context.

SUMMARY

MRD assessment is an important tool to evaluate the long-term prognosis in patients with MCL. For this reason, it is currently included as a strategic secondary end point in most clinical trials. This information will enable a more precise evaluation of the treatment efficacy in the near future. For these purposes, it will be necessary to develop more accurate and reproducible techniques. NGS could add to the current portfolio of methods and could not only increase the number of patients with a sensitive MRD marker but also allow a more precise MRD quantification. However, validation of NGS with respect to reproducible sensitivity and identification of prognostic subgroups is needed in clinical trials. In the EuroClonality-NGS consortium, comparative analysis of different MRD methods is already underway and regular quality controls for NGS-based MRD detection will be part of the Euro-MRD network activities.

In conclusion, MRD over more than 20 years has contributed to the understanding of the natural history of MCL, and has helped clinicians to precisely monitor benefits and limits of available treatments. However, the most important step forward would be that of implementing MRD diagnostics in the therapeutic algorithm of MCL, as already happens in acute lymphoblastic leukemia. The task is not easy. First, clinicians must recognize that even sustained MRD negativity is not equivalent to cure in MCL, because late molecular relapses frequently occur and, therefore, it might not wise to avoid effective nontoxic treatments such as rituximab maintenance, even in the best responders. In contrast, treatment intensification for high-risk subgroups might be an attractive option, if an innovative treatment has the potential of effectively modifying the clinical history of the disease. This approach would potentially help in maximizing the benefit of treatments, which can too toxic or too expensive if applied to broad, unselected, standard-risk populations. The portfolio of available therapeutic agents in MCL is rapidly expanding, and it is possible that well-designed MRD-tailored treatments could represent ideal settings to challenge these novel agents in the clinical arena.

REFERENCES

1. Lenz G, Dreyling M, Hoster E, et al. Immunochemotherapy with rituximab and cyclophosphamide, doxorubicin, vincristine, and prednisone significantly improve response and time to treatment failure, but not long-term outcome in patients with previously untreated mantle cell lymphoma: results of a prospective randomized trial of the German Low-Grade Lymphoma Study Group (GLSG). J Clin Oncol 2005;23(9):1984–92.

2. Hoster E, Unterhalt M, Pfreundschuh M, et al. The addition of rituximab to CHOP improves failure-free and overall survival of mantle-cell lymphoma patients—a pooled trials analysis of the German Low-Grade Lymphoma Study Group (GLSG) [abstract]. Blood 2014;124(21) [Abstract: 1752].

3. Geisler CH, Kolstad A, Laurell A, et al. Nordic Lymphoma Group. Long-term progression-free survival of mantle cell lymphoma after intensive front-line immunochemotherapy with in vivo-purged stem cell rescue: a nonrandomized phase 2 multicenter study by the Nordic Lymphoma Group. Blood 2008;112(7):2687–93.

4. Hermine O, Hoster E, Walewski J, et al. Alternating Courses of 3x CHOP and 3x DHAP Plus Rituximab Followed by a High Dose ARA-C Containing Myeloablative Regimen and Autologous Stem Cell Transplantation (ASCT) Is Superior to 6 Courses CHOP Plus Rituximab Followed by Myeloablative Radiochemotherapy and ASCT In Mantle Cell Lymphoma: Results of the MCL Younger Trial of the European Mantle Cell Lymphoma Network (MCL net). Blood 2010;116(21):110.

5. Andersen NS, Pedersen L, Elonen E, et al. Nordic Lymphoma Group. Primary treatment with autologous stem cell transplantation in mantle cell lymphoma: outcome related to remission pretransplant. Eur J Haematol 2003;71(2):73–80.

6. Dreyling M, Lenz G, Hoster E, et al. Early consolidation by myeloablative radiochemotherapy followed by autologous stem cell transplantation in first remission significantly prolongs progression-free survival in mantle-cell lymphoma: results of a prospective randomized trial of the European MCL Network. Blood 2005; 105(7):2677–84.

7. Kluin-Nelemans HC, Hoster E, Hermine O, et al. Treatment of older patients with mantle-cell lymphoma. N Engl J Med 2012;367(6):520–31.

8. Le Gouill S, Beldi-Ferchiou A, Cacheux V, et al. Obinutuzumab plus DHAP followed by ASCT plus Obinutuzumab maintenance provides a high MRD response rate in untreated patients with MCL, results of the LYMA-101 trial, a LYSA group study. Abstract S103. 24th European Hematology Association Congress, Amsterdam, NL, June 14, 2019.

9. Li W, Wei Q, Yu-Jia H, et al. Advances in targeted therapy for malignant lymphoma. Signal Transduct Target Ther 2020;5:15.

10. Hoster E, Dreyling M, Klapper W, et al. German Low-Grade Lymphoma Study Group (GLSG); European Mantle Cell Lymphoma Network. A new prognostic index (MIPI) for patients with advanced-stage mantle cell lymphoma. Blood 2008; 111(2):558–65.

11. Hoster E, Rosenwald A, Berger F, et al. Prognostic value of Ki-67 index, cytology, and growth pattern in mantle-cell lymphoma: results from randomized trials of the european mantle cell lymphoma network. J Clin Oncol 2016;34(12):1386–94.

12. Ferrero S, Rossi D, Rinaldi A, et al. KMT2D mutations and TP53 disruptions are poor prognostic biomarkers in mantle cell lymphoma receiving high-dose therapy: a FIL study. Haematologica 2020;105(6):1604–12.

13. Pott C. Minimal residual disease detection in mantle cell lymphoma: technical aspects and clinical relevance. Semin Hematol 2011;48:172–84.

14. Galimberti S, Luminari S, Ciabatti E, et al. Minimal residual disease after conventional treatment significantly impacts on progression-free survival of patients with follicular lymphoma: the FIL FOLL05 trial. Clin Cancer Res 2014;20:6398–405.

15. Hoster E, Pott C. Minimal residual disease in mantle cell lymphoma: Insights into biology and impact on treatment. Hematology Am Soc Hematol Educ Program 2016;2016(1):437–45.

16. Dongen JJM, der Velden JV, Brüggemann M, et al. Minimal residual disease diagnostics in acute lymphoblastic leukemia: need for sensitive, fast, and standardized technologies. Blood 2015;125(26):3996–4009.

17. Ladetto M, Bruggemann M, Monitillo L, et al. Next-generation sequencing and real-time quantitative PCR for minimal residual disease detection in B-cell disorders. Leukemia 2014;28:1299–307.

18. Drandi D, Kubiczkova-besse L, Ferrero S, et al. Minimal residual disease detection by droplet digital PCR in multiple myeloma , mantle cell lymphoma , and follicular lymphoma a comparison with real-time PCR. J Mol Diagn 2015;17: 652–60.

19. Pott C, Brüggemann M, Ritgen M, et al. MRD detection in B-cell non-hodgkin lymphomas using Ig gene rearrangements and chromosomal translocations as targets for real-time quantitative PCR. Methods Mol Biol 2013;971:175–200.

20. Brüggemann M, Kotrová M, Knecht H, et al. Standardized next-generation sequencing of immunoglobulin and T-cell receptor gene recombinations for MRD marker identification in acute lymphoblastic leukaemia; a EuroClonality-NGS validation study. Leukemia 2019;33:2241–53.

21. Cheminant M, Touzart DA, Schmit S, et al. Minimal residual disease monitoring by 8-color flow cytometry in mantle cell lymphoma: An EU-MCL and LYSA study. Haematologica 2016;101:336–45.

22. Ferrero S, Drandi D, Mantoan B, et al. Minimal residual disease detection in lymphoma and multiple myeloma: impact on therapeutic paradigms. Hematol Oncol 2011;29:167–76.

23. Böttcher S, Ritgen M, Buske S, et al, EU MCL MRD Group. Minimal residual disease detection in mantle cell lymphoma: methods and significance of four-color flow cytometry compared to consensus IGH-polymerase chain reaction at initial staging and for follow-up examinations. Haematologica 2008;93(4):551–9.

24. Chovancová J, Bernard T, Stehlíková O, et al. Detection of minimal residual disease in mantle cell lymphoma-establishment of novel eight-color flow cytometry approach. Cytometry B Clin Cytom 2015;88(2):92–100.

25. van Dongen JJM, Lhermitte L, Bottcher S, et al. EuroFlow antibody panels for standardized n-dimensional flow cytometric immunophenotyping of normal, reactive and malignant leukocytes. Leukemia 2012;26(9):1908–75.

26. Kalina T, Flores-Montero J, van der Velden VHJ, et al. EuroFlow standardization of flow cytometer instrument settings and immunophenotyping protocols. Leukemia 2012;26:1986–2010.

27. Theunissen P, Mejstrikova E, Sedek L, et al. Standardized flow cytometry for highly sensitive MRD measurements in B-cell acute lymphoblastic leukemia. Blood 2017;129:347–57.

28. Kalina T, Flores-Montero J, Lecrevisse Q, et al. Quality assessment program for EuroFlow protocols: Summary results of four-year (2010-2013) quality assurance rounds. Cytometry A 2015;87:145–56.

29. Flores-Montero J, Sanoja-Flores L, Paiva B, et al. Next Generation Flow for highly sensitive and standardized detection of minimal residual disease in multiple myeloma. Leukemia 2017;31(10):2094–103.

30. Rimokh R, Berger F, Delsol G, et al. Detection of the chromosomal translocation t(11;14) by polymerase chain reaction in mantle cell lymphomas. Blood 1994;83: 1871–5.

31. Kuiper RP, van Reijmersdal SV, Simonis M, et al. Targeted locus amplification & next generation sequencing for the detection of recurrent and novel gene fusions for improved treatment decisions in pediatric acute lymphoblastic leukemia. Blood 2015;126(23):696. Abstract.

32. Genuardi E, Klous P, Drandi D, et al. Targeted Locus Amplification (TLA): A Novel Next Generation Sequencing (NGS) Technology to Detect New Molecular Markers and Monitoring Minimal Residual Disease (MRD) in Mantle Cell and Follicular Lymphoma. Abstract. Blood 2017;30(Supplement 1):2742.

33. Ferrero S, Barbero S, Lo Schirico M, et al. Comprehensive Minimal Residual Disease (MRD) analysis of the fondazione italiana linfomi (FIL) MCL0208 clinical trial for younger patients with mantle cell lymphoma: a kinetic model ensures a more refined risk stratification. Blood 2018;132. abstract 920.

34. Ladetto M, Magni M, Pagliano G, et al. Rituximab induces effective clearance of minimal residual disease in molecular relapses of mantle cell lymphoma. Biology of blood and marrow transplantation. Biol Blood Marrow Transplant 2006;12(12): 1270–6.

35. Andersen NS, Donovan JW, Zuckerman A, et al. Real-time polymerase chain reaction estimation of bone marrow tumor burden using clonal immunoglobulin heavy chain gene and bcl-1/JH rearrangements in mantle cell lymphoma. Exp Hematol 2002;30(7):703–10.

36. Ladetto M, Sametti S, Donovan JW, et al. A validated real-time quantitative PCR approach shows a correlation between tumor burden and successful ex vivo purging in follicular lymphoma patients. Exp Hematol 2001;29:183–93.

37. Bruggemann M, Droese J, Bolz I, et al. Improved assessment of minimal residual disease in B cell malignancies using fluorogenic consensus probes for real-time quantitative PCR. Leukemia 2000;14(8):1419–25.

38. van der Velden VHJ, Cazzaniga G, Scrauder A, et al. Analysis of minimal residual disease by Ig/TCR gene rearrangements: guidelines for interpretation of real-time quantitative PCR data. Leukemia 2007;21:604–11.

39. Faham M, Zheng J, Moorhead M, et al. Deep-sequencing approach for minimal residual disease detection in acute lymphoblastic leukemia. Blood 2012;120: 5173–80.

40. Martinez-Lopez J, Lahuerta JJ, Pepin F, et al. Prognostic value of deep sequencing method for minimal residual disease detection in multiple myeloma. Blood 2014;123:3073–9.

41. Scheijen B, Meijers RWJ, Rijntjes J, et al. on behalf of the EuroClonality-NGS Working Group. Next-generation sequencing of immunoglobulin gene rearrangements for clonality assessment: a technical feasibility study by EuroClonality-NGS. Leukemia 2019;33:2227–40.

42. Geisler CH, Kolstad A, Laurell A, et al. Long-term progression-free survival of mantle cell lymphoma after intensive front-line immunochemotherapy with in vivo-purged stem cell rescue: a non-randomized phase 2 multicenter study by the Nordic Lymphoma Group. Blood 2008;112(7):2687–93.

43. Albertsson-Lindblad A, Kolstad A, Laurell A, et al. Lenalidomide-bendamustine-rituximab in untreated mantle cell lymphoma > 65 years, the Nordic Lymphoma Group phase I+II trial NLG-MCL4. Blood 2016. https://doi.org/10.1182/blood-2016-03-704023.

44. Andersen NS, Pedersen LB, Laurell A, et al. Pre-emptive treatment with rituximab of molecular relapse after autologous stem cell transplantation in mantle cell lymphoma. J Clin Oncol 2009;27(26):4365–70.

45. Pott C, Macintyre E, Delfau-Larue MH, et al. MRD eradication should be the therapeutic goal in mantle cell lymphoma and may enable tailored treatment approaches: results of the intergroup trials of the European MCL Network [abstract]. Blood 2014;124(21) [Abstract: 147].

46. Corradini P, Ladetto M, Zallio F, et al. Long-term follow-up of indolent lymphoma patients treated with high-dose sequential chemotherapy and autografting: evidence that durable molecular and clinical remission frequently can be attained only in follicular subtypes. J Clin Oncol 2004;22(8):1460–8.

47. Pott C, Schrader C, Gesk S, et al. Quantitative assessment of molecular remission after high-dose therapy with autologous stem cell transplantation predicts long-term remission in mantle cell lymphoma. Blood 2006;107:2271–8.

48. Ferrero S, Dreyling M, on behalf of the European Mantle Cell Lymphoma Network. Minimal residual disease in mantle cell lymphoma: are we ready for a personalized treatment approach? Haematologica 2017;102(7):1133–6.

49. Callanan M, Delfau MH, Thieblemont ME, et al. Predictive Power of Early, Sequential MRD monitoring in peripheral blood and bone marrow in patients with mantle cell lymphoma following autologous stem cell transplantation with or without rituximab maintenance; interim results from the LyMa-MRD Project. Blood 2015;126 [Abstract: 338].

50. Howard OM, Gribben JG, Neuberg DS, et al. Rituximab and CHOP induction therapy for newly diagnosed mantle-cell lymphoma: molecular complete responses are not predictive of progression-free survival. J Clin Oncol 2002; 20(5):1288.

51. Gianni AM, Magni M, Martelli M, et al. Long-term Remission in Mantle Cell Lymphoma Following High-Dose Sequential Chemotherapy and in Vivo Rituximab-Purged Stem Cell Autografting (R-HDS Regimen). Blood 2003;102(2):749–55.

52. Magni M, Di Nicola M, Devizzi L, et al. Successful in vivo purging of CD34-containing peripheral blood harvests in mantle cell and indolent lymphoma: evidence for a role of both chemotherapy and rituximab infusion. Blood 2000;96(3):864–9.

53. Kolstad A, Laurell A, Jerkeman M, et al. Nordic MCL3 study: 90Y-ibritumomab-tiuxetan added to BEAM/C in non-CR patients before transplant in mantle cell lymphoma. Blood 2014;123:2953–9.

54. Pott C, Hoster E, Beldjord K, et al. R-CHOP/R-DHAP Compared to R-CHOP Induction Followed by High Dose Therapy with Autologous Stem Cell Transplantation Induces Higher Rates of Molecular Remission In MCL: Results of the MCL Younger Intergroup Trial of the European MCL Network. Blood 2010;116(21):965.

55. Pott C, Delfau-Larue M, Beldjord K, et al. R-CHOP vs R-FC followed by maintenance with rituximab or IFN: First results of MRD assessment within the randomized trial for elderly patients with MCL [abstract]. Ann Oncol 2011;22(suppl 4) [Abstract: 233].

56. Armand P, Redd R, Bsat J, et al. A phase 2 study of Rituximab-Bendamustine and Rituximab-Cytarabine for transplant-eligible patients with mantle cell lymphoma. Br J Haematol 2016;173(1):89–95.

57. Gressin R, Callanan M, Daguindau N, et al. Frontline Therapy with the Ribvd Regimen Elicits High Clinical and Molecular Response Rates and Long PFS in Elderly Patients Mantle Cell Lymphoma (MCL); Final Results of a Prospective Phase II Trial by the Lysa Group. Blood 2014;124(21):148.

58. Visco C, Chiappella A, Nassi L, et al. Rituximab, bendamustine, and low-dose cytarabine as induction therapy in elderly patients with mantle cell lymphoma: a multicentre, phase 2 trial from Fondazione Italiana Linfomi. Lancet Haematol 2017;4(1):e15–23.

59. Gribben JG, Freedman AS, Neuberg D, et al. Immunologic purging of marrow assessed by PCR before autologous bone marrow transplantation for B-cell lymphoma. N Engl J Med 1991;325:1525–33.

60. Pott C, Hoster E, Delfau-Larue MH, et al. Molecular remission is an independent predictor of clinical outcome in patients with mantle cell lymphoma after combined immunochemotherapy: a European MCL intergroup study. Blood 2010;115:3215–23.

61. Kolstad A, Pedersen LB, Eskelund CW, et al. Nordic Lymphoma Group. Molecular monitoring after autologous stem cell transplantation and preemptive rituximab treatment of molecular relapse; Results from the nordic mantle cell lymphoma studies (MCL2 and MCL3) with median follow-up of 8.5 years. Biol Blood Marrow Transplant 2017;23:428–35.

62. Gressin R, Daguindau N, Tempescul A, et al. A phase 2 study of rituximab, bendamustine, bortezomib and dexamethasone for first-line treatment of older patients with mantle cell lymphoma. Haematologica 2019;104:138–46.

63. Kaplan LD, Maurer MJ, Stock W, et al. Bortezomib maintenance (BM) or consolidation (BC) following aggressive immunochemotherapy and autologous stem cell transplant (ASCT) for untreated mantle cell lymphoma (MCL): 8 year follow up of CALGB 50403 (alliance). Blood 2018;132:146.

64. Klener P, Fronkova E, Kalinova M, et al. R Potential loss of prognostic significance of minimal residual disease assessment after R-CHOP-based induction in elderly patients with mantle cell lymphoma in the era of rituximab maintenance. Hematol Oncol 2018;36(5):773–8.

65. Ferrero S, Monitillo L, Mantoan B, et al. Rituximab-based pre-emptive treatment of molecular relapse in follicular and mantle cell lymphoma. Ann Hematol 2013; 92(11):1503–11.
66. Federico M, Mannina D, Versari A, et al. Response oriented maintenance therapy in advanced follicular lymphoma. Results of the interim analysis of the FOLL12 TRIAL conducted by the Fondazione Italiana Linfomi. Abstract (2019). https://doi.org/10.1002/hon.110_2629.
67. Kobrinski DA, Smith SE, Al-Mansour Z, et al. Allogeneic hematopoietic stem cell transplantation for mantle cell lymphoma in a heavily pretreated patient population. J Clin Oncol 2017;35(15 suppl):7558. Abstract.
68. Magnusson EA, Cao Q, Linden LA, et al. Autologous and allogeneic donor transplantation for mantle cell lymphoma in rituximab era: impact of pre-transplant burden on survival. clinical allogenic and autologous transplantation –poster II. Blood 2012;120(21):3092.

Current Role and Emerging Evidence for Bruton Tyrosine Kinase Inhibitors in the Treatment of Mantle Cell Lymphoma

David A. Bond, MD[a],*, Kami J. Maddocks, MD[b]

KEYWORDS

- Therapy • BTKi • Acalabrutinib • Ibrutinib • Zanubrutinib • Tirabrutinib
- Orelabrutinib

KEY POINTS

- Acalabrutinib, ibrutinib, and zanubrutinib are each highly active as monotherapy in mantle cell lymphoma (MCL) and are currently approved for treating patients with relapsed or refractory disease.
- Combination treatment with ibrutinib and venetoclax in the relapsed setting shows promising depth of response, and current clinical trials are further evaluating this and other combination treatment approaches.
- Ibrutinib and rituximab has a high response rate in patients with previously untreated MCL, and ongoing studies are investigating combinations of BTKi with chemoimmunotherapy or targeted therapies as frontline treatment.

INTRODUCTION

Mantle cell lymphoma (MCL) is a heterogeneous non-Hodgkin lymphoma subtype with a wide range in clinical and biological behavior resulting in treatment approaches at diagnosis varying from initial observation in select patients to aggressive chemoimmunotherapy (CIT) and consolidation with autologous hematopoietic cell transplant (AHCT) in others. Although response rates to frontline CIT are generally high, relapse occurs in nearly all patients and chemoresistance generally increases with increasing prior lines of treatment. The median age at diagnosis of MCL is 67 years, resulting in many patients not being candidates for intensive treatment approaches such as AHCT

a Division of Hematology, The Ohio State University, 320 West 10th Avenue, A340 Starling Loving Hall, Columbus, OH 43210, USA; b Division of Hematology, The Ohio State University, 320 West 10th Street, A350C Starling Loving Hall, Columbus, OH 43210, USA
* Corresponding author.
E-mail address: David.Bond@osumc.edu
Twitter: @kmaddmd (K.J.M.)

Hematol Oncol Clin N Am 34 (2020) 903–921
https://doi.org/10.1016/j.hoc.2020.06.007
0889-8588/20/© 2020 Elsevier Inc. All rights reserved.

hemonc.theclinics.com

consolidation due to age and comorbid illness.[1] Developing less toxic treatment approaches suitable for older patients is a priority. The development of drugs targeting Bruton tyrosine kinase (BTK), a key component in B-cell receptor signaling, has been a major development in the treatment of relapsed and refractory (R/R) MCL and provides a highly active treatment generally well tolerated by both younger and older patients. In this review, the authors summarize the evidence for the use of the 3 currently approved BTK inhibitors (BTKi), acalabrutinib, ibrutinib, and zanubrutinib, for relapsed MCL and discuss emerging evidence for the use of BTKi in combination for both salvage and frontline treatment.

CURRENTLY APPROVED AGENTS AND INDICATIONS

Currently, 3 BTKi, acalabrutinib, ibrutinib, and zanubrutinib, have been granted accelerated approval by the US Food and Drug Administration (FDA) for the treatment of adult patients with MCL. All 3 are covalent, irreversible BTKi approved for the treatment of patients with MCL after at least one prior line of therapy. Ibrutinib was the first BTKi to be clinically developed and provided proof of principle for the activity of this class of treatments.[2] Head to head prospective data regarding the comparative toxicity and efficacy of these agents are not currently available. A review of the evidence to date for the safety and efficacy of each of these BTKi is presented in the following section and summarized in **Table 1**.

IBRUTINIB

Ibrutinib is a first in class BTKi, which also irreversibly inhibits structurally related kinases including the TEC family kinase ITK resulting in immunomodulatory properties.[3,4] After demonstrating clinical activity in MCL and other B-cell malignancies in a phase 1 study,[2] ibrutinib was studied in the PCYC-1104 study, a phase 2 study of ibrutinib in 111 adult patients with R/R MCL.[5] Baseline patient characteristics included a median age of 68 years, median of 3 prior lines of treatment, and 54 patients (49%) with high-risk Mantle Cell Lymphoma Prognostic Index (MIPI) score. Common adverse events (AEs) of any grade included diarrhea (50%), fatigue (41%), and nausea (31%), and grade 3 or greater toxicities included neutropenia (16%), thrombocytopenia (11%), anemia (10%), and bleeding (5%). The overall response rate (ORR) was 69% including 21% complete response (CR) with a median estimated progression-free survival (PFS) of 13.9 months, and with extended follow-up the median duration of response (DOR) was 17.5 months with 2-year overall survival (OS) of 47%.[6] A subsequent international randomized phase 3 study (MCL-3001) was performed in which 280 patients with R/R MCL were randomized to ibrutinib or temsirolimus.[7] Ibrutinib treatment resulted in an improved PFS (15 vs 6 months) with a significant reduction in the risk for progression or death (hazard ratio 0.4).

   With 370 patients with R/R MCL treated with ibrutinib across 3 published studies (PCYC-1104, MCL-2001, and MCL-3001), the efficacy of ibrutinib monotherapy for relapsed MCL is the best characterized of the BTKi. In a pooled analysis of patients treated across these studies, the ORR was 66%, with 20% CR, the median PFS was 13 months, and median OS was 25 months.[8] With 3.5 years follow-up, the median duration of response was significantly longer at 22 months for patients receiving ibrutinib second-line versus 8 months for those with 2 or more prior lines of therapy, supporting the use of BTKi as first salvage therapy in most of the patients.[9] Among 20 patients with mutations in TP53, the ORR was 55%, median PFS was 4 months, and median OS was 12 months,[9] which suggests that responses to single-agent BTKi treatment in TP53 mutated patients are brief and alternative treatment

Table 1
Summary of phase 2/3 study results for Bruton tyrosine kinase inhibitors in relapsed mantle cell lymphoma

BTKi	Patients Enrolled	Rate of Common AE Any Grade	Rate of AEs of Interest	ORR (CR)	Median PFS (mo)	Ref
Ibrutinib	370	Diarrhea 40%, cough 22%, nausea 22%, peripheral edema 20%	A-fib 5%, major bleeding 5%	66% (20%)	13	Rule et al,[8] 2017
Acalabrutinib	124	Headache 38%, diarrhea 31%, myalgia 21%, cough 19%, nausea 18%	A-fib 0%, major bleeding 2%	80% (40%)	20	Wang et al,[31] 2018; Wang et al,[32] 2019
Zanubrutinib	86	Rash 34%, URI 34%, diarrhea 15%	A-fib 0%, major bleeding 2%	84% (59%)	N.E.	Song et al,[37] 2018
Zanubrutinib	43	Diarrhea 30%, bleeding or bruising 30%, rash 16%	A-fib 5%, major bleeding 5%	80% (20%)	N.E.	Tam et al,[36] 2018

Abbreviations: AE, adverse event; A-fib, atrial fibrillation; CR, complete response; N.E., not evaluable; ORR, overall response rate; PFS, progression-free survival; Ref, reference; URI, upper respiratory tract infection.
Data from Refs.[8,31,32,36,37]

approaches are needed for this high-risk population. In contrast, patients receiving ibrutinib second-line who previously achieved a DOR of 2 years or greater after front-line treatment experienced high response rates (87% ORR, 47% CR) and prolonged PFS (median 58 months), suggesting that lower risk patients (chemosensitive disease, fewer lines of treatment) may experience superior outcomes with BTKi monotherapy.

The toxicity profile of ibrutinib monotherapy is well characterized from results of both prospective and observational studies. In the pooled analysis, common AEs of any grade included diarrhea (40%), fatigue (35%), cough (22%), nausea (22%), edema (20%), and rash (15%).[8] Major bleeding occurred in 18 patients (5%) and grade 3 or greater atrial fibrillation in 17 patients (5%). Of the toxicities associated with ibrutinib, bleeding and cardiovascular toxicities deserve particular mention. BTK plays a physiologic role in mediating glycoprotein Ib and glycoprotein VI (GPVI) platelet signaling regulating collagen-mediated platelet activation and Von Willebrand factor (vWF) signaling, and the related kinase TEC also plays a role in GPVI signaling.[10–12] High rates of low-grade bleeding events were reported in early studies of ibrutinib, and grade 3 or greater bleeding events were noted in 5% of patients, including life-threatening bleeding in patients receiving antiplatelet or anticoagulant therapies, leading to prohibition of patients receiving warfarin from subsequent ibrutinib studies.[2,5,13] In vitro studies demonstrated that ibrutinib inhibits collagen-induced platelet aggregation and vWF adhesion, supporting platelet dysfunction as the explanation for this bleeding phenotype.[14] These alterations in platelet function do not seem to be due exclusively to BTK inhibition, as functional studies performed ex vivo demonstrated abnormal thrombus formation occurring in ibrutinib but not acalabrutinib-treated patients relative to untreated controls.[15] Work by a separate group demonstrated impaired thrombus formation ex vivo in ibrutinib but not zanubrutinib-treated patients, and in mice both ex vivo and in vivo impairment in thrombus formation and hemostasis occur in ibrutinib but not zanubrutinib-treated mice.[16] Most of the bleeding events seen with ibrutinib are minor and self-limited. A systematic review and meta-analysis demonstrated an increased overall bleeding incidence in patients treated with ibrutinib compared with patients in control arms but no significant difference in the incidence of major bleeding,[17] and thus the magnitude and relevance of differences in bleeding risk between ibrutinib and the more selective BTKi acalabrutinib or zanubrutinib are uncertain. The second category of ibrutinib-associated toxicities of specific interest is cardiovascular toxicity. Atrial fibrillation was observed in early studies of ibrutinib, and a meta-analysis established an increased rate of atrial fibrillation with ibrutinib relative to controls in randomized clinical trials.[18] In a pooled analysis of patients treated with ibrutinib for lymphoid malignancies across 4 large randomized studies, the incidence of atrial fibrillation was 6.5% at the median follow-up of 16.6 months and was estimated at 13.8% after 36 months of follow-up.[19] Ventricular arrhythmia and sudden cardiac death have also been reported in patients receiving ibrutinib therapy[20–25]; these life-threatening events are less common and in cases of cardiac arrest leading to death may be difficult to ascertain, making a precise estimate of the magnitude of risk and association with ibrutinib difficult to establish. Inhibition of BTK or TEC have been hypothesized to mediate the risk for cardiac arrhythmia with ibrutinib,[26] and although the rates of atrial fibrillation seem to be lower with more selective BTKi, it remains to be established to what extent off- versus on-target kinase inhibition leads to the risk for cardiac arrhythmia. More common than cardiac arrhythmia, hypertension has recently been recognized to occur at an increased rate in patients treated with ibrutinib, with new hypertension occurring in 72% of ibrutinib-treated patients in a single-center study and associated with an increased risk for major adverse cardiovascular events.[27,28]

ACALABRUTINIB

Acalabrutinib is an oral irreversible BTKi, with significantly less off-target inhibition of structurally similar TEC, SRC, and ERBB family kinases in comparison to ibrutinib.[29,30] The efficacy of acalabrutinib in MCL was established in the pivotal phase II ACE-LY-004 trial in which 124 patients with previously treated MCL were enrolled and treated with acalabrutinib, 100 mg, twice daily.[31] Baseline characteristics included a median of 2 prior lines of treatment, median age of 68 years, 26 patients (21%) with blastoid or pleomorphic histology, 32 patients (33% of evaluable patients) with a Ki67 index greater than or equal to 50%, and 21 patients (17%) with high-risk MIPI score. The ORR was 80%, including 40% CR.[31] Common AEs and AEs of interest are summarized in **Table 1** and included headache (38%), diarrhea (31%), myalgia (21%), and nausea (18%). After a median follow-up of 26 months, the estimated median PFS was 20 months and the estimated OS at 24 months was 72%.[32] Among 29 patients evaluable for minimal residual disease (MRD), 8 patients (28%) (all in CR) had undetectable MRD. The safety profile in this study is consistent with that reported in a pooled analysis of 610 patients treated with acalabrutinib for assorted hematologic malignancies, which reported a 2.3% rate of atrial fibrillation and 2.5% rate of major bleeding.[33] The reported rates of cardiac events including atrial fibrillation and bleeding observed with acalabrutinib in studies is lower than that observed with ibrutinib, and the more selective BTKi may be preferred in patients with cardiac or bleeding risk factors, but longer duration of follow-up with ibrutinib may contribute to these differences and conclusions cannot be reached by cross-trial comparison. A head-to-head study of acalabrutinib versus ibrutinib in patients with chronic lymphocytic leukemia (CLL) is ongoing (NCT02477696) and will provide randomized prospective data regarding differences in rates of toxicities between drugs.

ZANUBRUTINIB

Zanubrutinib is a second-generation BTKi with greater selectivity for BTK relative to ibrutinib and a longer half-life than acalabrutinib.[34,35] In a phase 1 study, rapid and complete peripheral blood BTK occupancy was demonstrated at all studied dose levels and a dosing schedule of 160 mg twice daily achieved greater than 95% nodal BTK occupancy in 89% of patients and was established as the recommended phase 2 dose.[35] Preliminary results for patients with MCL enrolled in the dose expansion phase of this study (AU-003) have been presented in abstract form, including 38 patients with R/R MCL and 5 treatment-naïve (TN) patients.[36] Treatment emergent AEs and AEs of interest are summarized in **Table 1**. The ORR was 90% including 20% CR. In the pivotal phase II BGB-3111-206 study, 86 patients with R/R MCL were treated with zanubrutinib, 160 mg, twice daily. Baseline patient characteristics included a median age of 61 years, median of 2 prior lines of treatment, 12 (14%) patients with blastoid histology, and 72 patients (84%) with intermediate or high MIPI-b score. Common reported AEs and AEs of interest are summarized in **Table 1** and included rash in 29%, respiratory infection in 29%, and bleeding in 6% (including 1.2% major hemorrhage). With regard to efficacy, the ORR was 84%, including 59% CR.[37] In BGB-3111-206, response assessments were primarily performed by PET in contrast to AU-003 that used computed tomographic imaging, which may explain the disparate CR rates between these studies. The rates of some toxicities, such as atrial fibrillation, seem lower with the more specific zanubrutinib in comparison to ibrutinib, although comparison of AEs between trials should be interpreted with caution, and ongoing head to head trials of ibrutinib versus zanubrutinib (NCT03734016 and NCT03053440) in B-cell malignancies will better delineate differences in toxicity profiles.

ALTERNATIVE BRUTON TYROSINE KINASE INHIBITORS

In addition to the 3 currently approved BTKi, the irreversible BTKi, tirabrutinib and ore-labrutinib, have been studied in R/R MCL. Both tirabrutinib and orelabrutinib are second-generation BTKi designed for improved BTK specificity. Tirabrutinib was studied in patients with B-cell malignancies in a phase 1/2 study that enrolled 90 patients, including 16 with MCL, in cohorts treated with escalating dosages ranging from 20 to 600 mg/d.[38] Efficacy was observed across all dose levels and the maximum tolerated dose (MTD) was not reached. Common AEs included diarrhea in 16 patients (18%), petechiae in 13 patients (14%), rash in 16 patients (18%), neutropenia in 11 patients (12%), and hematoma in 9 patients (10%). New onset atrial fibrillation and grade 3 bleeding occurred in one patient each. With extended follow-up and intrapatient dose escalation, the ORR among patients with MCL treated with tirabrutinib was 69%, including 6 patients who achieved CR and 5 patients with partial response (PR).[39] The estimated median PFS was 26 months. Orelabrutinib was investigated in patients with R/R MCL in a phase 1/2 study conducted in China. In the phase 1 portion of this study, 2 cohorts of 20 patients were treated at dose levels of 100 mg twice daily or 150 mg daily, with the 150 mg daily dose chosen for phase 2 study to allow for once daily dosing, given similar response rates between cohorts.[40] One hundred six patients with R/R MCL were enrolled between the phase 1 and 2 study, with 99 evaluable for efficacy. AEs included bleeding in 30 patients (28%, none grade ≥3), diarrhea in 7 patients (7%), and grade 3 or greater hypertension in 4 patients (4%). No cases of grade 3 or greater atrial fibrillation were reported. The ORR was 86%, including 29% CR. Orelabrutinib and tirabrutinib, similar to acalabrutinib and zanubrutinib, seem to have lower observed rates of select toxicities, such as atrial fibrillation, and orelabrutinib seems to have comparable efficacy to currently approved BTKi in a large phase 2 study. With similar efficacy and toxicity profiles to current FDA-approved second-generation BTKi, the role for tirabrutinib or orelabrutinib in health care systems where other second-generation BTKi are already available is uncertain.

Irreversible covalent BTKi are widely used in MCL and other B-cell malignancies, and now early phase studies also show activity with a class of drugs targeting BTK via noncovalent, reversible inhibition. Unlike the irreversible BTKi, this class does not bind BTK at the C481 residue and thus would be expected to be unaffected by BTK binding site mutations.[41] Mutations within the BTK binding site (most commonly C481S) are a well-characterized resistance mechanism to ibrutinib and second-generation BTKi.[42–45] BTK binding site mutations are more frequently observed as a resistance mechanism in CLL[46] but occur in MCL in a minority of BTKi resistant cases.[44,47,48] Noncovalent, reversible BTKi represent a potential option to overcome BTK binding site mutations, and individual drugs within the class offer various potential advantages such as high selectivity for BTK obviating off-target toxicities[49] or broad kinase inhibition beyond BTK potentially resulting in additional therapeutic activity.[50] Preliminary results from phase 1 studies have been presented for 3 drugs within this class, LOXO-305, ARQ-531, and vecabrutinib, and support clinical activity in B-cell malignancies with further study ongoing.[51–53]

OPTIONS FOR PROGRESSION AFTER BRUTON TYROSINE KINASE INHIBITORS

Treatment of patients with progression of MCL while receiving BTKi therapy remains an unmet need, with an aggressive disease course and relatively short survival frequently observed in this setting.[47,48,54,55] TP53 mutations frequently occur in patients with progression on BTKi[47] resulting in chemoresistance and seem to be a factor in the aggressive disease course. Although alternative drugs have activity in this setting, the DOR is generally short and allogeneic hematopoietic cell transplant consolidation (HCT) or other emerging cellular therapy approaches should be considered in transplant eligible patients, particularly those with *TP53* mutations.[56] Lenalidomide as monotherapy or in combination had a 29% ORR in patients with MCL with prior BTKi treatment in a multicenter observational study, with a median DOR of 20 weeks.[57] A small observational series reported promising activity (3 CR, 2 PR among 5 patients) with the combination of lenalidomide, bortezomib, rituximab, and dexamethasone in patients with relapsed MCL post-BTKi,[58] and this regimen is an option in patients without prior lenalidomide treatment. The CIT regimen R-BAC (rituximab, bendamustine, and cytarabine) has been studied both as a frontline and salvage therapy for patients with MCL,[59,60] and promising results were recently reported from a multicenter observational study of 35 patients with R/R MCL treated with R-BAC after prior BTKi treatment.[61] The ORR with R-BAC was 83% (56% CR), the median PFS was 9 months, and median OS was 12 months.[61] The BCL-2 inhibitor venetoclax had single-agent activity in patients with MCL without prior BTKi treatment in a phase 1 study, generating enthusiasm for venetoclax after BTKi treatment[62]; however, limited data are available regarding the efficacy of venetoclax post-BTKi. In a recent report of 20 patients with relapsed MCL and prior BTKi treatment treated with venetoclax on a compassionate use protocol in the United Kingdom, 11 objective responses were seen (55% ORR, 15% CR); however the median PFS was only 3 months.[63] More promising, results were recently presented for the use of CD19-directed chimeric antigen receptor (CAR)-T therapy for the treatment of MCL post-BTKi, which may lead to a change in the future treatment paradigm of R/R MCL. In the ZUMA-2 study presented by Wang and colleagues[64] at the 2019 American Society of Hematology Annual Meeting, 68 patients with R/R MCL with prior BTKi treatment were treated with the CD19-directed CAR-T product KTE-X19. Baseline characteristics included a median age of 65 years, 25% with blastoid morphology, 69% with Ki67 proliferation index greater than or equal to 50%, and a median of 3 prior lines of therapy. AEs occurring during treatment included grade 3 or greater cytokine release syndrome in 10 patients (15%, median onset 2 days), grade 3 or greater neurologic events in 21 patients (31%, median onset 7 days, median duration 12 days), and 2 grade 5 events (organizing pneumonia and Staphylococcal septicemia in one patient each).[64] The ORR was 93%, including 67% CR, and at a median follow-up of 12 months, the median PFS and OS had not been reached. Despite the serious potential toxicities associated with CAR-T therapy, the activity of KTE-X19 in this high-risk population is unprecedented. Longer follow-up is needed to determine if responses remain durable, as seen after CD19 CAR-T therapy in DLBCL,[65,66] providing long-term disease control outside of allogeneic HCT.

COMBINATION THERAPY RELAPSED AND REFRACTORY
Bruton Tyrosine Kinase Inhibitors with CD20 Monoclonal Antibodies

Monoclonal antibodies targeting CD20 have favorable toxicity profiles and improve on the efficacy of conventional cytotoxic chemotherapy. The combination of ibrutinib and rituximab (IR) was studied in patients with R/R MCL in a phase 2 study, which enrolled 50 patients with a median of 3 prior therapies.[67] Toxicities with IR were comparable to those with single-agent ibrutinib and are summarized in **Table 2**. The ORR was 88%, including 44% CR, with a median event-free survival of 16 months and median DOR of 46 months.[68] Although the response rate and proportion of responding patients achieving CR was higher in this study than reported with ibrutinib monotherapy, the proportion of patients with high-risk MIPI score was relatively low (12%), and baseline

Table 2
Summary of published Bruton tyrosine kinase inhibitor combination studies for relapsed/refractory mantle cell lymphoma

BTKi	Combination Drug	Patients Enrolled	ORR	CR Rate	Rate of AEs of Interest
Ibrutinib	Rituximab	50	88%	44%	G3 bleeding 4%, G3 a-fib 12%, G3 hypertension 2%
Ibrutinib	Rituximab and lenalidomide	50	76%	56%	G3 GI toxicity 12%, G3 infection 22%, G3 rash 14%, G5 sepsis 4%
Ibrutinib	Venetoclax	24	71%	71%	G3 diarrhea 13%, G2 bleeding 4%, G3 a-fib 8%
Ibrutinib	Venetoclax	35	83%	41%	G3 neutropenia 29%, G3 a-fib 9%
Ibrutinib	Palbociclib	27	67%	37%	G3 neutropenia 41%, G3 thrombocytopenia 30%, G3 hypertension 15%, G3 rash 7%
Acalabrutinib	Bendamustine and rituximab	18	85%	65%	G4 neutropenia 22%, major bleeding 6%

Abbreviations: a-fib, atrial fibrillation; CR, complete response; G3, grade 3; G4, grade 4; G5, grade 5; Ref, reference.
Data from Refs.[67,77,83,86,89,91]

patient characteristics could contribute to the differences in response rate. Further, response rates seemed lower for patients with a Ki-67 greater than or equal to 50% (50% ORR) in comparison to patients with a lower Ki67% (ORR 100%), suggesting greater benefit in lower risk patients. Whether and to what extent rituximab or other CD20 antibodies improve on the efficacy of ibrutinib or other BTKi in R/R MCL should ideally be evaluated in the context of a randomized phase 3 study, although this combination may be most appealing in the frontline setting for patients without prior rituximab exposure. Preclinical models suggest that ibrutinib diminishes antibody-dependent cell-mediated cytotoxicity (ADCC),[69,70] potentially via off-target inhibition of ITK, and more selective BTKi such as acalabrutinib inhibit cellular cytotoxicity less, providing a rationale for studying second-generation BTKi in combination with CD20 antibodies.[71,72]

Bruton Tyrosine Kinase Inhibitors with Immunomodulatory Drugs

The immunomodulatory drug lenalidomide exerts direct antilymphoma toxicity,[73] enhances immune response including augmenting ADCC,[73] and has activity as single agent or in combination with rituximab in R/R MCL.[74–76] The combination of lenalidomide, rituximab, and ibrutinib was studied in R/R MCL in the multicenter phase 2 PHILEMON study.[77] Baseline characteristics of the 50 enrolled patients included a median age of 69 years, high-risk MIPI score in 23 patients (46%), a median of 2 prior lines of treatment, and mutated TP53 in 11 patients (22%). AEs are summarized in **Table 2** and included 3 treatment-related deaths (6%, 2 cases of sepsis and 1 embolic stroke), grade 3 rash in 14%, and grade 3 gastrointestinal toxicity in 10%. The ORR was 76%, including CR in 56%; however, most of the patients were not previously treated with BTKi, and it is not clear that this combination improves on BTKi monotherapy in an unselected relapsed patient population sufficiently to warrant the increased toxicities, including rash, gastrointestinal toxicity, and thromboembolism risk. However, the response rate among patients with TP53 mutations (79% ORR, 55% CR) was similar to the overall population, suggesting a role for BTKi and immunomodulatory drug combinations in these high-risk patients who fare poorly with CIT or single-agent BTKi.[9,78]

Bruton Tyrosine Kinase Inhibitors with BCL-2 Inhibitor

As previously discussed, venetoclax, a selective BCL-2 inhibitor,[79] demonstrated single-agent activity in a phase 1 study, with an ORR of 75% among 28 patients with MCL and a median PFS of 14 months.[62] Preclinical studies have shown synergy with combined BTK and BCL-2 inhibition,[80–82] prompting clinical studies exploring this combination in MCL. In the phase 2 ABT-199 (Venetoclax) and Ibrutinib in Mantle-Cell Lymphoma study, 23 patients with R/R MCL and 1 TN patient were treated with ibrutinib and venetoclax with ibrutinib administered for 4 weeks as lead-in therapy and venetoclax administered thereafter with ramp-up dosing.[83] Baseline patient characteristics included a median age of 68 years, a median of 2 prior lines of treatment, high-risk MIPI score in 75%, and mutated TP53 in 50% of patients. The ORR by PET was 71%, with 2 of the nonresponding patients not receiving venetoclax due to progression during ibrutinib lead-in. All responding patients achieved CR by PET as best response. Among 19 patients evaluable for MRD in the bone marrow, 16 (84%) achieved MRD negativity on at least one evaluation. Toxicities observed with the combination included diarrhea of any grade in 83% of patients, nausea in 71%, bleeding or bruising in 54%, and mucositis in 21%. Other AEs of interest are summarized in **Table 2**. With extended follow-up, the median PFS was 29 months, and the median OS was 32 months.[84] Among patients with TP53 mutations, the ORR by PET was

50%, and 4 responding patients were without progression more than 24 months after starting treatment. Correlative studies revealed enrichment for deleterious mutations in the SWI-SNF chromatin-remodeling complex leading to BCL-XL upregulation in nonresponding patients,[85] findings that suggest that mutations to these chromatin remodeling genes may be predictive of a lack of response. A second early phase study of ibrutinib and venetoclax has been reported, a phase 1/1b study in R/R MCL using an alternate dosing strategy. Thirty-five patients with MCL were enrolled with a median age of 63 years.[86] The best ORR was 83%, including 41% CR, with no clear relationship between dose level and response observed. AEs included diarrhea in 40% (6% grade $\geq$2), nausea in 37%, arthralgia in 31%, and grade 3 or greater neutropenia in 29%. Three patients discontinued treatment due to toxicity. Collectively, the efficacy of the combination of ibrutinib and venetoclax in these studies is promising, and the randomized phase 3 SYMPATICO study (NCT03112174) is underway comparing single-agent ibrutinib to ibrutinib and venetoclax in R/R MCL. The combination of second-generation BTKi with venetoclax is also under investigation in a phase 2 study of acalabrutinib with venetoclax in R/R MCL (NCT03946878). Although early phase studies have shown that some patients may achieve MRD negativity with the combination of BTKi and venetoclax, at this time it is unclear whether the combination can be given for a limited duration or if indefinite therapy is required.

Bruton Tyrosine Kinase Inhibitors with CDK 4/6 Inhibitor

MCL is characterized by cell-cycle dysregulation due to cyclin D1 upregulation, which in complex with CDK4 and CKD6 causes loss of G1 to S cell-cycle arrest and consequent tumor proliferation. Selective CDK4/CDK6 inhibitors have been studied in R/R MCL with single-agent activity seen in a phase 1b study of palbociclib[87] and cases of prolonged disease control observed with palbociclib monotherapy.[87,88] Targeting CDK4/6 in combination with BTK overcomes BTKi resistance in MCL cell lines, providing rationale for combining both agents at treatment onset to prevent the acquisition of BTKi resistance.[44] In a phase 1 study, 27 patients with R/R MCL were enrolled and treated with ibrutinib and palbociclib, with the MTD determined to be ibrutinib, 560 mg, and palbociclib, 100 mg, (days 1–21, 28-day cycle).[89] Toxicities of interest are summarized in **Table 2**. The ORR was 67%, including 37% CR, with similar response rates in patients with baseline Ki67 index greater than or equal to 30% compared with the overall patient population, a finding of note, given the mechanism of action of palbociclib and negative association between high Ki67 index and response to BTKi treatment in other studies.[67] AFT-32, a phase 2 study evaluating the combination of ibrutinib and palbociclib in patients with R/R MCL (NCT03478514) is currently underway and will further characterize the safety and efficacy of this combination in relapsed MCL.

Bruton Tyrosine Kinase Inhibitors with Chemoimmunotherapy

Bendamustine and rituximab (BR) has been studied in combination with either ibrutinib or acalabrutinib in phase 1b and 2 studies that included patients with R/R MCL. In a phase 1/1b study of BR and ibrutinib, an MTD of 560 mg ibrutinib daily in combination with BR given at standard dosing was determined, with BR given for 6 cycles and ibrutinib continued until progression or intolerance.[90] Observed toxicities were primarily hematologic, including grade 4 neutropenia in 21% and grade 3 or greater thrombocytopenia in 19%, as well as rash in 25% of patients. In terms of efficacy, among 17 patients with MCL (5 TN), the ORR was 94%, including 76% CR, with a median PFS not reached. In the LY-106 study, 18 patients with R/R and 18 patients with TN MCL were treated with acalabrutinib in combination with BR given for 6 cycles with acalabrutinib continued thereafter as well as rituximab maintenance for TN patients.[91] Toxicities included grade 4 neutropenia in 22% of patients and one major bleeding event (alveolar hemorrhage) leading to treatment discontinuation. The ORR in the relapsed cohort was 85%, including 65% CR, with a median PFS of 17 months, and the ORR in the TN cohort was 94% (72% CR) with the median PFS not reached. The combination of BTKi with CIT is of interest in the frontline setting, as discussed in the following section.

Frontline Therapy

A wide range of studies are currently investigating the use of BTKi in combination as frontline treatment of MCL, with preliminary evidence emerging from multiple studies. Current ongoing studies are highlighted, and preliminary results are summarized in **3** and discussed in the following section.

Bruton Tyrosine Kinase Inhibitors with CD20 Antibody

The combination of rituximab and ibrutinib has been studied as frontline treatment in 3 studies, with preliminary results showing promising activity. In a phase 2 study presented by Gine and colleagues[92] conducted by the Spanish GELTAMO, previously untreated patients with MCL considered to be clinically indolent as defined by Ki67 index less than 30%, largest lymph node diameter less than 3 cm, and at least 3 months of observation after diagnosis were treated with daily ibrutinib for at least 2 years in combination with 8 total doses of rituximab. Of 33 evaluable patients, the median age was 66 years and median time from diagnosis to treatment was 8 months. The ORR was 82%, including 75% CR, and among 23 patients with CR evaluable for MRD by peripheral blood after 12 cycles, 87% achieved MRD negativity. The estimated 15-month PFS was an impressive 96%, although one limitation is the lack of a comparator population in patients with indolent disease, some of whom may be expected to remain progression free without treatment. Two single-center studies, both from MD Anderson, have been reported studying the combination of IR in the frontline setting. Jain and colleagues[93] presented results from a phase 2 study enrolling patients aged 65 years or older with TN MCL to receive treatment with IR until disease progression or intolerance. Baseline characteristics included a Ki67 index less than 30% in 76%, high-risk MIPI score in 16%, and a median age of 71 years; patients with blastoid morphology or Ki67 greater than or equal to 50% were excluded. Among 49 evaluable patients, the ORR was 98%, with CR rate of 68% (CR in 84% of PET evaluable patients), and 21 of 26 patients (81%) evaluable for MRD were MRD negative. After a median follow-up of 28 months, only 4 patients had progressed. In a separate study presented by Wang and colleagues,[94] patients aged 65 years or younger with untreated MCL were treated with IR for up to 12 cycles until achieving CR followed by up to 4 cycles of R-Hyper CVAD alternating with R-methotrexate and cytarabine. Of 131 enrolled patients, including 49% with a Ki67 index greater than or equal to 30%, the ORR to IR lead-in treatment was 100% including 88% CR. Although the durability of response is difficult to interpret as patients went on to receive R-Hyper CVAD consolidation (3-year PFS was 85%), this study raises the intriguing possibility of a chemotherapy-free approach among young and fit patients, which would thereby avoid the toxicities associated with more intensive frontline treatments.

Bruton Tyrosine Kinase Inhibitors with Immunomodulatory Drug

Given the relevance of immune response and ADCC to the efficacy of lenalidomide and rituximab, results with this approach may be best in the frontline setting with an intact host immune system. In a phase 2 study, the combination of lenalidomide

Table 3
Frontline trials with Bruton tyrosine kinase inhibitor combination treatment

Study Name	Investigational Treatment	Phase	Control Treatment	Estimated Enrollment	ClinicalTrials.gov Identifier
OASIS	Ibrutinib, venetoclax, obinutuzumab	1/2	N/A	15	NCT02558816
Phase 2 Study of acalabrutinib-lenalidomide-rituximab	Acalabrutinib, lenalidomide, rituximab	2	N/A	24	NCT03863184
ACE-LY-106	Acalabrutinib, venetoclax, rituximab	1b	N/A	32	NCT02717624
EA4181	Acalabrutinib and BR followed by high-dose cyatarabine (Arm 2) or acalabrutinib and BR (Arm 3)	2	BR followed by high dose cytarabine (Arm 1)	369	NCT04115631
SHINE	Ibrutinib and BR followed by ibrutinib maintenance	3	BR	523	NCT01776840
ACE-LY-308	Acalabrutinib and BR	3	BR	546	NCT02972840
TRIANGLE	Ibrutinib and R-CHOP alternating with R-DHAP with (Arm A + I) or without (Arm I) AHCT consolidation followed by ibrutinib maintenance	3	R-CHOP alternating with R-DHAP with AHCT consolidation (Arm A)	870	NCT02858258

Abbreviations: BR, bendamustine and rituximab; R-CHOP, rituximab, cyclophosphamide, vincristine, doxorubicin, and prednisone; R-DHAP, rituximab, dexamethasone, cytarabine, and cisplatin.

and rituximab showed promising activity as frontline treatment, with an ORR of 92%, including 64% CR, a 2-year PFS of 85%, and with extended follow-up and estimated 5-year PFS of 64%.[95,96] As previously reviewed, the combination of ibrutinib with lenalidomide and rituximab has been studied in R/R MCL and was active regardless of *TP53* mutational status, making this combination of interest as frontline treatment in patients with mutated *TP53*. A multicenter phase 2 study is currently ongoing studying acalabrutinib with lenalidomide and rituximab as frontline treatment of MCL (NCT03863184), with preliminary results awaited.

Bruton Tyrosine Kinase Inhibitors with BCL-2 Inhibitor

Phase 1/2 trials of the combination of venetoclax and ibrutinib have shown promising depth of response, generating interest in using this combination frontline. Preliminary results from the phase 1/1b OASIS trial have been reported, in which TN patients with MCL were treated with obinutuzumab, venetoclax, and ibrutinib. Of 15 patients evaluable for response at data cutoff, the ORR was 100% after cycle 2, including CR or unconfirmed CR in 7 of 15 patients. Eight patients were assessed for MRD status after cycle 3 and all were MRD negative. Full results from the OASIS study and phase 2 frontline studies of rituximab, ibrutinib, and venetoclax (NCT03710772) and rituximab, acalabrutinib, and venetoclax (NCT02717624) will guide further study of this approach in the frontline setting.

Bruton Tyrosine Kinase Inhibitors with Chemoimmunotherapy

As previously reviewed, the combination of BTKi with BR has been studied in phase 1b/2 studies as both frontline and salvage MCL treatment and 2 currently ongoing phase 3 studies evaluating this combination in TN patients aged 65 years and older. The SHINE study (NCT01776840) is a randomized, placebo-controlled, double-blinded phase 3 study comparing BR with rituximab maintenance with BR plus ibrutinib followed by IR maintenance in patients with untreated MCL aged 65 years and older. The SHINE study has completed accrual, and follow-up for the primary outcome of PFS is currently ongoing. The randomized, placebo-controlled, double-blinded phase 3 ACE-LY-308 study is also ongoing, randomizing patients aged 65 years or older with TN MCL to treatment with either BR or BR plus acalabrutinib (NCT02972840) without maintenance therapy. Frontline trials enrolling younger patients are also ongoing, studying BTKi in combination with CIT. In the US Intergroup EA4181 study (NCT04115631), patients aged 70 years or older are randomized to 1 of 3 arms: BR and acalabrutinib for 6 cycles, BR for 3 cycles followed by high-dose cytarabine for 3 cycles, or acalabrutinib and BR for 3 cycles followed by high-dose cytarabine and acalabrutinib for 3 cycles. Concurrently, the European MCL Network Triangle study (NCT02858258) is a randomized 3-arm phase 3 study, with patients randomized to either the control arm of R-CHOP alternating with R-DHAP followed by AHCT or 1 of 2 arms receiving ibrutinib and R-CHOP alternating with R-DHAP followed by ibrutinib maintenance either with (Arm A + I) or without (Arm I) AHCT consolidation. Therefore, this study will not only evaluate whether BTKi can improve on a current intensive treatment approach in younger patients but also determine whether AHCT may be omitted with the addition of BTKi.

SUMMARY

BTKi are now the preferred therapy in most of the patients with relapsed MCL, with remarkable single-agent activity and a generally manageable side-effect profile. Three BTKi are now approved in the United States—acalabrutinib, ibrutinib, and zanubrutinib—each of which have high response rates, with potential differences in side-effect profile between the first-generation ibrutinib and the more selective second-generation acalabrutinib or zanubrutinib. BTKi-based combination therapy has been shown to be feasible in MCL and may further improve depth and duration of response, but results from phase 3 studies are needed to further define the role of combination therapy including the potential for limited duration therapy, given the cost and toxicities of indefinite treatment. Early evidence for BTKi combinations in TN patients is promising, and studies are currently underway evaluating whether incorporating BTKi into frontline MCL treatment may allow for AHCT consolidation to be eliminated in younger patients, improve length of response with CIT, or allow for a chemotherapy-free approach to treatment.

DISCLOSURE

D.A. Bond has nothing to disclose. K.J. Maddocks has received advisory honoraria from Astra-Zeneca, Pharmacyclics, and Celgene.

REFERENCES

1. Epperla N, Hamadani M, Fenske TS, et al. Incidence and survival trends in mantle cell lymphoma. Br J Haematol 2018;181(5):703–6.
2. Advani RH, Buggy JJ, Sharman JP, et al. Bruton tyrosine kinase inhibitor ibrutinib (PCI-32765) has significant activity in patients with relapsed/refractory B-cell malignancies. J Clin Oncol 2013;31(1):88–94.
3. Dubovsky JA, Beckwith KA, Natarajan G, et al. Ibrutinib is an irreversible molecular inhibitor of ITK driving a Th1-selective pressure in T lymphocytes. Blood 2013;122(15):2539–49.
4. Honigberg LA, Smith AM, Sirisawad M, et al. The Bruton tyrosine kinase inhibitor PCI-32765 blocks B-cell activation and is efficacious in models of autoimmune disease and B-cell malignancy. Proc Natl Acad Sci U S A 2010;107(29): 13075–80.
5. Wang ML, Rule S, Martin P, et al. Targeting BTK with ibrutinib in relapsed or refractory mantle-cell lymphoma. N Engl J Med 2013;369(6):507–16.
6. Wang ML, Blum KA, Martin P, et al. Long-term follow-up of MCL patients treated with single-agent ibrutinib: updated safety and efficacy results. Blood 2015; 126(6):739–45.
7. Dreyling M, Jurczak W, Jerkeman M, et al. Ibrutinib versus temsirolimus in patients with relapsed or refractory mantle-cell lymphoma: an international, randomised, open-label, phase 3 study. Lancet 2016;387(10020):770–8.
8. Rule S, Dreyling M, Goy A, et al. Outcomes in 370 patients with mantle cell lymphoma treated with ibrutinib: a pooled analysis from three open-label studies. Br J Haematol 2017;179(3):430–8.
9. Rule S, Dreyling M, Goy A, et al. Ibrutinib for the treatment of relapsed/refractory mantle cell lymphoma: extended 3.5-year follow up from a pooled analysis. Haematologica 2019;104(5):e211–4.
10. Quek LS, Bolen J, Watson SP. A role for Bruton's tyrosine kinase (Btk) in platelet activation by collagen. Curr Biol 1998;8(20):1137–40.
11. Atkinson BT, Ellmeier W, Watson SP. Tec regulates platelet activation by GPVI in the absence of Btk. Blood 2003;102(10):3592–9.
12. Liu J, Fitzgerald ME, Berndt MC, et al. Bruton tyrosine kinase is essential for botrocetin/VWF-induced signaling and GPIb-dependent thrombus formation in vivo. Blood 2006;108(8):2596–603.

13. Byrd JC, O'Brien S, James DF. Ibrutinib in relapsed chronic lymphocytic leukemia. N Engl J Med 2013;369(13):1278–9.
14. Levade M, David E, Garcia C, et al. Ibrutinib treatment affects collagen and von Willebrand factor-dependent platelet functions. Blood 2014;124(26):3991–5.
15. Bye AP, Unsworth AJ, Desborough MJ, et al. Severe platelet dysfunction in NHL patients receiving ibrutinib is absent in patients receiving acalabrutinib. Blood Adv 2017;1(26):2610–23.
16. Dobie G, Kuriri FA, Omar MMA, et al. Ibrutinib, but not zanubrutinib, induces platelet receptor shedding of GPIb-IX-V complex and integrin alphaIIbbeta3 in mice and humans. Blood Adv 2019;3(24):4298–311.
17. Caron F, Leong DP, Hillis C, et al. Current understanding of bleeding with ibrutinib use: a systematic review and meta-analysis. Blood Adv 2017;1(12):772–8.
18. Leong DP, Caron F, Hillis C, et al. The risk of atrial fibrillation with ibrutinib use: a systematic review and meta-analysis. Blood 2016;128(1):138–40.
19. Brown JR, Moslehi J, O'Brien S, et al. Characterization of atrial fibrillation adverse events reported in ibrutinib randomized controlled registration trials. Haematologica 2017;102(10):1796–805.
20. Lampson BL, Yu L, Glynn RJ, et al. Ventricular arrhythmias and sudden death in patients taking ibrutinib. Blood 2017;129(18):2581–4.
21. Cheng C, Woronow D, Nayernama A, et al. Ibrutinib-associated ventricular arrhythmia in the FDA adverse event reporting system. Leuk Lymphoma 2018; 59(12):3016–7.
22. Guha A, Derbala MH, Zhao Q, et al. Ventricular arrhythmias following ibrutinib initiation for lymphoid malignancies. J Am Coll Cardiol 2018;72(6):697–8.
23. Tomcsanyi J, Nenyei Z, Matrai Z, et al. Ibrutinib, an approved tyrosine kinase inhibitor as a potential cause of recurrent polymorphic ventricular tachycardia. JACC Clin Electrophysiol 2016;2(7):847–9.
24. Wallace N, Wong E, Cooper D, et al. A case of new-onset cardiomyopathy and ventricular tachycardia in a patient receiving ibrutinib for relapsed mantle cell lymphoma. Clin Case Rep 2016;4(12):1120–1.
25. Beyer A, Ganti B, Majkrzak A, et al. A perfect storm: tyrosine kinase inhibitor-associated polymorphic ventricular tachycardia. J Emerg Med 2017;52(4): e123–7.
26. McMullen JR, Boey EJ, Ooi JY, et al. Ibrutinib increases the risk of atrial fibrillation, potentially through inhibition of cardiac PI3K-Akt signaling. Blood 2014;124(25): 3829–30.
27. Dickerson T, Wiczer T, Waller A, et al. Hypertension and incident cardiovascular events following ibrutinib initiation. Blood 2019;134(22):1919–28.
28. Caldeira D, Alves D, Costa J, et al. Ibrutinib increases the risk of hypertension and atrial fibrillation: systematic review and meta-analysis. PLoS One 2019; 14(2):e0211228.
29. Byrd JC, Harrington B, O'Brien S, et al. Acalabrutinib (ACP-196) in relapsed chronic lymphocytic leukemia. N Engl J Med 2016;374(4):323–32.
30. Herman SEM, Montraveta A, Niemann CU, et al. The bruton tyrosine kinase (BTK) inhibitor acalabrutinib demonstrates potent on-target effects and efficacy in two mouse models of chronic lymphocytic leukemia. Clin Cancer Res 2017;23(11): 2831–41.
31. Wang M, Rule S, Zinzani PL, et al. Acalabrutinib in relapsed or refractory mantle cell lymphoma (ACE-LY-004): a single-arm, multicentre, phase 2 trial. Lancet 2018;391(10121):659–67.

32. Wang M, Rule S, Zinzani PL, et al. Durable response with single-agent acalabrutinib in patients with relapsed or refractory mantle cell lymphoma. Leukemia 2019;33(11):2762–6.
33. Byrd JC, Owen R, O'Brien S. Pooled analysis of safety data from clinical trials evaluating acalabrutinib monotherapy in hematologic malignancies. Blood 2017;130:4326.
34. Guo Y, Liu Y, Hu N, et al. Discovery of zanubrutinib (BGB-3111), a novel, potent, and selective covalent inhibitor of bruton's tyrosine kinase. J Med Chem 2019; 62(17):7923–40.
35. Tam CS, Trotman J, Opat S, et al. Phase 1 study of the selective BTK inhibitor zanubrutinib in B-cell malignancies and safety and efficacy evaluation in CLL. Blood 2019;134(11):851–9.
36. Tam CS, Wang M, Simpson D. Updated safety and activity of the investigational bruton tyrosine kinase inhibitor zanubrutinib (BGB-3111) in patients with mantle cell lymphoma. Blood 2018;132(Suppl 1):1592 [Abstract].
37. Song Y, Zhou K, Zou D. Safety and activity of the investigational bruton tyrosine kinase inhibitor zanubrutinib (BGB-3111) in patients with mantle cell lymphoma from a phase 2 trial. Blood 2018;132(Suppl 1):148 [Abstract].
38. Walter HS, Rule SA, Dyer MJ, et al. A phase 1 clinical trial of the selective BTK inhibitor ONO/GS-4059 in relapsed and refractory mature B-cell malignancies. Blood 2016;127(4):411–9.
39. Rule SA, Cartron G, Fegan C, et al. Long-term follow-up of patients with mantle cell lymphoma (MCL) treated with the selective Bruton's tyrosine kinase inhibitor tirabrutinib (GS/ONO-4059). Leukemia 2020;34(5):1458–61.
40. Song Y, Song Y, Liu L, et al. Safety and efficacy of orelabrutinib monotherapy in chinese patients with relapsed or refractory mantle cell lymphoma: a multicenter, open-label, phase II study. Blood 2019;134:755.
41. Johnson AR, Kohli PB, Katewa A, et al. Battling Btk mutants with noncovalent inhibitors that overcome Cys481 and Thr474 mutations. ACS Chem Biol 2016; 11(10):2897–907.
42. Furman RR, Cheng S, Lu P, et al. Ibrutinib resistance in chronic lymphocytic leukemia. N Engl J Med 2014;370(24):2352–4.
43. Woyach JA, Furman RR, Liu TM, et al. Resistance mechanisms for the Bruton's tyrosine kinase inhibitor ibrutinib. N Engl J Med 2014;370(24):2286–94.
44. Chiron D, Di Liberto M, Martin P, et al. Cell-cycle reprogramming for PI3K inhibition overrides a relapse-specific C481S BTK mutation revealed by longitudinal functional genomics in mantle cell lymphoma. Cancer Discov 2014;4(9):1022–35.
45. Woyach J, Huang Y, Rogers K, et al. Resistance to acalabrutinib in CLL is mediated primarily by BTK mutations. Blood 2019;134:504.
46. Woyach JA, Ruppert AS, Guinn D, et al. BTK(C481S)-mediated resistance to ibrutinib in chronic lymphocytic leukemia. J Clin Oncol 2017;35(13):1437–43.
47. Jain P, Kanagal-Shamanna R, Zhang S, et al. Long-term outcomes and mutation profiling of patients with mantle cell lymphoma (MCL) who discontinued ibrutinib. Br J Haematol 2018;183(4):578–87.
48. Martin P, Maddocks K, Leonard JP, et al. Postibrutinib outcomes in patients with mantle cell lymphoma. Blood 2016;127(12):1559–63.
49. Reiff SD, Muhowski EM, Guinn D, et al. Noncovalent inhibition of C481S Bruton tyrosine kinase by GDC-0853: a new treatment strategy for ibrutinib-resistant CLL. Blood 2018;132(10):1039–49.
50. Reiff SD, Mantel R, Smith LL, et al. The BTK inhibitor ARQ 531 targets ibrutinib-resistant CLL and richter transformation. Cancer Discov 2018;8(10):1300–15.

51. Allan JN, Patel K, Mato A, et al. Ongoing results of a phase 1B/2 dose-escalation and cohort-expansion study of the selective, noncovalent, reversible bruton's tyrosine kinase inhibitor, vecabrutinib, in B-cell malignancies. Blood 2019;134: 3041.

52. Mato A, Flinn I, Pagel JM, et al. Results from a first-in-human, proof-of-concept phase 1 trial in pretreated B-cell malignancies for Loxo-305, a next-generation, highly selective, non-covalent BTK inhibitor. Blood 2019;134:501.

53. Woyach J, Stephens DM, Flinn I, et al. Final results of phase 1, dose escalation study evaluating ARQ 531 in patients with relapsed or refractory B-cell lymphoid malignancies. Blood 2019;134:4298.

54. Epperla N, Hamadani M, Cashen AF, et al. Predictive factors and outcomes for ibrutinib therapy in relapsed/refractory mantle cell lymphoma-a "real world" study. Hematol Oncol 2017;35(4):528–35.

55. Cheah CY, Chihara D, Romaguera JE, et al. Patients with mantle cell lymphoma failing ibrutinib are unlikely to respond to salvage chemotherapy and have poor outcomes. Ann Oncol 2015;26(6):1175–9.

56. Lin RJ, Ho C, Hilden PD, et al. Allogeneic haematopoietic cell transplantation impacts on outcomes of mantle cell lymphoma with TP53 alterations. Br J Haematol 2019;184(6):1006–10.

57. Wang M, Schuster SJ, Phillips T, et al. Observational study of lenalidomide in patients with mantle cell lymphoma who relapsed/progressed after or were refractory/intolerant to ibrutinib (MCL-004). J Hematol Oncol 2017;10(1):171.

58. Srour SA, Lee HJ, Nomie K, et al. Novel chemotherapy-free combination regimen for ibrutinib-resistant mantle cell lymphoma. Br J Haematol 2018;181(4):561–4.

59. Visco C, Finotto S, Zambello R, et al. Combination of rituximab, bendamustine, and cytarabine for patients with mantle-cell non-Hodgkin lymphoma ineligible for intensive regimens or autologous transplantation. J Clin Oncol 2013;31(11): 1442–9.

60. Tisi MC, Paolini R, Piazza F, et al. Rituximab, bendamustine and cytarabine (R-BAC) in patients with relapsed-refractory aggressive B-cell lymphoma. Am J Hematol 2018;93(12):E386–9.

61. McCulloch R, Visco C, Frewin R, et al. R-BAC maintains high response rate in mantle cell lymphoma following relapse on BTK inhibitor therapy. Blood 2019; 134:3989.

62. Davids MS, Roberts AW, Seymour JF, et al. Phase I first-in-human study of venetoclax in patients with relapsed or refractory non-Hodgkin lymphoma. J Clin Oncol 2017;35(8):826–33.

63. Eyre TA, Walter HS, Iyengar S, et al. Efficacy of venetoclax monotherapy in patients with relapsed, refractory mantle cell lymphoma after Bruton tyrosine kinase inhibitor therapy. Haematologica 2019;104(2):e68–71.

64. Wang M, Munoz J, Goy A, et al. KTE-X19, an anti-CD19 chimeric antigen receptor T cell therapy, in patients with relapsed/refractory mantle cell lymphoma: results of the phase 2 ZUMA-2 study. Blood 2019;134:754.

65. Neelapu SS, Locke FL, Bartlett NL, et al. Axicabtagene ciloleucel CAR T-cell therapy in refractory large B-cell lymphoma. N Engl J Med 2017;377(26):2531–44.

66. Schuster SJ, Bishop MR, Tam CS, et al. Tisagenlecleucel in adult relapsed or refractory diffuse large B-cell lymphoma. N Engl J Med 2019;380(1):45–56.

67. Wang ML, Lee H, Chuang H, et al. Ibrutinib in combination with rituximab in relapsed or refractory mantle cell lymphoma: a single-centre, open-label, phase 2 trial. Lancet Oncol 2016;17(1):48–56.

68. Jain P, Romaguera J, Srour SA, et al. Four-year follow-up of a single arm, phase II clinical trial of ibrutinib with rituximab (IR) in patients with relapsed/refractory mantle cell lymphoma (MCL). Br J Haematol 2018;182(3):404–11.

69. Kohrt HE, Sagiv-Barfi I, Rafiq S, et al. Ibrutinib antagonizes rituximab-dependent NK cell-mediated cytotoxicity. Blood 2014;123(12):1957–60.

70. Da Roit F, Engelberts PJ, Taylor RP, et al. Ibrutinib interferes with the cell-mediated anti-tumor activities of therapeutic CD20 antibodies: implications for combination therapy. Haematologica 2015;100(1):77–86.

71. VanDerMeid KR, Elliott MR, Baran AM, et al. Cellular cytotoxicity of next-generation CD20 monoclonal antibodies. Cancer Immunol Res 2018;6(10): 1150–60.

72. Golay J, Ubiali G, Introna M. The specific Bruton tyrosine kinase inhibitor acalabrutinib (ACP-196) shows favorable in vitro activity against chronic lymphocytic leukemia B cells with CD20 antibodies. Haematologica 2017;102(10):e400–3.

73. Gribben JG, Fowler N, Morschhauser F. Mechanisms of action of lenalidomide in B-cell Non-Hodgkin lymphoma. J Clin Oncol 2015;33(25):2803–11.

74. Goy A, Sinha R, Williams ME, et al. Single-agent lenalidomide in patients with mantle-cell lymphoma who relapsed or progressed after or were refractory to bortezomib: phase II MCL-001 (EMERGE) study. J Clin Oncol 2013;31(29):3688–95.

75. Trneny M, Lamy T, Walewski J, et al. Lenalidomide versus investigator's choice in relapsed or refractory mantle cell lymphoma (MCL-002; SPRINT): a phase 2, randomised, multicentre trial. Lancet Oncol 2016;17(3):319–31.

76. Wang M, Fayad L, Wagner-Bartak N, et al. Lenalidomide in combination with rituximab for patients with relapsed or refractory mantle-cell lymphoma: a phase 1/2 clinical trial. Lancet Oncol 2012;13(7):716–23.

77. Jerkeman M, Eskelund CW, Hutchings M, et al. Ibrutinib, lenalidomide, and rituximab in relapsed or refractory mantle cell lymphoma (PHILEMON): a multicentre, open-label, single-arm, phase 2 trial. Lancet Haematol 2018;5(3):e109–16.

78. Eskelund CW, Dahl C, Hansen JW, et al. TP53 mutations identify younger mantle cell lymphoma patients who do not benefit from intensive chemoimmunotherapy. Blood 2017;130(17):1903–10.

79. Souers AJ, Leverson JD, Boghaert ER, et al. ABT-199, a potent and selective BCL-2 inhibitor, achieves antitumor activity while sparing platelets. Nat Med 2013;19(2):202–8.

80. Axelrod M, Gordon VL, Conaway M, et al. Combinatorial drug screening identifies compensatory pathway interactions and adaptive resistance mechanisms. Oncotarget 2013;4(4):622–35.

81. Zhao X, Bodo J, Sun D, et al. Combination of ibrutinib with ABT-199: synergistic effects on proliferation inhibition and apoptosis in mantle cell lymphoma cells through perturbation of BTK, AKT and BCL2 pathways. Br J Haematol 2015; 168(5):765–8.

82. Li Y, Bouchlaka MN, Wolff J, et al. FBXO10 deficiency and BTK activation upregulate BCL2 expression in mantle cell lymphoma. Oncogene 2016;35(48): 6223–34.

83. Tam CS, Anderson MA, Pott C, et al. Ibrutinib plus venetoclax for the treatment of mantle-cell lymphoma. N Engl J Med 2018;378(13):1211–23.

84. Handunnetti S, Anderson MA, Burbury K, et al. Three year update of the phase II ABT-199 (venetoclax) and ibrutinib in mantle cell lymphoma (AIM) study. Blood 2019;134:756.

85. Agarwal R, Chan YC, Tam CS, et al. Dynamic molecular monitoring reveals that SWI-SNF mutations mediate resistance to ibrutinib plus venetoclax in mantle cell lymphoma. Nat Med 2019;25(1):119–29.
86. Portell C, Wages NA, Kahl B, et al. Multi-institution phase I/Ib continual re-assessment study to identify the optimal dose of ibrutinib and venetoclax in relapsed or refractory mantle cell lymphoma. Blood 2019;134:1535.
87. Leonard JP, LaCasce AS, Smith MR, et al. Selective CDK4/6 inhibition with tumor responses by PD0332991 in patients with mantle cell lymphoma. Blood 2012; 119(20):4597–607.
88. Martin P, Ruan J, Furman R, et al. A phase I trial of palbociclib plus bortezomib in previously treated mantle cell lymphoma. Leuk Lymphoma 2019;60(12):2917–21.
89. Martin P, Bartlett NL, Blum KA, et al. A phase 1 trial of ibrutinib plus palbociclib in previously treated mantle cell lymphoma. Blood 2019;133(11):1201–4.
90. Maddocks K, Christian B, Jaglowski S, et al. A phase 1/1b study of rituximab, bendamustine, and ibrutinib in patients with untreated and relapsed/refractory non-Hodgkin lymphoma. Blood 2015;125(2):242–8.
91. Phillips TJ, Smith SD, Jurczak W. Safety and efficacy of acalabrutinib plus bend-amustine and rituximab (BR) in patients with treatment-naive (TN) or relapsed/re-fractory (R/R) mantle cell lymphoma (MCL). Blood 2018;132(Suppl 1):4144.
92. Gine E, De La Cruz M, Grande C, et al. Efficacy and safety of ibrutinib in combi-nation with rituximab as frontline treatment for indolent clinical forms of mantle cell lymphoma: preliminary results of geltamo IMCL-2015 phase II trial. Blood 2019; 134:752.
93. Jain P, Lee HJ, Steiner RE, et al. Frontline treatment with ibrutinib with rituximab (IR) combination is highly effective in elderly patients with mantle cell lymphoma - results from a phase II trial. Blood 2019;134:3988.
94. Wang M, Jain P, Lee H, et al. Frontline treatment with ibrutinib plus rituximab fol-lowed by short course R-hypercvad/MTX is extremely potent and safe in patients with mantle cell lymphoma - results of phase-II window-1 clinical trial. Blood 2019; 134:3987.
95. Ruan J, Martin P, Shah B, et al. Lenalidomide plus rituximab as initial treatment for mantle-cell lymphoma. N Engl J Med 2015;373(19):1835–44.
96. Ruan J, Martin P, Christos P, et al. Five-year follow-up of lenalidomide plus ritux-imab as initial treatment of mantle cell lymphoma. Blood 2018;132(19):2016–25.

What Causes Bruton Tyrosine Kinase Inhibitor Resistance in Mantle Cell Lymphoma and How Should We Treat Such Patients?

Rory McCulloch, MD[a], Toby A. Eyre, MD[b], Simon Rule, MD[c],*

KEYWORDS

- Mantle cell lymphoma • Resistance mechanisms • Bruton tyrosine kinase inhibitor
- Chimeric antigen receptor T-cell therapy

KEY POINTS

- The early dismal outcomes observed following BTKi failure were in heavily pre-treated patients and are improving the earlier the drugs are used.
- There are multiple mechanisms of BTK inhibitor resistance including mutations in, the alternative NF-KB pathway, B cell receptor signalling and cell cycle signalling.
- There is currently no clear optimal therapeutic approach post BTKi failure, although bendamustine based therapy looks the most active of the conventional therapies.
- The use of CAR-T cell therapy post BTKi looks highly promising albeit with limited data to date.

INTRODUCTION

The past decade has seen several significant therapeutic advances in mantle cell lymphoma (MCL), but none has had greater impact on patient outcomes than the emergence of Bruton tyrosine kinase inhibitors (BTKi). The oral medications ibrutinib and acalabrutinib are established in clinical practice for relapsed MCL with clinical studies demonstrating impressive response rates in heavily pretreated patients and notable for favorable side-effect profiles.[1,2] However, approximately a third of patients do not respond to treatment and durable responses are mainly limited to a minority of

a Department of Haematology, Peninsula Medical School, University of Plymouth, Plymouth, UK; b Department of Haematology, Oxford University Hospitals, Oxford, UK; c Department of Haematology, Peninsula Medical School, University of Plymouth, John Bull Building, Plymouth PL6 8BU, UK
* Corresponding author.
E-mail address: simon.rule@plymouth.ac.uk

Hematol Oncol Clin N Am 34 (2020) 923–939
https://doi.org/10.1016/j.hoc.2020.06.008
0889-8588/20/Crown Copyright © 2020 Published by Elsevier Inc. All rights reserved.

patients achieving complete response (CR). At progression, disease is often aggressive and resistant to further therapy and patient outcomes are invariably poor.[3] Effective management of patients with BTKi resistance is currently the greatest unmet clinical need in MCL.

In this review, we explore insights into the pathophysiology of BTKi resistance in MCL, and consider potential therapeutic targets. We review the possible clinical benefits of giving BTKis alongside other novel therapies, and evaluate clinical data for treatment strategies post-BTKi progression that may help guide current practice. We conclude by considering future approaches, including the potential role of chimeric antigen receptor T-cell (CAR-T) therapy.

BRUTON TYROSINE KINASE INHIBITOR OUTCOMES IN MANTLE CELL LYMPHOMA

The landmark phase II study of ibrutinib monotherapy at a dose of 560 mg once daily provided unprecedented responses in 111 heavily pretreated patients with MCL (median of 3 prior lines of therapy).[1] The overall response rate (ORR) was 68% with CR, defined by computed tomography (CT) imaging, 21%. The median progression-free survival (PFS) was 13.9 months and 18-month overall survival (OS) 58%. A subsequent randomized phase III trial compared ibrutinib monotherapy with temsirolimus (n = 280) with cross-over of therapy permitted at progression.[4] A significant PFS advantage was seen in the ibrutinib arm (median PFS 14.6 months vs 6.2 months; hazard ratio 0.43; $P<.0001$). Tolerance was also superior. Outcomes of these studies, and others assessing BTKi combination therapies are summarized in **Tables 1** and **2**.

Acalabrutinib is a second-generation BTKi with less "off-target" kinase inhibition, and possibly an improved safety profile. In a phase II trial of 124 patients with relapsed MCL (median of 2 prior lines therapy) the documented ORR, as assessed by PET/CT, was 81% (CR 40%).[2] The use of PET/CT may account for the higher CR rates seen with acalabrutinib as compared with Ibrutinib where conventional CT assessments were used. The 12-month estimated PFS was 67% (95% confidence interval [CI] 58%–75%) and OS was 87% (95% CI 79%–92%). The median PFS across all patients was 20 months.

The Food and Drug Administration (FDA) has granted an accelerated approval to the next-generation BTKi zanubrutinib for previously treated MCL based on 2 studies presented at the 15th International Conference on Malignant Lymphoma.[5,6] A summary of key clinical findings is provided in the FDA prescribing information.[7] In BGB-3111 to 206, a phase 2 study undertaken at sites across China, 86 patients with previously treated MCL received zanubrutinib 160 mg twice daily. The ORR was 84%, with CR, defined by PET/CT, 59%. The median duration of response (DOR) was 19.5 months (95% CI 16.6–not estimable [NE]). In BGB-3111-AU-003, an international multicenter phase I/2 study that included 32 patients with previously treated MCL, patients received zanubrutinib 160 mg twice daily or 320 mg once daily.[7] The ORR was 84% and CR, which did not require PET/CT, was 22%. The median DOR was 18.5 months (95% CI 12.6–NE).

Post hoc analyses have shown that the traditional adverse-risk markers in MCL appear predictive for BTKi responses, with blastoid histology, Ki-67 levels $\geq$50% by immunohistochemistry (IHC) and *TP53* mutations all risk factors for BTKi failure.[8–10] *TP53* mutation status was known in 39% (144/370) of patients in the pooled trial analysis.[11] Of these patients 13.9% (20/144) had *TP53* mutated MCL and this was associated with a significantly inferior ORR (mutated: 55.0% vs 70.2% in unmutated), median PFS (mutated: 4.0 [95% CI 2.1–8.3] vs 12.0 [95% CI 7.1–15.6] months in unmutated), and median OS (mutated: 10.3 [95% CI 2.5–12.6] vs 33.6 months [95% CI 18.3–NR (not reached)] in unmutated).

Table 1
Selective prospective trials assessing response to BTKi monotherapy and BTKi combination therapies in relapsed MCL

Treatment	Study	Patients, n	Median Age, y	Median High Risk[a,b]	Median Prior Lines (Range)	Response	Outcome (95% CI)	Grade 3/4 Adverse Events ≥10%	Reference
Ibrutinib monotherapy	Phase 2	111	68	49%	3 (1–5)	ORR 68% CR 21%	Median PFS 13.9 mo (7.0–NE)	Neutropenia 16% Thrombocytopenia 11%	Wang et al,[1] 2013
Ibrutinib monotherapy	Phase 3 RCT	139	67	22%	2 (1–9)	ORR 72% CR 19%	Median PFS 14.6 mo (10.4–NR)	Neutropenia 13%	Dreyling et al,[4] 2015
Ibrutinib monotherapy	Pooled trials analysis	370	68	32%	2 (1–9)	ORR 70% CR 27%	Median PFS 12.5 mo (9.8–16.6)	Neutropenia 16.5% Thrombocytopenia 11%	Rule et al,[9] 2017, Rule et al,[11] 2019
Acalabrutinib monotherapy	Phase 2	124	68	17%	2 (1–2)	ORR 81% CR 40%	Median PFS 20 mo (16.5–27.7) 2-y OS 72.4% (63.5–79.5)	Neutropenia 11%	Wang et al,[2] 2018, Wang et al,[10] 2019
Zanubrutinib monotherapy	Phase 2	86	60	13%	2 (1–4)	ORR 84% CR 59%	Median DOR 19.5 mo (16.6–NE)	Neutropenia 15% Pneumonia 10%	FDA,[7] 2019
Zanubrutinib monotherapy	Phase 1/2	32	70	31%	NA	ORR 84% CR 22%	Median DOR 18.5 mo (12.6–NE)		
Ibrutinib plus rituximab	Phase 2	50	67	12%	3 (1–9)	ORR 88% CR 44%	1-y PFS 75% (63–88)	Atrial fibrillation 12%	Wang et al,[8] 2016
Ibrutinib, lenalidomide plus rituximab	Phase 2	50	69	46%	2 (1–7)	ORR 76% CR 56%	Median PFS 16.0 mo (13.7–20.5) Median OS 22 mo (19.5–23.8)	Neutropenia 36% Infections 22% Cutaneous 14% Gastrointestinal 12% Thrombocytopenia 12% Vascular 10%	Jerkeman et al,[35] 2018

(continued on next page)

Table 1
(continued)

Treatment	Study	Patients, n	Median Age, y	Median High Risk[a,b]	Median Prior Lines (Range)	Response	Outcome (95% CI)	Grade 3/4 Adverse Events ≥10%	Reference
Ibrutinib plus venetoclax	Phase 2	24	68	75%	2 (0–6)	ORR 71% CR 71%	Median PFS 29 mo (13–NE) Median OS 32 mo (27–NE)	Neutropenia 33% Thrombocytopenia 17% Diarrhea 12% Anemia 12%	Tam and Handunnetti et al,[40,42] 2018
Ibrutinib plus umbralisib	Phase 2	21	68	Unknown	2 (2–3)	ORR 67% CR 27%	Median PFS 10.5 mo Median OS 29.7 mo	Infection 17%[a] Neutropenia 12%[a] Bruising 12%[a] Diarrhea 10%[a]	Davids et al,[46] 2019
Ibrutinib plus palbociclib	Phase 1	27	69	26%	1 (1–5)	ORR 67% CR 37%	2-y PFS 59.4%	Neutropenia 41% Thrombocytopenia 30% Hypertension 15% Febrile neutropenia 15% Lung infection 11%	Martin et al,[47] 2019

Abbreviations: BTKi, Bruton tyrosine kinase inhibitor; CI, confidence interval; CR, complete response; DOR, duration of response; FDA, Food and Drug Administration; MCL, mantle cell lymphoma; NE, not estimable; NR, not reached; ORR, overall response rate; OS, overall survival; PFS, progression-free survival; RCT, randomized controlled trial.

[a] Defined by MCL international prognostic index (MIPI) or sMIPI (simplified MIPI).

Data from Refs.[1,2,4,7–11,35,40,42,46,47]

Table 2
Selective studies assessing patient outcomes receiving therapy for MCL following relapse on BTKi

Treatment	Study	Patients, n	Median Age, y	High Risk[a]	Median Prior Lines Therapy	Response to Prior BTKi	Response to Treatment	Transplant Consolidation	Outcomes	Reference
Assorted (including lenalidomide 26%, cytarabine 18%, bendamustine 16%, bortezomib 10%)	Retrospective multicenter	73	67	48%	4 (1–11)	ORR 50% CR 11% Median DOI 4.7 mo	ORR 26% CR 7%	5 (6.8%)	Median OS 5.8 mo (3.7–10.4)	Martin et al,[3] 2016
Assorted (including. hyperCVAD 17%, bendamustine 14%, lenalidomide 11%)	Retrospective single center	36	69	63%	3 (1–11)	Median DOI 7.1 mo	ORR 27%	2 (5.5%)	Median survival 9 mo[b]	Jain et al,[13] 2018
Lenalidomide ± chemotherapy	Observational multicenter[c]	58	71	NA	4 (1–13)	ORR 45% CR 14% Median DOI 4.3 mo	ORR 29% CR 14%	NA	Median DOR 5 mo	Wang et al,[49] 2017
Venetoclax monotherapy	Retrospective multicenter	20	69	55%	3 (2–5)	ORR 55% CR 15% Median	ORR 53% CR 18%	1 (5.0%)	Median PFS 3.2 mo (1.2–	Eyre et al,[50] 2019

(continued on next page)

Table 2
(continued)

Treatment	Study	Patients, n	Median Age, y	High Risk[a]	Median Prior Lines Therapy	Response to Prior BTKi	Response to Treatment	Transplant Consolidation	Outcomes	Reference
						DOI 4.8 mo			11.3) Median OS 9.4 (1.5–NR)	
R-BAC	Retrospective multicenter	36	66	58%	2 (1–6)	ORR 68% CR 32% Median PFS 9.2 mo	ORR 83% CR 60%	12 (33.3%)	Median PFS 10.1 mo (6.9–13.3) Median OS 12.5 mo (11.0–14.0)	McCulloch et al,[52] 2020
KTE-X19 (CAR-T therapy)	Phase 2	28	65	NA	4 (1–5)	NA	ORR 86% CR 57%	-	1-y PFS 71% (50–84) 1-y OS 83% (60–93)	Wang et al,[59] 2019 (abstract only)

Abbreviations: BTKi, Bruton's tyrosine kinase inhibitor; CAR-T, chimeric antigen receptor T-cell; CR, complete response; DOI, duration of ibrutinib; DOR, duration of response; NA, not available; ORR, overall response rate; OS, overall survival; PFS, progression-free survival; R-BAC, rituximab, bendamustine, cytarabine.
[a] Defined by Mantle cell lymphoma international prognostic index (MIPI) or sMIPI (simplified MIPI).
[b] Survival time taken from date of last ibrutinib, not start of next line therapy.
[c] All but one patient enrolled retrospectively.
Data from Refs.[3,13,49,50,52,59]

OUTCOMES IN PATIENTS WITH BRUTON TYROSINE KINASE INHIBITOR RESISTANCE

The early reports on BTKi discontinuation largely involved patient groups with primary resistance or short responses to ibrutinib and here outcomes tended to be dismal. Studies highlighted a group of patients with disease progression so rapid that further systemic treatment was not possible. For example, one study of successive patients treated with ibrutinib at 8 US academic centers over a 3-year period observed that 20 (44%) of 45 patients stopping ibrutinib for progressive disease were not deemed fit for further therapy and rapidly died.[12] Sixteen of these patients (80%) had primary resistance to ibrutinib. In 29 patients receiving further systemic treatment, including 4 stopping ibrutinib due to toxicity, the ORR was 42% and median DOR to treatment only 3 months. The median OS for all patients following ibrutinib discontinuation was only 2.5 months.

In the largest available dataset, the outcomes of 104 patients were described.[3] Patients received a median 3 lines of therapy before ibrutinib. ORR to ibrutinib was 55%, with a median duration on treatment of only 4.7 months (95% CI 3.8–5.7), suggesting the study population was enriched for drug-resistant disease. Thirty-one patients (30%) received no further therapy due to rapid disease progression. Seventy-three patients received further treatment, of whom 61 were available for response assessment. The ORR to subsequent treatment was 30%, with CR rate only 7%. Median PFS from start of treatment following ibrutinib failure was only 1.9 months (95% CI 1.0–2.6) and median OS was 5.8 months (95% CI 3.7–10.4).

A report from MD Anderson detailed outcomes on all patients discontinuing ibrutinib for MCL over a 6-year period.[13] Eighty patients were included in the analysis, of whom 41 (51%) discontinued due to progressive disease. The median age of this group was 69 years, 63% were MCL international prognostic index (MIPI) high risk at time of ibrutinib initiation and median duration of ibrutinib was 8 months. Thirty-six of the relapsing patients (88%) went on to receive further therapy, and median OS from time of ibrutinib discontinuation was 9 months.

The studies described all incorporated numerous treatment regimens including lenalidomide, bortezomib, idelalisib, and various chemotherapy regimens; however, the numbers receiving individual therapies were too small to comment on the comparable efficacy.

The bleak outcomes have created concern that MCL relapses post BTKi are uniquely aggressive; however, these observations require some context. The studies were notable for a patient population exposed to multiple prior lines of therapy and a study design that focused disproportionately on patients with short responses to ibrutinib.[3] Diminishing returns with successive lines of therapy are well described in MCL across all therapeutic classes[14] and it is possible that the outcomes observed in these studies simply reflect the outcomes one might expect to see in a heavily pretreated group. Future phase III randomized controlled studies involving BTKis will help provide clarity to this issue.

MECHANISMS OF BRUTON TYROSINE KINASE INHIBITOR RESISTANCE

In MCL, and other B-cell malignancies, the B-cell receptor (BCR) pathway is frequently aberrantly upregulated.[15] Activation of the pathway triggers a signaling cascade involving several downstream proteins that include BTK, plus phosphatidylinositol 3-kinase (PI3K), protein kinase B (AKT), MAPK, and NF-κB (nuclear factor kappa-light-chain-enhancer of activated B cells), which lie more distal in the pathway, and leads to gene transcripts promoting cell survival, proliferation, and differentiation.

Ibrutinib binds covalently to the active site of BTK at cysteine 451, inhibiting BTK's enzymatic downstream signaling pathways.[16] In ibrutinib-sensitive MCL cell lines, knockout BTK models undergo apoptosis clarifying the importance of the ibrutinib-BTK interaction. However, in ibrutinib-resistant MCL cell lines, BTK-knockout models have shown ongoing survival and increased phosphorylation of downstream proteins in the BCR pathway, indicating resistance mechanisms that circumvent the role of BTK.[17]

Small series have examined in more detail additional driver mechanisms associated with ibrutinib resistance and a range of mutational aberrations have been described. These include the important role of the alternative or "noncanonical" NF-κB pathway including TRAF2 or BIRC3 inactivating mutations,[18] BCR-signaling including gain-of-function CARD11 mutations,[19] and aberrant cell cycle signaling via CCND1 mutations[20] and MYC activation.[21] BTK binding site mutations (C481S), a relatively common mechanism of ibrutinib resistance in chronic lymphocytic leukemia (CLL),[22] are also described in acquired BTKi resistance in MCL. The tumor microenvironment plays a key role in maintaining disease and represents a key therapeutic target[23] and a recent study also suggests differences in MCL cellular metabolism may contribute to ibrutinib resistance.[24]

Alternative or "Noncanonical" Nuclear Factor-κB Pathway

Rahal and colleagues[18] were the first to describe the importance of NF-κB pathway mutations in ibrutinib-resistant MCL. Cell line models identify subsets of MCL cell lines that are highly sensitive to BCR inhibition and exhibit chronic BCR-activation driving activation of the classic or "canonical" NF-κB pathway. Insensitive cell lines typically display activation of the alternative NF-κB pathway in a mutually exclusive fashion. Rahal and colleagues[18] performed transcriptome sequencing of ibrutinib-insensitive cell lines from 165 archived MCL tumor samples. Recurrent mutations in TRAF2, BIRC3, and MAP3K14, key regulators of the alternative NF-κB pathway were found in approximately 17% of cases.

B-cell Receptor-Signaling

The cysteine-to-serine (C481S) BTK binding site mutations, well described with BTK resistance in relapsed CLL[25] are notably less common in MCL but do occur in some patients, typically following initial ibrutinib responses.[3] PLCγ2 mutations have not been described to date in ibrutinib-resistant MCL.

Early evidence for the cysteine-to-serine mutation at the BTK binding site of ibrutinib (BTK C481S) was observed following serial biopsies before and after MCL progression on ibrutinib after initial partial responses in 2 patients by longitudinal integrative whole-exome and whole-transcriptome sequencing and targeted sequencing.[26] The C481S mutation limits the covalent binding affinity of ibrutinib and in the cases described, the mutation enhanced BTK and AKT activation. The mutation was not present in 6 cases of primary ibrutinib resistance within this series, suggesting other mechanisms of resistance are present in these cases. Further additional cases of BTK binding mutations have also been described in small numbers of patients who have initial response to ibrutinib and subsequently relapse.[3]

Wu and colleagues[19] performed whole-exome sequencing on 27 MCL samples from 13 patients. Eighteen genes recurrently mutated were found including those previously well described in MCL, such as ATM, MEF2B, and MLL2. Novel mutations in S1PR1 and CARD11 were found. Following this initial finding, an additional 173 MCL samples were screened for CARD11 mutations, a scaffold protein downstream of BTK, known to induce BCR pathway–mediated NF-κB activation. CARD11 mutations were found in 5.5% of cases. Further in vitro cell line–based experiments confirmed that activating mutations of *CARD11*, and subsequent BCR/NF-κB activation conferred resistance to ibrutinib in a subset of MCL.

Cell Cycle Signaling Defects

The characteristic hallmark of MCL pathophysiology is the t(11;14) translocation, which leads to deregulated overexpression of the cell cycle regulatory protein cyclin D1 (CCND1). Mohanty and colleagues[20] have reported that *CCND1* mutations can increase CCND1 protein levels via the mechanism of defective proteolysis. This mechanism has been shown to invoke ibrutinib resistance in MCL cell lines. The same group went on to show that Y44D CCND1 mutant cell lines are resistant to ibrutinib at supraphysiological concentrations (5–10 μM) and that primary MCL tumors with CCND1 mutations (sequence of CCND1 exon 1 as determined by Sanger sequencing) were less sensitive to ibrutinib by Cell Titer-Glo Luminescent assay.

Recently, Lee and colleagues[21] examined transcriptome changes in MCL cell lines that were either ibrutinib-sensitive and ibrutinib-resistant cell lines. They noted that a *MYC* gene signature was suppressed in ibrutinib-sensitive cell lines but not in cases that were resistant. *MYC* knockdown with RNA interference inhibited cell growth in both ibrutinib-sensitive and resistant cell lines, inferring the influence of MYC expression in ibrutinib resistance. Finally they showed that heat shock protein 90 (HSP90), a chaperon protein of MYC, can be inhibited directly by PU-H71. This mechanism can directly overcome ibrutinib resistance in MCL cell lines.

Tumor Microenvironment

The development of drug resistance in MCL appears dependent on evolving genetic and epigenetic alterations that stem from preexisting clonal heterogeneity that responds to selective pressure of therapy and a critical interplay with the surrounding tumor microenvironment (TME).[27,28] Stromal adhesion of MCL cells triggers c-Myc activation and histone deacetylase 6 induction, which modulate epigenetic regulation and confer drug resistance and clonogenicity.[29] When exposed to high concentrations of TME agonists, including interleukin-10 and CD40 L, drug-sensitive MCL cell lines have demonstrated acquired resistance to the drug combination of ibrutinib and venetoclax, linked to enhanced activation of the alternative NF-κB pathway.[30]

In an ex vivo study, SOX11, characteristically overexpressed in classic MCL, has been shown to upregulate expression of CXCR4 and FAK, which have important roles in TME signaling.[31] Enhanced expression promotes stromal interaction and increases cell-adhesion mediated drug resistance. The study demonstrated that specific FAK inhibition blocked downstream PI3K/AKT activation, indicating that therapeutic inhibition of this pathway may represent a strategy to overcome stroma-mediated therapy refractoriness.

Metabolic Reprogramming

A recent study in mouse models has found that ibrutinib resistance in MCL can be associated with metabolic reprogramming within cancer cells and a shift to reliance on glutaminolysis and oxidative phosphorylation. It was demonstrated that these drug-resistant cells could be effectively targeted with a small-molecule inhibitor of oxidative phosphorylation, showing promise for future clinical research.[24]

In summary, the key pathways documented to date that are important in BTKi resistance are (1) BCR-signaling, (2) the alternative NF-κB pathway, and (3) cell cycle signaling, and these pathways appear to be supported by important interactions with the TME and potentially aided by alterations in metabolic pathways. Although understanding remains incomplete, these findings provide a platform to rationalize potential therapeutic targets that may overcome BTKi resistance in the clinical setting.

THERAPEUTIC APPROACHES TO COMBAT BRUTON TYROSINE KINASE INHIBITOR RESISTANCE

Bruton Tyrosine Kinase Inhibitor Combination Therapies

In an effort to reduce primary resistance and improve DOR to BTKi monotherapy, a plethora of clinical studies have investigated the clinical efficacy of various combination therapies that combine BTKis with other active novel agents targeting complementary disease-signaling pathways (see **Tables 1** and **2** for details).

The anti-CD20 monoclonal antibody rituximab is an established component of standard immunochemotherapy with low associated toxicity making it an attractive partner for BTK inhibition. Ibrutinib (560 mg once daily) plus rituximab (IR) was investigated in 50 patients with relapsed, refractory disease in phase II trial.[8] The ORR was 88% (CR 44%) and the only grade 3 to 4 adverse event occurring in ≥10% of patients was atrial fibrillation. Results suggest the addition of rituximab may improve response rate without increased toxicity, although this study had a low proportion of high-risk patients relative to other trials. A phase III randomized controlled trial is currently recruiting that compares IR as upfront therapy in older patients against standard immunochemotherapy (ENRICH: NCT01880567).

Lenalidomide, a second-generation immunomodulatory drug, exerts antilymphoma effects through multiple mechanisms that include stimulation of dendritic cells and modification of the cytokine microenvironment[32] and has demonstrated clinical efficacy in non–ibrutinib-exposed patients with MCL.[33,34] The PHILEMON trial assessed the combination of ibrutinib (560 mg once daily), lenalidomide (15 mg once daily days 1–21 of 28-day cycle) plus rituximab in 50 patients with relapsed or refractory MCL.[35] ORR was 76%, including 56% with CR measured by PET/CT and the median PFS was 16.0 months (95% CI 13.7–20.5). Although the response rates appear modestly improved compared with ibrutinib monotherapy, the potential benefits were offset by higher toxicity with rates of grade 3 to 4 neutropenia 38% and infections 22%. Of note, 8 of 11 patients harboring TP53 mutations (73%) responded to therapy, suggesting this combination may be effective in this adverse-risk population although patient numbers were too low to make definitive conclusions. Overall, the results do not clearly indicate that this combination significantly improves on ibrutinib monotherapy.

Venetoclax is a highly selective BCL-2 inhibitor with potent activity against MCL cell lines[36] and demonstrated high response rates in 28 patients with ibrutinib-naïve, relapsed MCL (ORR 75%, CR 21%).[37] Ex vivo cellular models of ibrutinib plus venetoclax demonstrate synergistic cytotoxicity, and ibrutinib dependent inhibition of chemokine-mediated stromal adhesion, which results in characteristic egress of malignant cells into peripheral circulation,[38] appears to help overcome venetoclax resistance mechanisms that depend on stromal mediated CD40 stimulation.[39]

These preclinical findings are supported by the landmark phase II clinical trial in which 24 patients with MCL (23 patients with relapsed or refractory MCL) received ibrutinib 560 mg once daily plus venetoclax, given in stepwise, weekly increasing doses to 400 mg once daily[40] Half of patients had TP53 aberrations and 75% had a high-risk prognostic score. The rate of CR, measured by PET/CT according to Lugano classification,[41] was 71%. Cytopenias were problematic (grade 3–4 neutropenia 33%, thrombocytopenia 17%) and grade 1 to 2 diarrhea and nausea and vomiting exceeded 50%. Tumor lysis syndrome occurred in 2 patients. A recent update reported a median PFS of 29 months (95% CI 13–NR), and median OS of 32 months (95% CI 27–NR).[42]

The CR rate at week 16 of treatment, reported by CT to allow comparison with historical data, was 42%, compared with the result of 9% with ibrutinib. Elective treatment interruption was undertaken in 5 patients with minimal residual disease negative CRs. So far, there has been only one relapse, with ongoing responses exceeding 12 months off therapy in 3 cases. Although preliminary, these findings raise the appealing prospect of limited duration therapy.

The frequent finding of BTK-independent activation of the PI3K-AKT pathway in ibrutinib resistance suggests concurrent BCR pathway inhibition with a PI3Kδ inhibitor may reduce resistance and preclinical study of this combination has shown potential for synergistic cytotoxicity.[43] Concerns regarding excessive immune-related toxicity and limited efficacy in non–ibrutinib-exposed MCL have limited use of first-in-class idelalisib.[44] The second-generation PI3Kδ inhibitor umbralisib has demonstrated single-agent efficacy, with less off-target activity and reduced inhibitory activity of T-regulatory cells.[45] A phase I-Ib dose finding study assessed the combination of ibrutinib with umbralisib and included 21 patients with relapsed, refractory MCL (median 2 prior lines of therapy).[46] ORR was 67%, and 19% achieved CR with median PFS 10.5 months and median OS 29.7 months. Adverse event reporting did not separate from 21 patients on study with CLL, but suggested an increased risk of infection, with grade 3 to 4 events reported in 17%. The responses in MCL patients do not appear to improve on BTKi monotherapy.

Palbociclib, an oral, specific CDK4/6 inhibitor, in combination with ibrutinib was recently reported in a phase I trial.[47] The ORR was 67% and CR rate 37%. Response rates do not suggest a significant improvement on ibrutinib monotherapy and grade 3 to 4 neutropenia (41%) and febrile neutropenia (15%) appeared increased. A phase II multicenter clinical trial assessing this combination is ongoing (NCT03478514).

Proteasome inhibitors primarily induce apoptosis in MCL through NF-κB inhibition[48] making them an attractive partner to BTK inhibition and a phase II trial assessing ibrutinib plus bortezomib in combination is currently open to recruitment (NCT01776840). The possible benefit of adding BTKis to standard frontline chemotherapy is also being assessed in the phase III trials SHINE, assessing rituximab and bendamustine plus ibrutinib or placebo (NCT01776840), and TRIANGLE, assessing high dose cytarabine-based induction plus autologous stem cell consolidation with and without ibrutinib, plus an additional ibrutinib arm that omits transplant (NCT02858258).

Treatment Strategies in Post Bruton Tyrosine Kinase Inhibitor Relapse

There are very few published studies assessing efficacy of specific treatments in post-BTKi MCL, and evidence to guide practice is limited to a small number of retrospective studies. One observational study assessed efficacy of lenalidomide-based therapy in the post-ibrutinib setting.[49] Fifty-eight patients, of whom 48 discontinued ibrutinib due to lack of efficacy, were included. The ORR to prior ibrutinib was 45% and median duration of treatment 4.3 months (range 0.5–47.6). Thirteen patients received lenalidomide monotherapy, 11 with rituximab, and 34 in other combination therapies. The ORR was 29% and median DOR only 5 months. The poor responses to lenalidomide are disappointing although occurred in a patient group with notably poor response to prior ibrutinib. Based on this evidence use of post-BTKi lenalidomide appears to provide limited efficacy.

A retrospective analysis of patients receiving post-BTK inhibitor venetoclax monotherapy in a UK-based compassionate access scheme assessed responses in 20 patients.[50] Eighteen patients stopped BTKi due to lack of efficacy. Median duration of prior BTKi exposure was 4.8 months and 55% were MIPI high risk. The ORR to venetoclax was 53% with CR in 18%. The median PFS was 3.2 months (95% CI 1.2–11.3) and median OS 9.4 months (95% CI 1.5–NR). Response to prior BTKi appears to be a strong predictor of post-BTKi survival,[3,9] and in this context results for venetoclax monotherapy are reasonable, with ORR exceeding that for prior BTKi; however, the modest activity suggest this agent may be best used in combination with a BTKi.

R-BAC (rituximab, bendamustine, and cytarabine) has shown impressive responses in a phase II clinical trial, including a small cohort of relapsed patients with no prior exposure to ibrutinib (ORR 80%, CR 75%).[51] A retrospective analysis of 36 patients treated with R-BAC in 22 centers in the United Kingdom and Italy has recently been reported.[52] All patients had progressed on prior BTKi and 58% of patients were MIPI high risk at start of R-BAC. The median PFS with prior BTKi was 9.2 months. ORR to R-BAC was 83%, and CR/CRu (complete response unconfirmed) was 60%. Eleven patients received consolidation with allogeneic stem cell transplantation (alloSCT) and 1 patient, with prior allograft, received donor lymphocyte infusion. Median PFS was 10.1 months (95% CI 6.9–13.3) and median OS was 12.5 months (95% CI 11.0–14.0). Those receiving consolidation with cellular therapies displayed durable responses. Treatment was notable for high levels of neutropenic fever (47%) and transfusion support during therapy (68%). This cohort achieved favorable responses to the prior BTKi relative to the other retrospective studies. Nevertheless, the high response rate is impressive and makes it an attractive option in clinical practice, especially for patients considered fit for alloSCT consolidation.

Prospective clinical trial data assessing novel agents in the post-BTKi setting is pending. A trial assessing the second-generation proteasome inhibitor carfilzomib was aborted early after the first 4 patients to receive study drug (3 with prior ibrutinib exposure) failed to respond.[53] The next-generation PI3Kδ inhibitors umbralisib[45] and parsaclisib[54] have demonstrated efficacy in relapsed, refractory B-cell malignancies and both are recruiting to phase II study in the post-BTKi setting (NCT02793583, NCT03235544).

LOXO-305 is a next-generation, highly selective, non–covalent-binding BTKi, which overcomes resistance in C481-mutated BTK that has demonstrated activity in phase I study for relapsed lymphoid malignancies, which included 5 patients with MCL.[55] Although the prevalence of this mutation appears to be lower in MCL, for some patients, particularly those with an initial response to BTKi, LOXO-305 may be very effective. Phase II clinical trial is ongoing (NCT03740529).

Cellular Therapies

A role for alloSCT in select patients with MCL is well established and evidence of graft versus lymphoma is well described.[56] AlloSCT consolidation in fit patients responding to ibrutinib is a plausible approach, and supported by a 1-year PFS of 76% in patients adopting this strategy.[57] However, real-world data suggest this approach is currently only used in 14% of patients receiving ibrutinib in the UK, perhaps reflecting concerns regarding treatment morbidity and patient fitness outside of clinical trials.[58] Given the short responses and limited survival described in post-BTKi MCL, consolidating responses with alloSCT should be the aim for transplant-eligible patients. This rationale is supported by favorable results described in the R-BAC cohort.[52] However, the future role of alloSCT in MCL is uncertain, and depends on the clinical success and general availability of chimeric antigen receptor T-cell (CAR-T) therapy.

Findings from the ZUMA-2 trial presented at ASH 2019 described clinical responses to KTE-X19, an autologous anti-CD19 CAR-T, in 28 patients with median age 65 years.[59] All patients had prior BTKi exposure and median of 4 prior lines of therapy. The ORR was 86% and CR 57%. At 12 months follow-up, OS was 86%. Toxicity included grade 3 or 4 encephalopathy in 25% and cytokine release syndrome in

18%. Although toxicity was notable, this was mainly reversible and the reported outcomes are very promising and potentially practice changing. Based on this preliminary data it is conceivable to envisage CAR-T therapy playing a central role in future management of patients with MCL; however, caution at this early stage is advised. Phase 2 data can be difficult to replicate when applied to general populations, and it is not established which patients will be suitable candidates for therapy. At this stage, the limits of CAR-T-cell therapy are difficult to estimate, and newer products will aim to obviate issues of delivering treatment in a timely manner. The potential in this area provides great hope to patients but fresh challenges to clinicians and is likely to occupy a central focus of clinical research in the coming decade.

SUMMARY

Using complementary novel agents alongside BTKis to reduce primary resistance follows sensible rationale supported by several preclinical studies demonstrating enhanced, synergistic cytotoxicity. Unfortunately, these have not necessarily translated to improved clinical outcomes, and results from clinical trials have been mainly disappointing. In the studies described, additional novel agents have not appreciably improved the response rate to BTKis, suggesting little additional impact on a highly drug-resistant cohort of patients. What is more, most combination therapies reported significant increase in toxicity, particularly grade 3 to 4 cytopenias and a problematic trend for increased infections observed with lenalidomide, umbralisib, and palbociclib. The addition of rituximab did not appear to increase toxicity, although enhanced efficacy is yet to be confirmed.

Outcome data for the combination of ibrutinib and venetoclax appears most promising. ORR was similar to ibrutinib monotherapy, but impressively all patients responding achieved CR. Deeper remissions appear to translate into prolonged disease control with median PFS of 29 months, appearing superior to BTKi monotherapy and reports of patients remaining in remission beyond 12 months from stopping therapy suggests limited duration therapy may be feasible. Although there is increased toxicity, with patients often requiring regular granulocyte - colony stimulating factor support to avoid neutropenia, the prolonged responses observed with this combination make it an appealing combination for future phase III trials.

MCL relapsing after BTKi represents a major therapeutic challenge with little evidence to help guide management. The UK and Italian experience of using R-BAC is promising and appears to offer a high chance of achieving clinical response, although these are often short-lived. Achieving long-term responses appear dependent on consolidation with cellular therapies. Traditionally this has been alloSCT; however, the impressive emerging trial data for CAR-T therapy in relapsed MCL suggests this approach may soon be superseded.

DISCLOSURE

R. McCulloch: Sanofi (France), research funding. T.A. Eyre: Roche, speaker honorarium; KITE, advisory board honorarium; Janssen, speaker honorarium, travel to scientific conferences; AbbVie, speaker honorarium, travel to scientific conferences, advisory board honorarium. S. Rule: Janssen, speaker's bureau, paid consultancy, paid travel, research funding; Pharmacyclics (USA), research funding; AstraZeneca, paid consultancy; KITE, paid consultancy.

REFERENCES

1. Wang ML, Rule S, Martin P, et al. Targeting BTK with ibrutinib in relapsed or refractory mantle-cell lymphoma. N Engl J Med 2013;369(6):507–16.
2. Wang M, Rule S, Zinzani PL, et al. Acalabrutinib in relapsed or refractory mantle cell lymphoma (ACE-LY-004): a single-arm, multicentre, phase 2 trial. Lancet 2018;391(10121):659–67.
3. Martin P, Maddocks K, Leonard JP, et al. Postibrutinib outcomes in patients with mantle cell lymphoma. Blood 2016;124(12):1559–63.
4. Dreyling M, Jurczak W, Jerkeman M, et al. Ibrutinib versus temsirolimus in patients with relapsed or refractory mantle-cell lymphoma: an international, randomised, open-label, phase 3 study. Lancet 2016;387(10020):770–8.
5. Song Y, Zhou K, Zou D, et al. Zanubrutinib in patients with relapsed/refractory mantle cell lymphoma. Hematol Oncol 2019;37(Suppl 2):45–6.
6. Tam CS, Wang M, Simpson D, et al. Updated safety and efficacy data in phase 1 trial of patients with mantle cell lymphoma (MCL) treated with Bruton tyrosine kinase (BTK) inhibitor zanubrutinib (BGB-3111). Hematol Oncol 2019;37(Suppl 2): 245–7.
7. BeiGene. Brukinsa™ (zanubrutinib) prescribing information. Available at: https://www.brukinsa.com/prescribing-information.pdf. Accessed April 3, 2020.
8. Wang ML, Lee H, Chuang H, et al. Ibrutinib in combination with rituximab in relapsed or refractory mantle cell lymphoma: a single-centre, open-label, phase 2 trial. Lancet Oncol 2016;17(1):48–56.
9. Rule S, Dreyling M, Goy A, et al. Outcomes in 370 patients with mantle cell lymphoma treated with ibrutinib: a pooled analyisis from three open-label studies. Br J Haematol 2017;179(3):430–8.
10. Wang M, Rule S, Zinzani PL, et al. Durable response with single-agent acalabrutinib in patients with relapsed or refractory mantle cell lymphoma. Leukemia 2019;33(11):2762–6.
11. Rule S, Dreyling M, Goy A, et al. Ibrutinib for the treatment of relapsed/refractory mantle cell lymphoma: extended 3.5-year follow up from a pooled analysis. Haematologica 2019;104(5):e211–4.
12. Epperla N, Hamadani M, Cashen AF, et al. Predictive factors and outcomes for ibrutinib therapy in relapsed/refractory mantle cell lymphoma-a "real world" study. Hematol Oncol 2017;35(4):528–35.
13. Jain P, Kanagal-Shamanna R, Zhang S, et al. Long-term outcomes and mutation profiling of patients with mantle cell lymphoma (MCL) who discontinued ibrutinib. Br J Haematol 2018;183(4):578–87.
14. Kumar A, Sha F, Toure A, et al. Patterns of survival in patients with recurrent mantle cell lymphoma in the modern era: progressive shortening in response duration and survival after each relapse. Blood Cancer J 2019;9(6):50.
15. Buggy JJ, Elias L. Bruton tyrosine kinase (BTK) and its role in B-cell malignancy. Int Rev Immunol 2012;31(2):119–32.
16. Cinar M, Hamedani F, Mo Z, et al. Bruton tyrosine kinase is commonly overexpressed in mantle cell lymphoma and its attenuation by ibrutinib induces apoptosis. Leuk Res 2013;37(10):1271–7.
17. Ma J, Lu P, Guo A, et al. Characterization of ibrutinib-sensitive and –resistant mantle lymphoma cells. Br J Haematol 2014;166(6):849–61.
18. Rahal R, Frick M, Romero R, et al. Pharmacological and genomic profiling identifies NF-κB-targeted treatment strategies for mantle cell lymphoma. Nat Med 2014;20(1):87–92.

19. Wu C, de Miranda NF, Chen L, et al. Genetic heterogeneity in primary and relapsed mantle cell lymphomas: Impact of recurrent CARD11 mutations. Oncotarget 2016;7(25):38180–90.

20. Mohanty A, Sandoval N, Das M, et al. CCND1 mutations increase protein stability and promote ibrutinib resistance in mantle cell lymphoma. Oncotarget 2016; 7(45):73558–72.

21. Lee J, Zhang LL, Wu W, et al. Activation of MYC, a bona fide client of HSP90, contributes to intrinsic ibrutinib resistance in mantle cell lymphoma. Blood Adv 2018; 2(16):2039–51.

22. Woyach JA, Ruppert AS, Guinn D, et al. BTK^{C481S}-mediated resistance to ibrutinib in chronic lymphocytic leukaemia. J Clin Oncol 2017;35(13):1437–43.

23. Shain KH, Dalton WS, Tao J. The tumor microenvironment shapes hallmarks of mature B-cell malignancies. Oncogene 2015;34(36):4673–82.

24. Zhang L, Yao Y, Zhang S, et al. Metabolic reprogramming toward oxidative phosphorylation identifies a therapeutic target for mantle cell lymphoma. Sci Transl Med 2019;11(491) [pii:eaau1167].

25. Woyach JA, Furman RR, Liu TM, et al. Resistance mechanisms for the Bruton's tyrosine kinase inhibitor ibrutinib. N Engl J Med 2014;370(24):2286–94.

26. Chiron D, Di Liberto M, Martin P, et al. Cell-cycle reprogramming for PI3K inhibition overrides a relapse-specific C481S BTK mutation revealed by longitudinal functional genomics in mantle cell lymphoma. Cancer Discov 2014;4(9):1022–35.

27. Medina DJ, Goodell L, Glod J, et al. Mesenchymal stromal cells protect mantle cell lymphoma cells from spontaneous and drug-induced apoptosis through secretion of B-cell activating factor and activation of the canonical and non-canonical nuclear factor κB pathways. Haematologica 2012;97(8):1255–63.

28. Zhao X, Lwin T, Silva A, et al. Unification of de novo and acquired ibrutinib resistance in mantle cell lymphoma. Nat Commun 2017;8:14920.

29. Lwin T, Zhao X, Cheng F, et al. A microenvironment-mediated c-Myc/miR-548m/HDAC6 amplification loop in non-Hodgkin B cell lymphomas. J Clin Invest 2013;123(11):4612–26.

30. Jayappa KD, Portell CA, Gordon VL, et al. Microenvironmental agonists generate de novo phenotypic resistance to combined ibrutinib plus venetoclax in CLL and MCL. Blood Adv 2017;1(14):933–46.

31. Balsas P, Palomer J, Eguileor Á, et al. SOX11 promotes tumor protective microenvironment interactions through CXCR4 and FAK regulation in mantle cell lymphoma. Blood 2017;130(4):501–13.

32. Reddy N, Hernandez-Ilizaliturri FJ, Deeb G, et al. Immunomodulatory drugs stimulate natural killer-cell function, alter cytokine production by dendritic cells, and inhibit angiogenesis enhancing the anti-tumour activity of rituximab in vivo. Br J Haematol 2008;140(1):36–45.

33. Goy A, Sinha R, Williams ME, et al. Single-agent lenalidomide in patients with mantle-cell lymphoma who relapsed or progressed after or were refractory to bortezomib: phase II MCL-001 (EMERGE) study. J Clin Oncol 2013;31(29):3688–95.

34. Ruan J, Martin P, Shah B, et al. Lenalidomide plus rituximab as initial treatment for mantle-cell lymphoma. N Engl J Med 2015;373(19):1835–44.

35. Jerkeman M, Eskelund CW, Hutchings M, et al. Ibrutinib, lenalidomide, and rituximab in relapsed or refractory mantle cell lymphoma (PHILEMON): a multicentre, open-label, single-arm, phase 2 trial. Lancet Haematol 2018;5(3):e109–16.

36. Souers AJ, Leverson JD, Boghaert ER, et al. ABT-199, a potent and selective BCL-2 inhibitor, achieves antitumour activity while sparing platelets. Nat Med 2013;19(2):202–8.

37. Davids MS, Roberts AW, Seymour JF, et al. Phase I first-in-human study of vene-toclax in patients with relapsed or refractory non-hodgkin lymphoma. J Clin Oncol 2017;35(8):826–33.

38. Chang BY, Francesco M, De Rooij MF, et al. Egress of CD19(+)CD5(+) cells into the peripheral blood following treatment with the Bruton tyrosine kinase inhibitor ibrutinib in mantle cell lymphoma patients. Blood 2013;122(14):2412–24.

39. Chiron D, Dousset C, Brosseau C, et al. Biological rational for sequential targeting of Bruton tyrosine kinase and Bcl-2 to overcome CD40-induced ABT-199 resis-tance in mantle cell lymphoma. Oncotarget 2015;6(11):8750–9.

40. Tam CS, Anderson MA, Pott C, et al. Ibrutinib plus venetoclax for the treatment of mantle-cell lymphoma. N Engl J Med 2018;378(13):1211–23.

41. Cheson BD, Fisher RI, Barrington SF, et al. Recommendations for initial evalua-tion, staging, and response assessment of Hodgkin and non-Hodgkin lymphoma: the Lugano classification. J Clin Oncol 2014;32(27):3059–68.

42. Handunnetti SM, Anderson MA, Burbury K, et al. Three year update of the phase II ABT-199 (venetoclax) and ibrutinib in mantle cell lymphoma (AIM) study. Blood 2019;134(Suppl. 1):756.

43. de Rooij MF, Kuil A, Kater AP, et al. Ibrutinib and idelalisib synergistically target BCR-controlled adhesion in MCL and CLL: a rationale for combination therapy. Blood 2015;125(14):2306–9.

44. Kahl BS, Spurgeon SE, Furman RR, et al. A phase 1 study of the PI3Kδ inhibitor idelalisib in patients with relapsed/refractory mantle cell lymphoma (MCL). Blood 2014;123(22):3398–405.

45. Burris HA 3rd, Flinn IW, Patel MR, et al. Umbralisib, a novel PI3Kδ and casein ki-nase-1ε inhibitor, in relapsed or refractory chronic lymphocytic leukaemia and lymphoma: an open-label, phase 1, dose-escalation, first-in-human study. Lancet Oncol 2018;19(4):486–96.

46. Davids MS, Kim HT, Nicotra A, et al. Umbralisib in combination with ibrutinib in patients with relapsed or refractory chronic lymphocytic leukaemia or mantle cell lymphoma: a multicentre phase 1-1b study. Lancet Haematol 2019;6(1): e38–47.

47. Martin P, Bartlett NL, Blum KA, et al. A phase 1 trial of ibrutinib plus palbociclib in previously treated mantle cell lymphoma. Blood 2019;133(11):1201–4.

48. Pham LV, Tamayo AT, Yoshimura LC, et al. Inhibition of constitutive NF-kappa B activation in mantle cell lymphoma B cells leads to induction of cell cycle arrest and apoptosis. J Immunol 2003;171(1):88–95.

49. Wang M, Schuster SJ, Phillips T, et al. Observational study of lenalidomide in pa-tients with mantle cell lymphoma who relapsed/progressed after or were refrac-tory/intolerant to ibrutinib (MCL-004). J Hematol Oncol 2017;10(1):171.

50. Eyre TA, Walter HS, Iyengar S, et al. Efficacy of venetoclax monotherapy in pa-tients with relapsed, refractory mantle cell lymphoma after Bruton tyrosine kinase inhibitor therapy. Haematologica 2019;104(2):e68–71.

51. Visco C, Finotto S, Zamebello R, et al. Combination of rituximab, bendamustine, and cytarabine for patients with mantle-cell non-Hodgkin lymphoma ineligible for intensive regimens or autologous transplantation. J Clin Oncol 2013;31(11): 1442–9.

52. McCulloch R, Visco C, Eyre TA, et al. Efficacy of R-BAC in relapsed, refractory mantle cell lymphoma post BTK inhibitor therapy. Br J Haematol 2020. https://doi.org/10.1111/bjh.16416.

53. Lee HJ, Badillo M, Romaguera J, et al. A phase II study of carfilzomib in the treatment of relapsed/refractory mantle cell lymphoma. Br J Haematol 2019;184(3): 460–2.
54. Forero-Torres A, Ramchandren R, Yacoub A, et al. Parsaclisib, a potent and highly selective PI3Kδ inhibitor, in patients with relapsed or refractory B-cell malignancies. Blood 2019;133(16):1742–52.
55. Mato AR, Flinn IW, Pagel JM, et al. Results from a first-in-human, proof-of-concept phase 1 trial in pretreated b-cell malignancies for LOXO-305, a next-generation, highly selective, non-covalent BTK inhibitor. Blood 2019;134(Suppl. 1):501.
56. Le Gouill S, Kroger N, Dhedin N, et al. Reduced-intensity conditioning allogeneic stem cell transplantation for relapsed/refractory mantle cell lymphoma: a multicenter experience. Ann Oncol 2012;23(10):2695–703.
57. Dreger P, Michaller M, Bosman P, et al. Ibrutinib for bridging to allogeneic hematopoietic cell transplantation in patients with chronic lymphocytic leukemia or mantle cell lymphoma: a study by the EBMT chronic malignancies and lymphoma working parties. Bone Marrow Transplant 2019;54(1):44–52.
58. McCulloch R, Rule S, Eyre TA, et al. Ibrutinib at first relapse for mantle cell lymphoma: a United Kingdom real world analysis of outcomes in 169 patients. Blood 2019;134(Suppl. 1):3993.
59. Wang ML, Munoz J, Goy A, et al. KTE-X19, an Anti-CD19 Chimeric Antigen Receptor (CAR) T cell therapy, in patients (Pts) With Relapsed/Refractory (R/R) Mantle Cell Lymphoma (MCL): Results of the Phase 2 ZUMA-2 Study. Blood 2019;134(Suppl. 1):754.

Blastoid Mantle Cell Lymphoma

Preetesh Jain, MBBS, MD, DM, PhD, Michael Wang, MD*

KEYWORDS

- Mantle cell lymphoma • Blastoid • Pleomorphic • Aggressive mantle cell lymphoma
- Transformation • *BTK* • Ibrutinib • Venetoclax

KEY POINTS

- Poor prognosis, aggressive disease course, and drug resistance observed in patients with blastoid mantle cell lymphoma (MCL) result from an interplay of complex pathogenic mechanisms, genomic profile, and aberrant cell signaling pathways distinct from the classic variant of MCL.
- De novo and transformed blastoid MCLs show distinct clinical and molecular patterns.
- Anti–CD 19 chimeric antigen receptor therapy induces significant responses in patients with relapsed blastoid MCL.

INTRODUCTION

Mantle cell lymphoma (MCL) is witnessing dramatic improvements[1,2] in the availability of newer therapeutic options (BTK inhibitors, venetoclax, anti–cluster of differentiation [CD] 19 chimeric antigen receptor T cell [CAR-T]), enhanced understanding of pathogenic mechanisms, the role of microenvironmental factors and the identification of chromosomal aberrations,[3] and coding and noncoding[4] genomic aberrations. Despite these advances, the disease continues to pose challenges.

Significant heterogeneity exists in patients with MCL, with a subset showing an indolent clinical course[5–8] (generally SOX-11 negative, mutated IGHV, CD200 positivity, and leukemic nonnodal MCL) and another subset generally considered as high-risk MCL[9,10] (high Ki-67%[11] in involved tissues, blastoid or pleomorphic histology, *TP53* mutations,[12–15] del17p, complex karyotype,[16,17] and MYC-positive MCL[18]) showing poor survival and frequent relapses. However, acquisition of secondary chromosomal abnormalities, del17p or *TP53* mutations,[19] in SOX-11–negative patients with MCL can lead to aggressive disease course. In a series[20] of 21 blastoid MCL cases, 13 out of 21 (62%) had unmutated IGHV sequence, whereas 8 out of 21 (38%) had

---

Department of Lymphoma/Myeloma, The University of Texas MD Anderson Cancer Center, 1515 Holcombe Boulevard, Unit 429, Houston, TX 77030, USA
* Corresponding author.
E-mail address: miwang@mdanderson.org

Hematol Oncol Clin N Am 34 (2020) 941–956
https://doi.org/10.1016/j.hoc.2020.06.009
0889-8588/20/© 2020 Elsevier Inc. All rights reserved.

mutated IGHV, and these patients had a better survival than patients with unmutated IGHV.

Because patients with both blastoid and pleomorphic variant MCL show aggressive clinical courses and differences between blastoid versus pleomorphic variants are not well understood, and blastoid variants are commoner then pleomorphic variants, this article focuses on recent advances and the status of blastoid MCL in 2020.

Histopathology

Expert hematopathology evaluation of involved tissue biopsies is critical in the initial assessment of patients with MCL. Most of these patients show a classic histology MCL, which can present with nodular, diffuse, or mantle zone cytomorphologic patterns, whereas a diagnosis of aggressive histology MCL is rendered when there is either blastoid or pleomorphic cytomorphology of MCL cells or even when there is evidence of high Ki-67% with aggressive morphologic features not fitting into blastoid or pleomorphic morphology. Blastoid MCL cells are a medium-sized, homogenous population of cells resembling lymphoblasts, with fine chromatin and round nuclei, and pleomorphic variant cells are large, anaplastic cells with irregular nuclei, resembling large B-cell lymphoma.[21] In a subset of patients, intermediate-form MCL is also described,[22] which shows a blend of features from classic and aggressive histologies with higher expression of CCND1 and Ki-67% compared with classic histology, and showed survival (31 months) inferior to classic MCL (77 months) but longer than aggressive MCL (18 months). The intermediate form of MCL is not considered a standard variant of MCL by the World Health Organization (WHO.[21] Infrequently, biopsies can also show in situ blastoid MCL, but the clinical relevance of this observation is unclear. In 1 report, among the 17 patients with blastoid MCL,[23] biopsies showed a diffuse pattern of distribution of follicular dendritic cells (FDCs) and this pattern correlated with poorer outcome compared with the nodular distribution of FDCs. In general, most of the patients with blastoid MCL showed SOX-11 positivity and high Ki-67% ($\geq$50%) in the involved tissues.[10]

In our opinion, the prognostic or mechanistic relationship of Ki-67%–rich areas, CD21+ FDCs, T-cell subsets, stromal cells, chemokine expression, and lymphoid tissue microenvironmental heterogeneity (lymph node vs spleen) in blastoid MCLs is not well understood and requires dedicated studies.

Clinical Features

Exact incidence and prevalence of aggressive histology MCL (blastoid or pleomorphic) remains unknown because of the smaller number of these patients and lack of prospective data; however, approximately 10% to 20% of newly diagnosed patients with MCL show blastoid or pleomorphic histologies. Clinically, these patients frequently present with extranodal involvement ranging from 20% to 72% of blastoid MCL[9,24,25]: bone marrow (50%–80%), skin[26] (72%), pulmonary (30%), gastrointestinal tract (20%–30%), and central nervous system (CNS) (5%–30%[27]; leptomeningeal involvement was predominant). Patients with blastoid MCL at initial diagnosis are de novo blastoid MCL, whereas those patients who evolved from classic variant MCL at initial diagnosis to blastoid/pleomorphic MCL are considered as transformed MCL.[10,25] Transformed MCL is clonally related to an initial MCL clone,[28] but unlike richter's transformation few reports have systematically evaluated the clonality in transformed MCL. Rarely, clonally related Hodgkin lymphoma in transformed blastoid MCL is also described.[29]

In the largest retrospective series of aggressive histology MCL from MD Anderson Cancer Center reported by Jain and colleagues,[10] among the 183 patients with aggressive histology MCL (152 blastoid and 31 pleomorphic variants), the median age was 65 years and most were men (75%). In this report, 60% of patients showed monoclonal kappa light chains on MCL cells, 67% had marrow involvement, 5% had CNS involvement, 27% had leukemic phase, median Ki-67% was 70% (range, 10%–100%), and 81% had positive SOX-11 expression.

Other Features Observed in Blastoid Mantle Cell Lymphoma

1. Immunophenotype: few reports on immunophenotypic aberrancies in blastoid MCL were noted, especially for the loss of CD5 expression. Among the 25 patients with CD5-negative MCL, 1 study[30] showed that 5 patients (25%) were blastoid, and, in another study[31] with 57 patients with CD5-negative MCLs, 16 patients (28%) were blastoid MCL. In another study on 103 patients with CD23-positive MCL,[32] 19% were blastoid. Rarely, cyclin D1-negative blastoid MCL is described.[33] In 1 study with 56 patients with cyclin D1–negative MCL, 10 (19%) were blastoid MCL and, among these 10 cases, 6 were cyclin D2+, 1 was cyclin D3+, but 3 patients were solely positive for cyclin E.

2. Karyotype: complex karyotype is frequently detected in patients with blastoid MCL. Tetraploidy was frequent in blastoid MCL.[34] Among 104 patients with MCL[16] (21 blastoid MCL), a mean of 8.8 additional chromosomal abnormalities were detected in blastoid MCL compared with 4.8 in classic MCL ($P = .01$). Deletion 13q and deletion 18q were observed in 50% and 27% of blastoid MCLs compared with 20% and 7% in classic MCL respectively. Another study[35] evaluated cytogenetics in 27 patients with blastoid/pleomorphic MCL and 24 out of 27 (88%) had complex karyotype. Aberrancies in chromosomes 13, 18, 8, and 9 were frequent in blastoid MCL (n = 12). Pleomorphic variant (n = 15) had a higher median number of chromosomal abnormalities (median, 10) with frequent abnormalities in chromosomes 13, 17, 3, and 9. Monosomy of chromosome 22 and abnormality of chromosome 11 were frequent in pleomorphic MCL. However, the prognostic relevance of abnormal karyotype in the context of newer agents (BTK inhibitors, CAR T cell) is unclear. Using whole-exome sequencing, Jain and colleagues have recently shown that patients with aggressive histology MCL (n = 42) show a significantly higher degree of aneuploidy compared with nonaggressive classic MCL (n = 39).[10]

3. Somatic mutations in certain genes: in TP53[12,13], NOTCH1, NOTCH2,[36] and NSD2, the incidence of mutations varies in different studies but these mutations are prevalent in blastoid MCL. In 1 recent study, among 20 patients with TP53 mutated MCL, 12 (60%) had blastoid MCL. In another study, 6 out of 21 (28%) blastoid MCLs had TP53 mutations. NOTCH1 mutations were predominant in patients with blastoid MCL, associated with poor outcome compared with NOTCH1 wild-type MCL and NOTCH2 mutations, which also predicted poor survival in MCL compared with wild-type NOTCH2 MCL. We have previously reported that, among the 4 patients who transformed to blastoid/pleomorphic histology after ibrutinib therapy, 3 patients developed NSD2 and TP53 mutations, suggesting the impact of epigenetic pathway alterations in blastoid MCL.[37] NSD2 mutations are associated with an increase in H3K36 and a decrease in H3K27 methylation across the genome, thereby promoting oncogenesis. Recently, our group[10] has shown a genomic profile comparison of aggressive histology MCL versus nonaggressive MCL, exclusively mutated genes in AH-MCL compared with nonaggressive MCL were NOTCH2, NOTCH3, UBR5, and the CCND1 mutations, which were 10 times more frequent in aggressive histology MCL. Among the aggressive histology MCL, we showed that those patients with Ki-67 greater than or equal to 50% had exclusive occurrence of mutations in CCND1, NOTCH1, TP53, SPEN, SMARCA4, RANBP2, KMT2C, NOTCH2, NOTCH3, and NSD2 compared with low Ki-67 less

than 50%, and these data suggest that morphology in conjunction with aberrant somatic mutation profile in high Ki-67% MCL identifies a subset of very-high-risk MCL with poor outcomes. Although clonal evolution leading to disease progression is considered the most probable reason for the pathogenesis of transformed blastoid MCL, in another study from Memorial Sloan Kettering Cancer Center, (abstract form)[38] it was reported that high-risk somatic mutations (TP53, KMT2D, CCND1, and SMARCA4) were observed in patients since the time of initial diagnosis of MCL, and clonal evolution may not be important in disease transformation.

4. MYC aberrations: frequently observed in patients with blastoid/pleomorphic MCL. In a series[39] of 27 patients with MYC gene rearrangement in MCL, 24 patients (89%) had blastoid/pleomorphic histology. MYC-rearranged patients (n = 27) had inferior survival compared with patients with extra copies of MYC (n = 21). In another report, MYC overexpression was significantly higher in 11 patients with blastoid/pleomorphic MCL[18] (mean 19% vs 1.9% in classic MCL; n = 54). Recently, gene set enrichment analyses in ibrutinib-resistant aggressive MCL showed that MYC gene pathway expression[40] was significantly higher in ibrutinib-resistant MCL compared with ibrutinib-sensitive MCL, and associated with an aggressive clinical course.

Factors Associated with the Evolution and the Pathogenesis of Blastoid Mantle Cell Lymphoma

Structure of aggressive histology MCL: using a novel approach, S-FTIR (Synchrotron Fourier transformed infrared microspectroscopy technique) and principal component analysis of lymphoid tissues, 1 study[41] with 18 patients with MCL showed for the first time the differences in the structural composition of classic (n = 9) versus aggressive MCL (n = 9). Higher degree of absorbance intensity of protein moiety in spectra in aggressive variant MCL was shown and the absorbance increase in peaks was attributed to the presence of amide I, amide II, and nucleic acids, much more pronounced in aggressive MCL. These findings further confirm that classic and blastoid MCL are distinct at structural, genomic, and biological levels.

Cyclin D1 alterations[42,43]: cell cycle dysregulation and cyclin-D1 overexpression are well known to play an instrumental role in the pathogenesis of MCL. Furthermore, aberrations in TP53 and CDKN2A genes and decreased expression of p16INK4a and p21waf1[44] are frequently seen in patients with MCL. Using gene expression profiling and real-time quantitative polymerase chain reaction, it was shown that the truncated form of cyclin-D1 messenger RNA (mRNA) (3′-untranslated region [UTR])[45] led to higher levels of cyclin D1 protein, more stable cyclin D1 protein, and is significantly associated with blastoid MCL[46] and MCL with higher Ki-67%. Therefore, these patients show an aggressive clinical course. Presence of 3′-UTR–deficient short isoforms of cyclin-D1 mRNA leads to removal of the destabilizing function of adenylate-uridylate-rich elements[47] at the 3′ end, and this in turn provides persistence of cyclin D1, and hence higher proliferation exists in these MCL cells. Point mutations[48] in cyclin D1 led to premature polyadenylation signals, which also contributed to 3′-UTR cyclin-D1 mRNA.

BACH2 downregulation and blastoid MCL[49]: Broad-Complex, Tramtrack, and Bric à brac and Cap'n'collar homology 2 is a B-cell transcription factor that plays an important role in somatic hypermutation of IGHV and oxidative stress–mediated drug resistance in MCL. Downregulation of BACH2 (repressed by hypoxia-inducible factors-alpha) was associated with increased proliferation; MCL dissemination to bone marrow, spleen, and gastrointestinal tract; and blastoid histology.

Akt pathway activation and blastoid MCL: preferential, constitutive activation of Akt and phosphorylation of multiple downstream pathways (p27kip1, FRKHL-1, MDM2,

Bad, mammalian target of rapamycin, and p70S6K) was noted in 12 patients with blastoid MCL.[50] Loss of *PTEN* can also contribute to Akt activation in blastoid MCL.

Methylation patterns: based on DNA methylation analysis,[51] 2 clusters of MCL were recognized, cluster 1 and cluster 2. Cluster 1 patients had unmutated IGHV and poor survival. Disease aggressiveness was worse in patients with cluster 1 methylation pattern with somatic mutations.

MiR-18b, miR-15b, and miR-17-92[52] overexpression: genomewide microRNA (miRNA) microarray profiling identified that increased levels of mi-18b[53] were significantly associated with poor outcome. Another study showed that increased levels of miR-15b[54] were associated with aggressive histology MCL. The clinical relevance of miRNAs in blastoid MCL is yet to be fully explored.

Mcl-1 overexpression: in 1 small study,[55] overexpression of antiapoptotic Mcl-1 (myeloid cell leukemia protein-1) was significantly associated with blastoid MCL and *TP53* mutations.

Pathogenesis of blastoid/pleomorphic MCL continues to evolve and the understanding of these variants of MCL is improving. The authors believe that, as the disease resistance and aggressive histologic patterns continue to develop after the advent of newer therapies in patients with MCL (BTK inhibitors, venetoclax, and anti-CD19-CAR-T-triple-resistant MCL), novel genomic aberrations, clonal evolution, and changes in microenvironmental milieu continue to evolve under different selection pressures, and overcoming these resistance mechanisms should be the next challenge in high-risk blastoid MCL.

Management of Patients with Blastoid Mantle Cell Lymphoma

It is important to recognize and differentiate blastoid MCL from other differential diagnoses such as CD5+ diffuse large B-cell lymphoma and aggressive high-grade large B-cell lymphomas by specific immunophenotypic, cytogenetic, and molecular features.[1] In the absence of clinical symptoms, the authors do not recommend performing cerebrospinal fluid analyses at the baseline on every patient with blastoid MCL. Staging work-up and follow-up evaluation of these patients is similar to classic variant of MCL; however, because of the high frequency of extranodal involvement, we recommend performing baseline gastrointestinal endoscopy and random biopsies.

Prospective clinical trials focusing on blastoid MCL variant are lacking because of the smaller number of this cohort of patients with MCL. **Table 1** summarizes the data obtained from various clinical trials and retrospective analyses on blastoid MCL. Patients with blastoid MCL are included in the high-risk category of MCL (in addition to patients with Ki-67% greater than or equal to 30%, *TP53* mutations, advanced stage, and high-risk MCL International Prognostic Index), and treatment of these patients poses a constant challenge to physicians. In general, various centers treat these patients with intensive chemoimmunotherapy followed by consolidation with autologous stem cell transplant (ASCT). The authors recommend enrolling these patients in clinical trials (if available). There is a considerable hope that, with the incorporation of ibrutinib, acalabrutinib, venetoclax, and anti-CD19 CAR-T therapies in the treatment of MCL, the outcomes, depth, and duration of response in patients with blastoid MCL will significantly improve compared with intensive chemoimmunotherapy.[1]

Previously untreated blastoid MCL: subset analyses on blastoid MCL were not clearly shown in the original frontline randomized clinical trials for young[56] and elderly[57] patients because the numbers of patients with blastoid MCL were small. In the phase 3 multicenter randomized study from the European MCL network in young (≤65 years of age) previously untreated patients,[56] 28 (9%) patients were blastoid

Table 1
Summary of pivotal clinical studies in blastoid/pleomorphic mantle cell lymphoma

Protocol Used	Number of Patients/ Overall Number	Median Follow-up	ORR (CR) %	TTF/PFS	OS	Comments
Frontline Single-arm Studies/Pooled Analyses						
MDACC: R-HCVAD/ Mtx-ara-C[62,75,76] (no ASCT)	14/97	13.4 y	NA/79	8 y 35%	8 y 43%	• In young or older patients with blastoid MCL, at 10 y and at 13.4 y median follow-up, the PFS and OS did not differ significantly between blastoid and nonblastoid MCL • Blastoid MCL did not significantly affect PFS or OS in multivariate analysis
Nordic MCL2- R-maxi-CHOP/R-HiDAC (with ASCT)[60,61,77]	31/160	6.8 y	NA/54[a]	44% (10 y)	51% (10 y)	• At 11.6-y follow-up, blastoid MCL showed a nonsignificant trend for inferior OS but no significant difference with respect to PFS compared with nonblastoid MCL • Blastoid MCL did not significantly affect PFS or OS in multivariate analysis
CALGB study. R-Mtx–augmented CHOP: high-dose cytarabine and etoposide with R and G-CSF then ASCT and 2 doses of rituximab[78]	12/78	4.7 y	NA/69[a]	56% (5 y)[a]	64% (5 y)[a]	• Small cohort of blastoid MCL, subset-specific responses not described • Reduced Mtx dose was required in a subset of patients because of renal toxicity without compromising the efficacy
BR and R high-dose cytarabine: ASCT[79]	11/88	33 mo	91/82	66% (3 y)	92% (3 y)[a]	• Pooled analysis of 2 phase II trials and 47 off-protocol patients • Blastoid MCL had inferior PFS compared with classic variant MCL ($P = .038$) • MRD testing was available in all patients with ctDNA-based detection of disease relapse 7.2 mo before clinical relapse

						Key Findings
Frontline Randomized Studies						
MCL Younger: R-CHOP-ASCT (n = 234) vs R-CHOP alternating with R-DHAP–ara-C ASCT (n = 232)[5,6]	28/466	6.1 y	81/23[58]	18 mo	32 mo	• 5-y OS was significantly inferior in blastoid MCL, 38% vs 75% in classic MCL (P = .0001), whereas PFS was borderline negative for blastoid MCL (P = .05) • TTF was significantly longer in the cytarabine group (median 9.1 y) than in the control group (3.9 y), albeit with higher rates of grade 3 and 4 hematologic toxicities • 79% MRD negative in cytarabine group
MCL Elderly: R-CHOP-ASCT (n = 234) vs R-CHOP alternating with R-DHAP–ara-C ASCT (n = 232)[57,59]	34/287	3 y	NA	19 mo	29 mo	• 5-y OS was significantly inferior in blastoid MCL: 29 mo vs 78 mo in nonblastoid MCL (P = .0085) • 5-y PFS was not significantly different between blastoid and nonblastoid MCL
Relapsed MCL						
Ibrutinib[63]	36/370	3.5 y	50/NA	5.1 mo	12.8 mo	• Time to best response was similar in blastoid vs nonblastoid MCL • Duration of response was 8.5 vs 18.8 mo in blastoid and nonblastoid MCL
Ibrutinib + rituximab[64]	7/49	4 y	71/43	21 mo	30 mo	Relapsed patients with blastoid MCL have inferior outcomes and lower response rates compared with nonblastoid MCL, albeit number of patients with blastoid MCL was small
Acalabrutinib[65]	26/124	2 y	77/35	15 mo	NA	Response rates and outcomes were inferior in blastoid compared with nonblastoid MCL

(continued on next page)

Table 1
(continued)

Protocol Used	Number of Patients/ Overall Number	Median Follow-up	ORR (CR) %	TTF/PFS	OS	Comments
Retrospective Studies (Miscellaneous Regimens)						
Jain et al,[10] 2020: Retrospective analysis of 183 patients with blastoid/pleomorphic MCL from a single center	183	19.6 mo	78/56	13	33 mo	• Largest study on blastoid (n = 152) and pleomorphic MCL (n = 31), combined as aggressive histology MCL • De novo blastoid MCL has superior outcomes compared with transformed blastoid MCL • Pleomorphic have inferior failure-free survival after first-line treatment compared with blastoid, but clinical features in blastoid and pleomorphic were similar • Response rates according to the treatment type (excluding SCT) were 86%, 75%, 69%, 50%, 50% in R-HCVAD–based regimens, R-chemotherapy, ibrutinib or other BTK inhibitors, R-lenalidomide–based regimens, and miscellaneous regimens respectively • ASCT after chemoimmunotherapy improved FFS not OS
Bhatt et al,[24] 2016 (pre-ibrutinib era)	—	31 (24) evaluable	58/45	16% (5 y)	24% (5 y)	Blastoid and diffuse classic MCL had inferior PFS compared with nodular classic MCL Addition of rituximab with HCVAD induced better PFS (2 y, 66%) 13 patients received rituximab-based therapies and 18 did not get rituximab
Bernard et al,[9] 2001 (pre-rituximab era), CHOP/CVP	24	33	NA/36	13	14.5	• Median OS was significantly shorter in blastoid MCL compared with classic MCL • Twelve patients (36%) entered a CR1 with a median duration of 11 mo. Fifteen patients (46%) failed to respond and rapidly died of progressive disease

Abbreviations: ara-C, cytarabine; ASCT, autologous stem cell transplant; CR, complete response rate; ctDNA, circulating tumor DNA; MRD, minimal residual disease; Mtx, methotrexate; NA, not available; ORR, overall response rate; OS, overall survival; PFS, progression-free survival; R-DHAP, rituximab with dexamethasone, cisplatin, ara-C; R-HCVAD/Mtx-ara-C, rituximab with hyperfractionated cyclophosphamide, vincristine, doxorubicin, dexamethasone alternating with high-dose methotrexate and cytosine arabinoside; TTF, time to treatment failure.

[a] Data not solely from blastoid MCL; these data are obtained from all patients in this study.

MCL. Patients were randomized to 6 courses of R-CHOP (rituximab plus cyclophosphamide, doxorubicin, vincristine, and prednisone) followed by myeloablative radiochemotherapy and ASCT (control group; n = 234), or 6 courses of alternating R-CHOP or R-DHAP (rituximab plus dexamethasone, high-dose cytarabine, and cisplatin) followed by a high-dose cytarabine conditioning regimen and ASCT (cytarabine group; n = 232). Addition of cytarabine prolonged the time to treatment failure (TTF) overall (9.1 years vs 3.9 years in the control group) as well in patients with high Ki-67% ($\geq$30%; 4.5 years in cytarabine vs 2 years in control group, as shown in figure S6B in Ref.[56]). From the overall aggregate of 28 patients with blastoid MCL in this study, 5-year overall survival (OS) was significantly inferior in blastoid MCL: 38% versus 75% in classic MCL (P = .0001; shown in Dreyling and colleagues[58] figure 2A).

In another randomized study from the European MCL network in elderly (>60 years of age), previously untreated patients with MCL,[57,59] 34 (12%) patients were blastoid MCL. Patients were randomized to 8 cycles of R-CHOP every 21 days or 6 cycles of rituximab, fludarabine, and cyclophosphamide (R-FC) every 28 days. Patients who had a response underwent a second randomization to rituximab or interferon alfa maintenance therapy until progression. R-CHOP induction was significantly better than R-FC induction, and rituximab maintenance significantly reduced the risk of disease progression or death compared with interferon alfa. From the overall aggregate of 34 patients with blastoid MCL in this study, 5-year OS was significantly inferior in blastoid MCL: 30% versus 60% in classic MCL (P = .0085; shown in Ref.[58] figure 2B). Significantly, inferior OS and progression-free survival (PFS) of patients with blastoid MCL compared with patients without blastoid MCL was further confirmed when a pooled analysis[11] from the European MCL network was performed in 620 patients, of whom 62 (10%) patients were blastoid MCL. However, the prognostic impact of Ki-67% was significantly higher compared with the blastoid variant MCL in this study.

The Nordic MCL2 study[60] was a single-arm multicenter study in 160 patients (31 with blastoid MCL) with previously untreated MCL (age<66 years). Patients received 6 cycles of rituximab with intensive induction chemotherapy, and an augmented CHOP regimen (R-maxi-CHOP) alternating with high-dose cytarabine was administered. All patients underwent high-dose chemotherapy with BEAM (carmustine, etoposide, cytarabine, melphalan) or BEAC (carmustine, etoposide, cytarabine, and cyclophosphamide) and ASCT. After a median observation time of 6.8[60] years, patients with blastoid MCL showed significantly inferior OS (10-year OS, 51% vs 61% in nonblastoid MCL; P = .01), whereas, at 11.4 years follow-up,[61] blastoid MCL had a trend toward inferior OS but it was not statistically significant.

Romaguera and colleagues[62] envisaged a single-center phase II trial of rituximab with hyper-CVAD (cyclophosphamide, vincristine, adriamycin and dexamethasone)(R-HCVAD) in previously untreated patients with MCL (n = 97). Fourteen patients had blastoid MCL, and complete response rate was 79% after 6 cycles of R-HCVAD; after subsequent follow-up,[62] PFS and OS were not significantly different in patients with blastoid versus nonblastoid MCL.

Previously treated relapsed blastoid MCL: BTK inhibitors (BTKi) such as ibrutinib, acalabrutinib, and zanubrutinib have significantly influenced the therapeutic armamentarium in MCL.[1] Ibrutinib is so far the most extensively studied BTKi. From a pooled analysis[63] of 370 patients treated with single-agent ibrutinib in 3 different clinical trials, 36 (10%) had blastoid MCL. Median lines of prior therapy were 2 (range, 1–9). In this analysis, it was shown that overall response rate in blastoid MCL was inferior: 50% compared with 68% in nonblastoid MCL. In addition, PFS, OS, and duration of response were significantly shorter in blastoid MCL compared with nonblastoid MCL (see **Table 1**). After a 4-year median follow-up of a phase II study with ibrutinib and rituximab combination[64] in relapsed MCL, blastoid (n = 7) versus nonblastoid MCL (n = 42) showed an inferior PFS (21 vs 48 months respectively; P = .16) and inferior OS (30 months vs not reached, respectively; P = .15). Response rates were 71% in blastoid versus 91% in nonblastoid MCL (P = .001). Furthermore, the authors have shown that, after a 38-month follow-up after discounting ibrutinib,[37] of the 41 patients who progressed on ibrutinib, 36% had blastoid MCL, indicating the refractoriness to ibrutinib in blastoid MCL variants.

Furthermore, 24-month follow-up on single-agent acalabrutinib[65] in 124 patients was reported: 26 patients (21%) were blastoid MCL. Overall response was similar in blastoid versus nonblastoid MCL (77% vs 82%), complete response rates were 35% and 45% respectively, PFS was 15 versus 25 months, and the duration of response was 14 versus 26 months respectively. Although these data were reported from relapsed patients with MCL, the real impact of BTKi on treatment-naive blastoid MCL is unclear at this time; however, BTKi have shown better efficacy and safety as a nonchemotherapeutic option for patients with blastoid MCL and therefore are a significant advance in managing elderly patients with blastoid MCL or patients with significant comorbidities.

The most recent advance in the treatment of refractory blastoid MCL is the development of anti-CD19 CAR-T therapy (KTE-X19).[66] In patients with refractory large B-cell lymphoma treated with axicabtagene ciloleucel, an autologous anti-CD19 CAR-T therapy containing a CD3ζ T-cell activation domain and CD28 signaling domain, 37% of patients had ongoing responses after 27.1 months of follow-up, and median survival was not yet reached.[67]

KTE-X19 (Brexucabtagene autoleucel) was recently investigated in patients with relapsed/refractory MCL (n = 68) in the ZUMA-2 study, which is a single-arm, international, multicenter, open-label, phase 2 trial, Patients had a median of 3 prior lines of therapy (range, 1–5 lines) and all patients had progressed on BTKi. Data were presented in the 2019 annual American Society of Hematology meeting. Patients were relapsed/refractory MCL (1–5 prior therapies) and all had progressed on BTKi. Patients underwent leukapheresis and conditioning chemotherapy followed by KTE-X19 infusion at a target dose of 2×10^6 CAR-T/kg. Seventeen patients (25%) had blastoid MCL. The overall response rate was 93% in patients with blastoid MCL. Significant responses (>90%) were observed across all high-risk categories of patients with MCL. At a median follow-up of 12.3 months (range, 7.0–32.3 months), 57% of all patients remained in remission. Median duration of response, PFS, and OS were not reached. Common grade 3 or greater adverse events were cytopenias (69%) and infections (32%). There were grade 3 or greater cytokine release syndrome and neurologic events in 15% and 31% of patients, respectively, and none were fatal. CAR-T therapy has further revolutionized the treatment options in blastoid MCL; longer follow-up data from this study would reveal the durability of responses in blastoid MCL. Advances in cellular therapy such as CD19 chimeric antigene receptor natural killer (CAR-NK) cells,[68] humanized binding domain in CD10 CAR-T cells (Hu19-CD828Z),[69] and proposals to combine CAR-T with BTKi and investigate them in the frontline setting are very promising strategies in the treatment of blastoid MCL.

In addition, the role of other agents, such as lenalidomide, bortezomib, and immunotherapies, for treating blastoid MCL remains unclear. Considering the benefit obtained from rituximab maintenance in high-risk MCL,[57] the authors also recommend rituximab maintenance in responding patients with blastoid MCL.

Another challenging question in patients with blastoid MCL is the role of CNS prophylaxis. It is clear from retrospective studies[27,70,71] that there are few baseline high-risk characteristics of patients with MCL (blastoid MCL, very high lactate dehydrogenase levels, high Ki-67%), which predisposes them for CNS involvement and it is known that the outcomes of CNS-MCL are very poor. The role of routine administration of CNS prophylaxis in blastoid MCL is controversial and is not investigated in a prospective randomized study (with/without CNS prophylaxis). Among the 57 patients who developed CNS involvement,[27] 20% had prior intrathecal chemotherapy and 18% had prior R-HCVAD; therefore, these strategies may not completely prevent CNS involvement in MCL. However, considering that almost a third of patients who developed CNS involvement had blastoid MCL, these patients are advised to receive prophylactic intrathecal chemotherapy, and the clinical relevance of CNS prophylaxis in blastoid MCL remains unclear. Another question that further complicates the matter is the relevance of CNS prophylaxis in the era of ibrutinib-based frontline therapies. Ibrutinib has been shown to penetrate the blood-brain barrier[72,73] and therefore the role of CNS prophylaxis in ibrutinib-treated patients with MCL is also unknown. In our frontline study, WINDOW-1,[74] induction treatment with ibrutinib-rituximab followed by 4 cycles of R-HCVAD/rituximab with hyperfractionated cyclophosphamide, vincristine, doxorubicin, and dexamethasone alternating with high-dose methotrexate and cytosine arabinoside was very effective: none of the patients received CNS prophylaxis and 1 patient had CNS relapse.

SUMMARY AND FUTURE DIRECTIONS

Blastoid and pleomorphic variants of MCL are high-risk, poor-prognostic variants of mantle cell lymphoma and these patients continue to pose a therapeutic challenge to treating physicians. These patients rarely achieve durable remissions and prolonged clinical outcome with the currently available chemotherapies and targeted therapies. Dedicated comprehensive studies are urgently needed to delineate their pathobiology and mechanisms of drug resistance, but, because of its rarity, it might take many years to conduct such studies. Therefore, leaders in this field should urgently discuss and reach a consensus to effectively manage these poor-prognostic patients. Although the understanding of these variants has increased, the problem of blastoid MCL is far from over. Certain aspects that require deeper understanding are the intricate relationship of blastoid MCL cells with their microenvironmental milieu (T-cell subsets, architectural patterns of Ki-67–rich areas in lymphoid tissues, FDCs, and macrophages), predisposition to extranodal sites (CNS), homing chemokine/inflammatory cytokine levels, adhesion molecules, genomic and multiomics profiling, epigenetic perturbations, and lymphoid tissue heterogeneity. Moreover, an accurate differentiation of blastoid and pleomorphic variants at cellular and clinical levels is required because the failure-free survival[10] was significantly shorter in pleomorphic variants compared with blastoid variant MCL. Considering the inferior responses to BTKi and venetoclax treatment in relapsed patients with blastoid MCL compared with patients without blastoid MCL, these patients need to be enrolled into clinical trials with newer agents and cellular therapy studies. Therapy options for blastoid MCL are improving and combinatorial approaches with incorporation of next-generation BTKi (LOXO-305) and venetoclax with anti-CD19 CAR-T therapy have a tremendous potential to provide durable and deep remissions in these patients. Detailed molecular analyses of sequential samples in patients with resistant blastoid MCL are required to explore the mutation dynamics and clonal evolution in blastoid MCLs resistant to BTKi, venetoclax, and CAR-T(triple-resistant MCL). The next generation of CAR-T cells, CAR-NK cells, humanized binding domain in CAR-T, and CAR-T against newer antigens (CD22, CD79b, and CD123) are still evolving but these cellular therapies hold great promise for the treatment of patients with blastoid MCL. Data on blastoid MCL, ASCT, and allogenic stem cell transplant are sparse; however, these approaches are used in nonclinical trial settings in conjunction with conventional intensive chemoimmunotherapy, and facility and experience with allogenic SCT is not available at all centers.

In conclusion, blastoid MCL is one of the worst prognostic variants of MCL, showing poor clinical outcomes with currently available therapies. Cellular therapies might bring hope to change the clinical course of this challenging harsh clinical reality. Although these are exciting times in the history of MCL, blastoid MCL remains a huge challenge and comprehensive, collaborative approaches are required to efficiently treat and understand more about blastoid MCL.

DISCLOSURE

P. Jain: none. M. Wang: *stock or othe ownership* in MoreHealth; *honoraria* from Pharmacyclics, Janssen, AstraZeneca/Acerta Pharma, Targeted Oncology, and OMI; *consultancy or advisory role* for Pharmacyclics, Celgene, Janssen, AstraZeneca/Acerta Pharma, MoreHealth, Loxo Oncology, Kite, a Gilead Company, and Pulse Biosciences; *research funding* from Pharmacyclics, Janssen, AstraZeneca/Acerta Pharma, BioInvent, Novartis, Kite, a Gilead Company, Juno, Celgene, Loxo Oncology, and VelosBio; *expert testimony* for AstraZeneca/Acerta Pharma; and *travel support* from Janssen, Pharmacyclics, Celgene, Targeted Oncology, and OMI.

REFERENCES

1. Jain P, Wang M. Mantle cell lymphoma: 2019 update on the diagnosis, pathogenesis, prognostication, and management. Am J Hematol 2019;94(6):710–25.
2. Monga N, Garside J, Quigley J, et al. Systematic literature review of the global burden of illness of mantle cell lymphoma. Curr Med Res Opin 2020;36(5): 843–52.
3. Nadeu F, Martin-Garcia D, Clot G, et al. Genomic and epigenomic insights into the origin, pathogenesis and clinical behavior of mantle cell lymphoma subtypes. Blood 2020. https://doi.org/10.1182/blood.2020005289.
4. Pararajalingam P, Coyle KM, Arthur S, et al. Coding and non-coding drivers of mantle cell lymphoma identified through exome and genome sequencing. Blood 2020. https://doi.org/10.1182/blood.2019002385.
5. Navarro A, Clot G, Royo C, et al. Molecular subsets of mantle cell lymphoma defined by the IGHV mutational status and SOX11 expression have distinct biologic and clinical features. Cancer Res 2012;72(20):5307–16.
6. Ondrejka SL, Lai R, Smith SD, et al. Indolent mantle cell leukemia: a clinicopathological variant characterized by isolated lymphocytosis, interstitial bone marrow involvement, kappa light chain restriction, and good prognosis. Haematologica 2011;96(8):1121–7.
7. Hu Z, Sun Y, Schlette EJ, et al. CD200 expression in mantle cell lymphoma identifies a unique subgroup of patients with frequent IGHV mutations, absence of SOX11 expression, and an indolent clinical course. Mod Pathol 2018;31(2): 327–36.
8. Ye H, Desai A, Zeng D, et al. Smoldering mantle cell lymphoma. J Exp Clin Cancer Res 2017;36(1):185.
9. Bernard M, Gressin R, Lefrere F, et al. Blastic variant of mantle cell lymphoma: a rare but highly aggressive subtype. Leukemia 2001;15(11):1785–91.
10. Jain P, Zhang S, Kanagal-Shamanna R, et al. Genomic profiles and clinical outcomes of de novo blastoid/pleomorphic MCL are distinct from those of transformed MCL. Blood Adv 2020;4(6):1038–50.

11. Hoster E, Rosenwald A, Berger F, et al. Prognostic value of Ki-67 index, cytology, and growth pattern in mantle-cell lymphoma: results from randomized trials of the european mantle cell lymphoma network. J Clin Oncol 2016;34(12):1386–94.

12. Eskelund CW, Dahl C, Hansen JW, et al. TP53 mutations identify younger mantle cell lymphoma patients who do not benefit from intensive chemoimmunotherapy. Blood 2017;130(17):1903–10.

13. Greiner TC, Moynihan MJ, Chan WC, et al. p53 mutations in mantle cell lymphoma are associated with variant cytology and predict a poor prognosis. Blood 1996;87(10):4302–10.

14. Hernandez L, Fest T, Cazorla M, et al. p53 gene mutations and protein overexpression are associated with aggressive variants of mantle cell lymphomas. Blood 1996;87(8):3351–9.

15. Halldorsdottir AM, Lundin A, Murray F, et al. Impact of TP53 mutation and 17p deletion in mantle cell lymphoma. Leukemia 2011;25(12):1904–8.

16. Sarkozy C, Terre C, Jardin F, et al. Complex karyotype in mantle cell lymphoma is a strong prognostic factor for the time to treatment and overall survival, independent of the MCL international prognostic index. Genes Chromosomes Cancer 2014;53(1):106–16.

17. Greenwell IB, Staton AD, Lee MJ, et al. Complex karyotype in patients with mantle cell lymphoma predicts inferior survival and poor response to intensive induction therapy. Cancer 2018;124(11):2306–15.

18. Choe JY, Yun JY, Na HY, et al. MYC overexpression correlates with MYC amplification or translocation, and is associated with poor prognosis in mantle cell lymphoma. Histopathology 2016;68(3):442–9.

19. Royo C, Navarro A, Clot G, et al. Non-nodal type of mantle cell lymphoma is a specific biological and clinical subgroup of the disease. Leukemia 2012;26(8): 1895–8.

20. Cogliatti SB, Bertoni F, Zimmermann DR, et al. IgV H mutations in blastoid mantle cell lymphoma characterize a subgroup with a tendency to more favourable clinical outcome. J Pathol 2005;206(3):320–7.

21. Swerdlow SH, Campo E, Pileri SA, et al. The 2016 revision of the World Health Organization classification of lymphoid neoplasms. Blood 2016;127(20):2375–90.

22. Kimura Y, Sato K, Arakawa F, et al. Mantle cell lymphoma shows three morphological evolutions of classical, intermediate, and aggressive forms, which occur in parallel with increased labeling index of cyclin D1 and Ki-67. Cancer Sci 2010; 101(3):806–14.

23. Schrader C, Meusers P, Brittinger G, et al. Growth pattern and distribution of follicular dendritic cells in mantle cell lymphoma: a clinicopathological study of 96 patients. Virchows Arch 2006;448(2):151–9.

24. Bhatt VR, Loberiza FR Jr, Smith LM, et al. Clinicopathologic features, management and outcomes of blastoid variant of mantle cell lymphoma: a Nebraska Lymphoma Study Group Experience. Leuk Lymphoma 2016;57(6):1327–34.

25. Jain P, Kanagal-Shamanna R, Zhang S, et al. Clinical and genomic characteristics in de novo blastoid/pleomorphic (dnMCL) and transformed blastoid/pleomorphic (t-MCL) mantle cell lymphoma (MCL) in the ibrutinib era: comprehensive analysis of 168 patients. Blood 2018;132(Suppl 1):1599.

26. Kim DH, Medeiros LJ, Aung PP, et al. Mantle cell lymphoma involving skin: a clinicopathologic study of 37 cases. Am J Surg Pathol 2019;43(10):1421–8.

27. Cheah CY, George A, Gine E, et al. Central nervous system involvement in mantle cell lymphoma: clinical features, prognostic factors and outcomes from the European Mantle Cell Lymphoma Network. Ann Oncol 2013;24(8):2119–23.

28. Yin CC, Medeiros LJ, Cromwell CC, et al. Sequence analysis proves clonal identity in five patients with typical and blastoid mantle cell lymphoma. Mod Pathol 2007;20(1):1–7.

29. Tashkandi H, Petrova-Drus K, Batlevi CL, et al. Divergent clonal evolution of a common precursor to mantle cell lymphoma and classic Hodgkin lymphoma. Cold Spring Harb Mol Case Stud 2019;5(6):843–52.

30. Liu Z, Dong HY, Gorczyca W, et al. CD5- mantle cell lymphoma. Am J Clin Pathol 2002;118(2):216–24.

31. Miao Y, Lin P, Saksena A, et al. CD5-negative mantle cell lymphoma: clinicopathologic correlations and outcome in 58 patients. Am J Surg Pathol 2019;43(8):1052–60.

32. Saksena A, Yin CC, Xu J, et al. CD23 expression in mantle cell lymphoma is associated with CD200 expression, leukemic non-nodal form, and a better prognosis. Hum Pathol 2019;89:71–80.

33. Martin-Garcia D, Navarro A, Valdes-Mas R, et al. CCND2 and CCND3 hijack immunoglobulin light-chain enhancers in cyclin D1(-) mantle cell lymphoma. Blood 2019;133(9):940–51.

34. Ott G, Kalla J, Ott MM, et al. Blastoid variants of mantle cell lymphoma: frequent bcl-1 rearrangements at the major translocation cluster region and tetraploid chromosome clones. Blood 1997;89(4):1421–9.

35. Khoury JD, Sen F, Abruzzo LV, et al. Cytogenetic findings in blastoid mantle cell lymphoma. Hum Pathol 2003;34(10):1022–9.

36. Bea S, Valdes-Mas R, Navarro A, et al. Landscape of somatic mutations and clonal evolution in mantle cell lymphoma. Proc Natl Acad Sci U S A 2013;110(45):18250–5.

37. Jain P, Kanagal-Shamanna R, Zhang S, et al. Long-term outcomes and mutation profiling of patients with mantle cell lymphoma (MCL) who discontinued ibrutinib. Br J Haematol 2018;183(4):578–87.

38. Joffe E, Kumar A, Zheng S, et al. Genomic profiling of mantle cell lymphoma suggests poor-risk profile is present at diagnosis and does not arise by tumor evolution. Blood 2019;134(Supplement_1):22.

39. Hu Z, Medeiros LJ, Chen Z, et al. Mantle cell lymphoma With MYC rearrangement: a report of 17 patients. Am J Surg Pathol 2017;41(2):216–24.

40. Zhang L, Yao Y, Zhang S, et al. Metabolic reprogramming toward oxidative phosphorylation identifies a therapeutic target for mantle cell lymphoma. Sci Transl Med 2019;11(491). eaau1167.

41. Kolodziej M, Jesionek-Kupnicka D, Braun M, et al. Classification of aggressive and classic mantle cell lymphomas using synchrotron Fourier Transform Infrared microspectroscopy. Sci Rep 2019;9(1):12857.

42. Jares P, Colomer D, Campo E. Molecular pathogenesis of mantle cell lymphoma. J Clin Invest 2012;122(10):3416–23.

43. Hedstrom E, Eriksson S, Zawacka-Pankau J, et al. p53-dependent inhibition of TrxR1 contributes to the tumor-specific induction of apoptosis by RITA. Cell Cycle 2009;8(21):3584–91.

44. Pinyol M, Hernandez L, Cazorla M, et al. Deletions and loss of expression of p16INK4a and p21Waf1 genes are associated with aggressive variants of mantle cell lymphomas. Blood 1997;89(1):272–80.

45. Chen RW, Bemis LT, Amato CM, et al. Truncation in CCND1 mRNA alters miR-16-1 regulation in mantle cell lymphoma. Blood 2008;112(3):822–9.

46. Slotta-Huspenina J, Koch I, de Leval L, et al. The impact of cyclin D1 mRNA isoforms, morphology and p53 in mantle cell lymphoma: p53 alterations and

blastoid morphology are strong predictors of a high proliferation index. Haematologica 2012;97(9):1422–30.

47. Espel E. The role of the AU-rich elements of mRNAs in controlling translation. Semin Cell Dev Biol 2005;16(1):59–67.

48. Wiestner A, Tehrani M, Chiorazzi M, et al. Point mutations and genomic deletions in CCND1 create stable truncated cyclin D1 mRNAs that are associated with increased proliferation rate and shorter survival. Blood 2007;109(11):4599–606.

49. Zhang H, Chen Z, Miranda RN, et al. Bifurcated BACH2 control coordinates mantle cell lymphoma survival and dispersal during hypoxia. Blood 2017; 130(6):763–76.

50. Rudelius M, Pittaluga S, Nishizuka S, et al. Constitutive activation of Akt contributes to the pathogenesis and survival of mantle cell lymphoma. Blood 2006; 108(5):1668–76.

51. Queiros AC, Beekman R, Vilarrasa-Blasi R, et al. Decoding the DNA methylome of mantle cell lymphoma in the light of the entire B cell lineage. Cancer Cell 2016; 30(5):806–21.

52. Rao E, Jiang C, Ji M, et al. The miRNA-17 approximately 92 cluster mediates chemoresistance and enhances tumor growth in mantle cell lymphoma via PI3K/AKT pathway activation. Leukemia 2012;26(5):1064–72.

53. Husby S, Ralfkiaer U, Garde C, et al. miR-18b overexpression identifies mantle cell lymphoma patients with poor outcome and improves the MIPI-B prognosticator. Blood 2015;125(17):2669–77.

54. Arakawa F, Kimura Y, Yoshida N, et al. Identification of miR-15b as a transformation-related factor in mantle cell lymphoma. Int J Oncol 2016;48(2): 485–92.

55. Khoury JD, Medeiros LJ, Rassidakis GZ, et al. Expression of Mcl-1 in mantle cell lymphoma is associated with high-grade morphology, a high proliferative state, and p53 overexpression. J Pathol 2003;199(1):90–7.

56. Hermine O, Hoster E, Walewski J, et al. Addition of high-dose cytarabine to immunochemotherapy before autologous stem-cell transplantation in patients aged 65 years or younger with mantle cell lymphoma (MCL Younger): a randomised, open-label, phase 3 trial of the European Mantle Cell Lymphoma Network. Lancet 2016;388(10044):565–75.

57. Kluin-Nelemans HC, Hoster E, Hermine O, et al. Treatment of Older Patients with Mantle-Cell Lymphoma. N Engl J Med 2012;367(6):520–31.

58. Dreyling M, Klapper W, Rule S. Blastoid and pleomorphic mantle cell lymphoma: still a diagnostic and therapeutic challenge! Blood 2018;132(26):2722–9.

59. Kluin-Nelemans HC, Hoster E, Hermine O, et al. Treatment of older patients with mantle cell lymphoma (MCL): long-term follow-up of the randomized european MCL elderly trial. J Clin Oncol 2020;38(3):248–56.

60. Geisler CH, Kolstad A, Laurell A, et al. Nordic MCL2 trial update: six-year followup after intensive immunochemotherapy for untreated mantle cell lymphoma followed by BEAM or BEAC + autologous stem-cell support: still very long survival but late relapses do occur. Br J Haematol 2012;158(3):355–62.

61. Eskelund CW, Kolstad A, Jerkeman M, et al. 15-year follow-up of the Second Nordic Mantle Cell Lymphoma trial (MCL2): prolonged remissions without survival plateau. Br J Haematol 2016;175(3):410–8.

62. Romaguera JE, Fayad L, Rodriguez MA, et al. High rate of durable remissions after treatment of newly diagnosed aggressive mantle-cell lymphoma with rituximab plus hyper-CVAD alternating with rituximab plus high-dose methotrexate and cytarabine. J Clin Oncol 2005;23(28):7013–23.

63. Rule S, Dreyling M, Goy A, et al. Outcomes in 370 patients with mantle cell lymphoma treated with ibrutinib: a pooled analysis from three open-label studies. Br J Haematol 2017;179(3):430–8.

64. Jain P, Romaguera J, Srour SA, et al. Four-year follow-up of a single arm, phase II clinical trial of ibrutinib with rituximab (IR) in patients with relapsed/refractory mantle cell lymphoma (MCL). Br J Haematol 2018;182(3):404–11.

65. Wang M, Rule S, Zinzani PL, et al. Durable response with single-agent acalabrutinib in patients with relapsed or refractory mantle cell lymphoma. Leukemia 2019;33(11):2762–6.

66. Wang M, Munoz J, Goy A, et al. KTE-X19 CAR T-Cell Therapy in Relapsed or Refractory Mantle-Cell Lymphoma. N Engl J Med 2020;382(14):1331–42.

67. Locke FL, Ghobadi A, Jacobson CA, et al. Long-term safety and activity of axicabtagene ciloleucel in refractory large B-cell lymphoma (ZUMA-1): a single-arm, multicentre, phase 1-2 trial. Lancet Oncol 2019;20(1):31–42.

68. Liu E, Marin D, Banerjee P, et al. Use of CAR-Transduced Natural Killer Cells in CD19-Positive Lymphoid Tumors. N Engl J Med 2020;382(6):545–53.

69. Brudno JN, Lam N, Vanasse D, et al. Safety and feasibility of anti-CD19 CAR T cells with fully human binding domains in patients with B-cell lymphoma. Nat Med 2020;26(2):270–80.

70. Chihara D, Asano N, Ohmachi K, et al. Ki-67 is a strong predictor of central nervous system relapse in patients with mantle cell lymphoma (MCL). Ann Oncol 2015;26(5):966–73.

71. Ferrer A, Bosch F, Villamor N, et al. Central nervous system involvement in mantle cell lymphoma. Ann Oncol 2008;19(1):135–41.

72. Bernard S, Goldwirt L, Amorim S, et al. Activity of ibrutinib in mantle cell lymphoma patients with central nervous system relapse. Blood 2015;126(14):1695–8.

73. Lionakis MS, Dunleavy K, Roschewski M, et al. Inhibition of B Cell Receptor Signaling by Ibrutinib in Primary CNS Lymphoma. Cancer Cell 2017;31(6):833–43.e5.

74. Wang M, Jain P, Zhang S, et al. Ibrutinib with rituximab (ir) and short course r-hypercvad/mtx is very efficacious in previously untreated young pts with mantle cell lymphoma (MCL). Hematol Oncol 2019;37(S2):42–3.

75. Romaguera JE, Fayad LE, Feng L, et al. Ten-year follow-up after intense chemoimmunotherapy with Rituximab-HyperCVAD alternating with Rituximab-high dose methotrexate/cytarabine (R-MA) and without stem cell transplantation in patients with untreated aggressive mantle cell lymphoma. Br J Haematol 2010;150(2):200–8.

76. Chihara D, Cheah CY, Westin JR, et al. Rituximab plus hyper-CVAD alternating with MTX/Ara-C in patients with newly diagnosed mantle cell lymphoma: 15-year follow-up of a phase II study from the MD Anderson Cancer Center. Br J Haematol 2016;172(1):80–8.

77. Geisler CH, Kolstad A, Laurell A, et al. Long-term progression-free survival of mantle cell lymphoma after intensive front-line immunochemotherapy with in vivo-purged stem cell rescue: a nonrandomized phase 2 multicenter study by the Nordic Lymphoma Group. Blood 2008;112(7):2687–93.

78. Damon LE, Johnson JL, Niedzwiecki D, et al. Immunochemotherapy and autologous stem-cell transplantation for untreated patients with mantle-cell lymphoma: CALGB 59909. J Clin Oncol 2009;27(36):6101–8.

79. Merryman RW, Edwin N, Redd R, et al. Rituximab/bendamustine and rituximab/cytarabine induction therapy for transplant-eligible mantle cell lymphoma. Blood Adv 2020;4(5):858–67.

Allogeneic Transplantation and Chimeric Antigen Receptor-Engineered T-Cell Therapy for Relapsed or Refractory Mantle Cell Lymphoma

Jordan Gauthier, MD, MSc[a,b,c,]*, David G. Maloney, MD, PhD[a,b,c]

KEYWORDS

- Mantle cell lymphoma • Allogeneic hematopoietic cell transplantation
- CAR-T cell therapy

KEY POINTS

- Ibrutinib treatment is a feasible and promising bridge to allogeneic hematopoietic cell transplantation (allo-HCT) for relapsed and refractory mantle cell lymphoma (MCL).
- Patients with MCL at high risk of short duration of response on ibrutinib (high MCL Lymphoma International Prognostic Index, high Ki67 index, blastoid variant, >2 lines of prior therapies) should be considered for an allo-HCT.
- Compared to HLA-matched allo-HCT, Haploidentical reduced-intensity conditioning allo-HCT with posttransplant cyclophosphamide are associated with comparable outcomes in patients with relapsed or refractory MCL.
- Preliminary data from the ZUMA-1 and the TRANSCEND-NHL-001 pivotal trials suggest high efficacy of CD19-targeted chimeric antigen receptor-engineered T-cell therapy for relapsed or refractory MCL after ibrutinib failure, which may challenge the role of allo-HCT.

INTRODUCTION

Mantle cell lymphoma (MCL) is a rare entity accounting for fewer than 10% of non-Hodgkin lymphoma worldwide.[1] MCL is more frequent in older patients with a median age of 60 at diagnosis, and is molecularly defined by the t(11;14) translocation. Poor prognostic factors, allowing calculation of the MCL Lymphoma International Prognostic Index[2] (MIPI), include age, Eastern Cooperative Oncology Group (ECOG)

[a] Clinical Research Division, Fred Hutchinson Cancer Research Center, 1100 Fairview Ave. N., Mail Stop D3-100, Seattle, WA 98109, USA; [b] Integrated Immunotherapy Research Center, Fred Hutchinson Cancer Research Center, Seattle, WA, USA; [c] Department of Medicine, University of Washington, Seattle, WA, USA
* Corresponding author.
E-mail address: jgauthier@fredhutch.org
Twitter: @drjgauthier (J.G.)

Hematol Oncol Clin N Am 34 (2020) 957–970
https://doi.org/10.1016/j.hoc.2020.06.010
hemonc.theclinics.com

performance status, lactate dehydrogenase serum concentration, white blood cell count, and the Ki-67 proliferation index. Patients with a high MIPI (≥6.2) have an estimated median overall survival (OS) of 37 months. Patients with the blastoid variant of MCL have a poor prognosis, with an estimated median OS of only 14 months.[3]

Despite the benefits of maintenance rituximab after autologous hematopoietic cell transplantation (auto-HCT) with an estimated 4-year progression-free survival (PFS) of 83%,[4] a significant subset of patient may not be transplant eligible; others will be refractory to front-line therapy or will relapse after auto-HCT. High rates of durable responses have been reported after ibrutinib treatment with or without rituximab in patients with relapsed and refractory (R/R) MCL[5–7] (overall response rates [ORR], 68% to 88%, median duration of response, 17.5 to 22 months), yet responses can be short-lived in patients with blastoid variant MCL, high MIPI, or high Ki-67 proliferation. Receiving ibrutinib later in the course of the disease is also associated with shorter duration of response; in patients responding to ibrutinib after their second line of treatment but not reaching a complete response (CR), the median duration of response was 8 months.[8] Prognosis is poor in patients with progressive disease after treatment with Bruton tyrosine kinase (BTK) inhibitors, with a median OS of 3 to 8 months on ibrutinib discontinuation.[9,10]

In the R/R and ibrutinib-refractory setting, allogeneic HCT (allo-HCT) remains the only treatment associated with long-term remissions and potential cure. In the first section of this article, we review the studies attempting to clarify the ideal timing of allo-HCT for R/R MCL. We will also inspect the comparative data investigating the role of conditioning intensity. In addition, we review the factors predictive of posttransplant outcomes, which can be useful to consider when referring patients for an allo-HCT. Next, we highlight some recent progress in the allo-HCT field, in particular the use of T-cell-replete haploidentical grafts with posttransplant cyclophosphamide (HAPLO PT-Cy). In spite of these advances, approximately 30% of patients with MCL will still relapse after allo-HCT. Moreover, the procedure remains limited by significant treatment-related mortality, which is largely due to graft-versus-host disease (GVHD) and infections.

In the second section, we discuss a novel promising approach using chimeric antigen receptor-engineered T (CAR-T) cells for R/R MCL. High rates of durable responses have been reported after CD19-targeted CAR-T cell therapy in patients with relapsed or refractory B-cell malignancies. This led to the recent approval by the Food and Drug Administration (FDA) of 2 commercial CD19-targeted CAR-T cell products for R/R large B-cell lymphoma. We review the preliminary safety and efficacy data of 2 pivotal clinical trials investigating the use of CD19 CAR-T cells for R/R MCL specifically. Last, we highlight ongoing clinical trials of CAR-T cell therapy aiming at antigens beyond the CD19 target.

ALLOGENEIC HEMATOPOIETIC STEM CELL TRANSPLANTATION FOR RELAPSED AND REFRACTORY MANTEL CELL LYMPHOMA

Evidence of a plateau in the PFS curves several years post allo-HCT suggest that MCL is sensitive to graft-versus-lymphoma (GVL) activity. In some patients this is associated with long-term disease control. The existence of a GVL effect is also strongly supported by the association between chronic GVHD and a lower risk of posttransplant relapse in patients with MCL.[11] Tempering its potential benefits, treatment-related or nonrelapse mortality and extensive chronic GVHD remain significant limitations of allo-HCT. Although guidelines have been proposed,[12,13] there is to date no firm consensus as to the indication, timing, and conditioning intensity of allo-HCT for MCL.

In the following section we review the optimal timing of allo-HCT relative to auto-HCT and ibrutinib treatment in patients with R/R MCL. Next, we discuss the role of conditioning intensity before allo-HCT, the factors impacting posttransplant outcomes, and the use of HAPLO PT-Cy allo-HCT.

Timing of Allogeneic Hematopoietic Stem Cell Transplantation for Relapsed and Refractory Mantel Cell Lymphoma

Prospective randomized trials comparing front-line auto-HCT with or without maintenance rituximab to allo-HCT in MCL are lacking, and most published studies consist of retrospective analyses of single center or registry data; most of these studies also pre-date the use of post-auto-HCT maintenance rituximab and the approval of BTK inhibitors. In 2009, Tam and colleagues[14] from the MD Anderson Cancer Center compared the outcomes of patients receiving an auto-HCT in first remission (n = 50) or in the R/R setting (n = 36), or after a non-myeloablative (NMA) allo-HCT in the R/R setting (n = 35). The investigators reported that long-term disease-free survival, after a median follow-up of 6 years, was only achieved in the following groups: (1) after auto-HCT in first remission with a rituximab-containing conditioning regimen; and (2) in the R/R setting after NMA allo-HCT. Fenske and colleagues[15] attempted to characterize the optimal timing of HCT by examining the data from 519 patients with MCL in the Center for International Blood and Marrow Transplant Research (CIBMTR) registry. Overall, they observed favorable outcomes after auto-HCT and reduced-intensity conditioning (RIC) allo-HCT when performed in first remission (5-year relapse probability, 32% and 15%, respectively). Using a time-dependent multivariable Cox model, they predicted in the early HCT cohort increased short-term mortality (within 2 years from diagnosis) after allo-HCT compared with auto-HCT (hazard ratio [HR] 4.69; 95% confidence interval [CI] 2.55–8.62, $P<.001$), while the effect on long-term mortality was undetermined (HR 0.63; 95% CI 0.25–1.57, $P = .32$). Compared with late RIC allo-HCT, early RIC allo-HCT was associated with higher short-term mortality (HR 2.34; 95% CI 1.17–4.70; $P = .02$), but lower long-term mortality (HR 0.31; 95% CI 0.12–0.81; $P = .02$). The investigators concluded that auto-HCT should remain the preferred option for patients with MCL in first remission.

Others hypothesized that early allo-HCT in first remission might only benefit patients with high-risk MCL and at low risk of treatment-related mortality, for example, younger patients without comorbidities. This approach has been evaluated prospectively by Rule and colleagues[8]; they reported the outcomes of 25 patients treated with BEAM-Campath-conditioned matched-related donor (MRD) or matched-unrelated donors (MUD) allo-HCT on a multicenter phase II trial. Patients were required to have had at least a partial response to their initial therapy. After a median follow-up of 60.5 months, the PFS and OS were 68% and 80% at 2 years, and 56% and 76% at 5 years. The investigators did not observe treatment-related mortality events by day 100. The results from this very small study suggest front-line BEAM-Campath allo-HCT is feasible in a highly selected population. Yet, validated predictive tools are lacking to identify patients likely to benefit from an upfront allo-HCT and this approach cannot be routinely recommended.

A key and unanswered question for the field is the following: what is the best timing of allo-HCT relative to treatment with ibrutinib? Although ibrutinib can lead to prolonged responses in patients with MCL, data suggest a very poor prognosis after disease progression on ibrutinib.[9,10] This suggests ibrutinib could be used as a bridge to allo-HCT, but the timing of transplantation while responding to ibrutinib remains difficult to identify. Dreger and colleagues[16] from the European Bone Marrow Transplant Society and the Lymphoma Working Party, investigated the safety and feasibility of pretransplant ibrutinib treatment in 22 patients with MCL. They speculated that the immune-modifying properties of ibrutinib might impact the GVL/GVHD effects. RIC was used in 73% of patients, whereas 27% received myeloablative conditioning (MAC) followed by a matched-related (27%) or unrelated (68%) allo-HCT. The 1-year TRM, relapse rate, PFS, and OS were 5%, 19%, 76%, and 86%, respectively. Prior ibrutinib failure was associated with significantly worse PFS (HR 0.03; 95% CI 0.04–0.26). Only 1 relapse was observed in the 16 ibrutinib-sensitive patients, with a 1-year PFS probability of 90%. The investigators concluded that ibrutinib could be a promising bridging strategy before a RIC allo-HCT if used before frank disease progression.

Choice of Conditioning Intensity Before Allogeneic Hematopoietic Stem Cell Transplantation in Patients with Mantel Cell Lymphoma

Conditioning intensity is a double-edged sword: MAC being invariably associated with fewer relapses but at the price of higher treatment-related mortality. Conversely, RIC or non-myeloablative conditioning (NMA) is better tolerated, but associated with higher relapse rates after allo-HCT. To further investigate the impact of conditioning intensity on post-allo-HCT outcomes in MCL, Kharfan-Dabaja and colleagues[17] performed a meta-analysis of 16 studies including a total of 710 patients. Importantly, many of these studies were single-arm cohorts with high heterogeneity across studies. Despite higher relapse rates after RIC allo-HCT (pooled rates, 29%; 95% CI 17%–43%) compared with MAC (pooled rates, 18%; 95% CI 3%–42%), the investigators estimated higher OS (53%; 95% CI 39%–67% vs 40%; 95% CI 28%–52%, respectively) and PFS (47%; 95% CI 32%–61% vs 34%; 95% CI 21%–50%) after RIC compared with MAC allo-HCT. MAC was associated with lower relapses rates after allo-HCT, but this was offset by the increased TRM compared with RIC allo-HCT (37%; 95% CI 23%–51% vs 24%; 95% CI 16%–33%, respectively). Although meta-analyses cannot replace randomized phase III trials, this study strongly suggests a potential survival advantage of RIC over MAC allo-HCT in MCL. Nevertheless, relapse rates post RIC allo-HCT remain high, stressing the need for complementary (eg, incorporating novel agents in the conditioning regimen, bridging therapies, maintenance therapy post RIC allo-HCT), or alternative therapeutic strategies. The feasibility of maintenance rituximab after allo-HCT has been reported,[18] but its role in preventing relapse remains unclear in the absence of controlled data.

Predictive Factors of Outcomes After Allogeneic Hematopoietic Stem Cell Transplantation for Mantel Cell Lymphoma

Prognostic factors could help us identify patients with MCL with a higher probability of benefiting from an allo-HCT. Unfortunately, robust multivariable modeling has been limited by small sample sizes, and most identified factors failed to replicate across independent cohorts.

We have previously reported promising long-term outcomes after allo-HCT following NMA conditioning with fludarabine and low-dose (2 Gy) total body irradiation in 70 patients with R/R MCL treated at the at the Fred Hutchinson Cancer Research Center.[19,20] Grafts were obtained from most HLA-matched-related (47%) or unrelated donors (41%). At the time of allo-HCT the median age was 57, 43% of patients had significant comorbidities with an HCT-CI ≥3, 36% had progressive disease (refractory or with untreated relapse), and bulky disease (≥5 cm) was observed in 17%. Forty percent had previously received an auto-HCT. The 5-year OS and PFS probabilities were 55% and 46%, respectively. The 5-year incidence of treatment-related mortality (TRM) was 28% and the relapse rate was

26%. Using multivariable regression, R/R disease at the time of allo-HCT was associated with relapse (HR 2.94; 95% CI 1.0–8.7). A high-risk cytomegalovirus (CMV) status (HR 2.02; 95% CI 1.0–4.3) and a low CD3+ dose ($<3 \times 10^8$/kg) predicted worse OS (HR 2.32; 95% CI 1.1–4.8).

Investigators at the Memorial Sloan Kettering Cancer Center conducted univariate analyses of outcomes to identify prognostic factors in 29 patients undergoing NMA or RIC allo-HCT for MCL. In a first report,[21] it was noted that both in vivo T-cell depletion with alemtuzumab and a second-line IPI ≥1 predicted worse PFS after allo-HCT. In a more recent publication from the same group,[22] the investigators observed comparable relapse rates regardless of the presence of absence of *TP53* alterations – suggesting allo-HCT might overcome its negative impact.

In a large registry study (n = 106) from the French Society of Bone Marrow Transplantation and Cellular Therapy, pretransplant disease status (partial versus complete response, stable or progressive disease vs CR) was the main factor associated with worse PFS and OS after RIC allo-HCT for MCL after auto-HCT failure.

In summary, pretransplant disease status remains the key determinant of post-allo-HCT outcomes. Ibrutinib appears to be a promising bridge to allo-HCT in MCL, with very favorable outcomes in ibrutinib-sensitive patients. These factors should be considered when evaluating a patient with R/R MCL for allo-HCT.

Haploidentical Grafts with Posttransplant Cyclophosphamide Reduced-Intensity Conditioning Allogeneic Hematopoietic Stem Cell Transplantation for Relapsed and Refractory Mantel Cell Lymphoma

The lack of an HLA-matched donor in a large subset of patients sparked the development of transplant modalities using alternative graft sources. A promising approach, pioneered by investigators at Johns Hopkins and our institution,[23] involves the use of haploidentical related donor with the administration of high-dose posttransplant cyclophosphamide (HAPLO PT-CY) to prevent GVHD. Two large retrospective studies from the CIBMTR compared HAPLO PT-CY RIC allo-HCT MRD,[24] and to MUD RIC allo-HCT with or without anti-thymocyte globulin[25] (ATG) in patients with relapsed or refractory lymphoma. Patients with MCL made for only 12% (n = 21) of the HAPLO cohort, 14% (n = 113) of the MRD cohort, and 16% (n = 118) of the MUD cohort. In a subgroup analysis restricted to patients with MCL, the investigators estimated comparable 3-year OS and PFS after HAPLO compared with MRD allo-HCT (60% vs 57%, P = .80, and 51% vs 43%, P = .47, respectively). When adjusting for key disease, patient, and transplant-related baseline characteristics (eg, lymphoma type, chemosensitivity, HCT-CI), the independent effect of HAPLO PT-Cy on OS and PFS compared with MRD was undetermined (HR 0.98, 0.77–1.23; HR 1.14, 0.87–1.49). There was a trend toward higher NRM (HR 1.52; 95% CI 0.99–2.34), and lower relapse rates (HR 0.80; 95% CI 0.61–1.04) associated with HAPLO PT-Cy compared with MRD. The 1-year cumulative incidence of chronic GVHD was significantly lower after HAPLO PT-Cy allo-HCT compared with MRD (12% vs 45%; P<.001), and this benefit was confirmed in multivariable analysis (HR 0.21; 95% CI 0.14–0.31; P<.001). Taken together, these results suggest comparable or higher GVL effect with lower risk of chronic GVHD after HAPLO PT RIC allo-HCT compared with MRD. Compared with MUD with or without ATG, the investigators estimated similar or higher 3-year OS and PFS in patients with MCL after HAPLO (OS, 49% and 54% vs 60%, P = .76; PFS, 33% and 41% vs 51%, P = .46, respectively). The independent effect on OS and PFS of HAPLO PT-Cy compared with MUD with or without ATG was also undetermined using multivariable regression in the entire dataset adjusting for lymphoma type and other relevant covariates. There was a trend toward higher NRM in MUD with ATG compared with HAPLO PT-Cy (HR 1.54; 95% CI 0.98–2.4), and also toward lower relapse rates with MUD without ATG compared with HAPLO (HR 0.8; 95% CI 0.59–1.08). In the entire dataset including all lymphoma types, the 1-year cumulative incidence of chronic GVHD at 1 year after HAPLO allo-HCT was 13% (95% CI 8–18) compared with 51% (95% CI 46–55) in MUD without ATG, and 33% (95% CI 27–39) in URD with ATG (P<.001). Multivariable analysis showed a higher risk of chronic GVHD in the recipients of MUD allo-HCT without ATG (HR 5.85; 95% CI 3.96–8.64; P<.0001) and MUD allo-HCT with ATG (HR 3.64; 95% CI 2.37–5.60; P<.0001).

According to a search on the clinicaltrial.gov Web site, there is currently no phase III randomized trial comparing HAPLO to MRD or MUD specifically for patients with lymphoma. The results of the BMT CTN 1101 study (NCT01597778), which compared HAPLO PT-Cy to double umbilical cord blood RIC allo-HCT in patients with refractory hematologic malignancies including MCL, have not, to our knowledge, been reported.

Although randomized data are needed to confirm the equivalence or superiority of HAPLO over HLA-matched donors, comparable "crude" outcomes were observed in terms of OS and PFS in several retrospective studies, with significantly lower rates of chronic GVHD in patients receiving a HAPLO PT-Cy RIC allo-HCT. Tied to the role of the graft source is the impact of PT-Cy outside of the HAPLO setting. The BMT CTN 1703/1801 study (NCT03959241) was designed to address this question. This study, currently enrolling patients with relapsed or refractory hematologic malignancies, is a randomized, phase III, multicenter trial comparing 2 GVHD prophylaxis regimens: tacrolimus/methotrexate versus PT-Cy/tacrolimus/mycophenolate mofetil in the setting of (RIC) allo-HCT with peripheral blood stem cell grafts.

CHIMERIC ANTIGEN RECEPTOR-ENGINEERED T-CELL THERAPY FOR RELAPSED AND REFRACTORY MANTEL CELL LYMPHOMA

We previously reported an early efficacy signal in patients with MCL treated on a phase I/II trial of CD19-targeted CAR-T cell therapy of defined composition.[26] Since this report, 2 CD19-targeted CAR-T cell products, axicabtagene ciloleucel (axi-cel) and tisagenlecleucel, have been approved by the FDA for the treatment of relapsed or refractory aggressive large B-cell lymphoma after 2 lines of therapy based on the results of the ZUMA-1[27,28] and JULIET[29] trials. Another CD19-targeted CAR-T cell product, lisacabtagene maraleucel (liso-cel or JCAR017), developed based on preliminary work performed at our institution,[26,30,31] is anticipated to be approved by the FDA in the near future in approximately the same indications based on the results of the TRANSCEND-NHL-001 trial.[32] Although these 3 products have similarities, key distinctive features should be highlighted: first, the axi-cel transgene includes the CD28 costimulatory domain. CD28 costimulation is associated with potent cytotoxic function, and interleukin-2 production, but potentially shorter in vivo persistence. In contrast, tisagenlecleucel and liso-cel CARs contain the 4-1BB costimulatory domain. 4-1BB costimulation has been described to stimulate CD8+ central memory T-cell generation and to favor CAR-T cell persistence.[33]

There is to date no FDA-approved CAR-T cell product for R/R MCL. We review in the following sections the preliminary results of 2 ongoing pivotal clinical trials that showed promise with high rates of durable responses in patients with R/R MCL (**Fig. 1**). Last, we discuss other CAR-T cell therapies currently being evaluated in phase I trials.

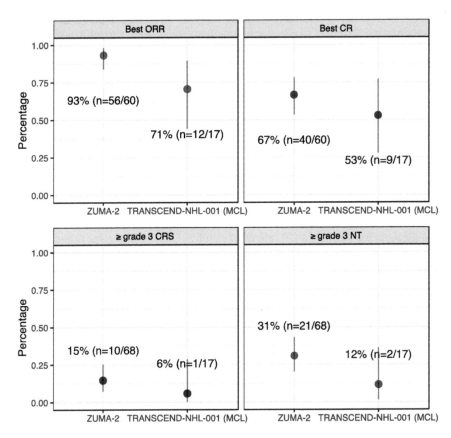

Fig. 1. Summary of the preliminary efficacy and toxicity data of 2 pivotal trials of CD19 CAR-T cell therapy for R/R MCL after ibrutinib failure. The ZUMA-2 data were obtained from the oral presentation by Wang and colleagues at the 2019 American Society of Hematology annual meeting (efficacy data, n = 60; toxicity analysis, n = 68; all patients received 2×10^6 KTE-X19 cells/kg). The TRANSCEND-NHL-001 data were obtained from the poster presentation by Wang and colleagues at the 2019 ASCO annual meeting (efficacy and toxicity analysis, n = 17, patients were treated at 2 dose levels: 50×10^6 CAR-T cells, n = 6; 100×10^6 CAR-T cells, n = 11). Vertical bars represent 95% CIs computed using the Copper-Pearson method. NT, neurologic toxicity.

KTE-X19 (ZUMA-2 Trial)

The CD19-targeted CAR-T cell product KTE-X19, which uses the same CAR trans-gene as axicabtagene ciloleucel (Yescarta) with a distinct cell manufacturing process, is being investigated in a phase 2, pivotal, multicenter ZUMA-2 study in patients with R/R MCL (NCT02601313). Preliminary results were presented at the 2019 American Society of Hematology annual meeting with a data cutoff on July 24, 2019.[34] Patients with MCL with progressive disease or stable disease after prior therapies were eligible. Prior therapies must have included an anthracycline or bendamustine-containing chemotherapy and an anti-CD20 monoclonal antibody therapy, and ibrutinib or aca-labrutinib. Patients with an ECOG performance status of 0 or 1, ALC $\geq$100 were included. Key exclusion criteria were prior allo-HCT, prior CD19-targeted therapy, prior CAR-T cell therapy, history of current central nervous system (CNS) involvement by MCL or other CNS disorders. Patients received lymphodepletion chemotherapy with fludarabine 30 mg/m^2/d with cyclophosphamide 500 mg/m^2/d for 3 days followed by the infusion of 2 × 10^6 KTE-X19 cells/kg. The primary endpoint was best ORR. KTE-X19 was successfully manufactured in 71 patients (96%) and administered to 68 (92%). The primary efficacy analysis was performed on the first 60 treated patient per protocol, while the safety analysis was conducted on all infused patients (n = 68). The median age was 65%, 85% of patients had stage IV disease, 56% an intermediate or high MIPI. Bone marrow involvement and extranodal disease were reported in 54% and 56% of patients, respectively. *TP53* mutation was reported in 17% of patients, while blastoid variant morphology was present in 25%. The median number of prior therapies was 3, with 81% having received ≥3 lines of therapies, and 56% were primary refractory to BTK inhibitors. Bridging therapy after leukapheresis was allowed with dexamethasone, ibrutinib, or acalabrutinib, and was used in 37% of patients.

In the 60 patients evaluated for response, the ORR after independent review was 93% (95% CI 84–98) with a CR rate of 67% (95% CI 53–78). Similar to the ZUMA-1 data, 24 (40%) of 60 patients converted from a PR/SD to a CR. Responses were durable, and the median duration of response was not reached after a median follow-up of 12.3 months; the estimated PFS was 57% in all responders and 78% in CR patients. The median OS and PFS were not reached in all 60 patients. Two grade 5 adverse events were reported (organizing pneumonia at day 37, and staphylococcal sepsis at day 134). Any grade cytokine release syndrome (CRS) was reported in 91% of patients, and 15% developed severe ≥ grade 3 CRS using the Lee and colleagues 2014 consensus criteria.[35] Median time to CRS onset was 2 days (range, 1–13). CRS was prolonged in many patients with a median duration of 11 days. Neurologic toxicity was also significant with 63% of patients developing any grade neurologic symptoms, including 31% of grade ≥3 events. One patient developed grade 4 cerebral edema, requiring intubation and treated with aggressive therapies including high-dose steroids, intrathecal cytarabine, ventriculostomy and IV ATG. This led to complete resolution of the neurotoxicity, and this patient remains in CR 24 months after CAR-T cell infusion. Overall, the investigator did not report any grade 5 CRS or neurologic toxicity. In line with previous reports in patients with aggressive lymphoma, higher CAR-T cell counts in the peripheral blood measured by flow cytometry were associated with both response,[28] higher severity of CRS,[36] and higher severity of neurologic toxicity.[27,36] The toxicity profile and kinetics of KTE-X19 were comparable to the ZUMA-1 data with axi-cel[27,28]; CRS and neurologic toxicity were common complications of KTE-X19 treatment, most events occurred early and were reversible in all cases. Yet CRS and neurologic toxicities were severe in a significant portion of patients. Given the extremely promising efficacy data, we anticipate in the future the approval by the FDA of KTE-X19 for R/R MCL. Further follow-up is mandated to better assess response durability.

Lisocabtagene Maraleucel (TRANSCEND-NHL-001 Trial)

Another CD19-targeted CAR-T cell product, liso-cel, is under investigation for patients with R/R MCL in the ongoing phase I/II TRANSCEND-NHL-001 trial (NCT02631044). In contrast with KTE-X19, JCAR017 is formulated with a 1:1 ratio of CD8+:CD4+ CAR-T cells, while KTE-X19 contains bulk CAR-T cells with a variable ratio of CD8+:CD4+. A preliminary analysis of the phase I data was reported at the 2019 American Society of Clinical Oncology (ASCO) annual meeting.[37] The main eligibility criteria were as follows: ≥1 line of prior therapy, ECOG performance

Table 1
List of active or recruiting clinical trials of chimeric antigen receptor-engineered T-cell immunotherapy enrolling patients with mantle cell lymphoma

National Cancer Institute ID	Study Title	Investigational Product Name	Phase	Status
NCT02601313	A Phase 2 Multicenter Study Evaluating Subjects With Relapsed/Refractory Mantle Cell Lymphoma	KTE-X19	Phase 2	Active, not recruiting
NCT00924326	CAR T Cell Receptor Immunotherapy for Patients With B-cell Lymphoma	CD19-CAR PBL + aldesleukin	Phase 1/2	Active, not recruiting
NCT03185494	Treatment of Relapsed and/or Chemotherapy Refractory B-cell Malignancy by Tandem CAR T Cells Targeting CD19 and CD22	anti-CD19/22-CAR vector-transduced T cells	Phase 1/2	Active, not recruiting
NCT04186520	CAR-20/19-T Cells in Patients With Relapsed Refractory B-Cell Malignancies	CAR-20/19-T Cells	Phase 1/2	Not yet recruiting
NCT04223765	Study of Kappa Chimeric Antigen Receptor (CAR) T Lymphocytes Co-Expressing the Kappa and CD28 CARs for Relapsed/Refractory Kappa + Non-Hodgkin Lymphoma	CAR.k.28	Phase 1	Not yet recruiting
NCT04176913	Study of LUCAR-20S in Patients With R/R NHL	LUCAR-20S CAR-T cells	Phase 1	Recruiting
NCT03676504	Treatment of Patients With Relapsed or Refractory CD19+ Lymphoid Disease With T Cells Expressing a Third-generation CAR	CD19.CAR T Cells	Phase 1/2	Recruiting
NCT02706392	Genetically Modified T-Cell Therapy in Treating Patients With Advanced ROR1+ Malignancies	ROR1 CAR-specific Autologous T-Lymphocytes	Phase 1	Recruiting
NCT04184414	The Clinical Application of Chimeric Antigen Receptor T Cells in the Treatment of CD19 Positive Recurrent Refractory B-Cell-derived Hematological Malignancies	CD19-CART	Phase 1	Recruiting
NCT04049513	ENABLE (Engaging Toll-like Receptor Signaling for B-cell Lymphoma Chimeric Antigen Receptor Therapy)	WZTL002-1 (1928T2z CAR-T cells)	Phase 1	Recruiting

(continued on next page)

| Table 1 *(continued)* | | | | |
National Cancer Institute ID	Study Title	Investigational Product Name	Phase	Status
NCT03097770	Treatment of Relapsed and/or Chemotherapy Refractory B-cell Malignancy by Tandem CAR T Cells Targeting CD19 and CD20	anti-CD19/20-CAR vector-transduced T cells	Phase 1/2	Recruiting
NCT04007029	Modified Immune Cells (CD19/CD20 CAR-T Cells) in Treating Patients With Recurrent or Refractory B-Cell Lymphoma or Chronic Lymphocytic Leukemia	Chimeric Antigen Receptor T-Cell Therapy	Phase 1	Recruiting

Data from the clinicaltrial.gov database; query date, February 6th, 2020

status ≤ 2. Patients with a history of auto-HCT or allo-HCT and those with secondary CNS involvement were still eligible. Enrolled subjects received lymphodepletion chemotherapy with fludarabine 30 mg/m^2 per day and cyclophosphamide 300 mg/m^2 per day for 3 days before liso-cel infusion. Of 25 enrolled patients and leukapheresed, 17 (68%) received liso-cel and were evaluable for safety analysis (1 patient who received a nonconforming liso-cel product was excluded from the analysis). Two doses were evaluated: 50 × 10^6 CAR-T cells (DL1, n = 6), or 100 × 10^6 CAR-T cells (DL2, n = 11). Of note, the latter dose was previously selected for the dose expansion stage in the other cohorts of this trial. The median age was 66, and the median number of prior therapies was 4, including ibrutinib and venetoclax in 94% and 12% of patients, respectively. Ibrutinib refractoriness was reported in 7 patients (41%). Ten patients (59%) received bridging chemotherapy between leukapheresis and CAR-T cell infusion. The toxicity profile was favorable; overall 7 patients developed CRS (41%), 6 having received DL2. The median time to CRS onset was 7 days (range, 2–10) and the median time to resolution was 4 days (range, 2–8). One patient developed grade 4 CRS in the DL2 cohort. The investigators noted neurologic toxicity in only 3 patients (18%) in DL2 cohort, with severe events (grade 3–4) occurring in 2 patients. The median time to onset of neurologic toxicity was 9 days (range, 7–25), and was of limited duration in most patients with a median time to resolution of 4 days 2 to 8. One patient died from tumor lysis syndrome in the DL2 cohort.

In the DL1 cohort, the best ORR was 67% with 2 patients in CR (33%). The median PFS and OS were 2.6 months and 10.9 months, respectively, after a median follow-up of 18 months. Higher efficacy was reported in the DL2 cohort, with a best ORR of 73%, CR 64%. The median PFS was 5.8 months and the median OS was not reached after a median follow-up of 6.2 months. When the 2 dose levels were pooled, the best ORR was 71%, CR 53%, and the estimated median PFS was 5.8 months with a median OS of 11.1 months. The median duration of response was not reached, with this limited follow-up, although durable responses were noted in the DL1 cohort, up to day 545 after CAR-T cell infusion. Seven patients (41%) were still in response at the data cutoff. In summary, this preliminary analysis shows promise, although more mature data are needed to assess both response rates and duration.

Future Directions Using Chimeric Antigen Receptor-Engineered T-Cell Therapies for Relapsed and Refractory Mantel Cell Lymphoma

CAR-T cell therapy for R/R MCL, and for R/R lymphoid malignancies more broadly, is currently an area of intense focus. **Table 1** lists 12 studies currently active or already enrolling patients with R/R MCL (clinicaltrial.gov database; query date, February 6th, 2020). One of these studies, currently enrolling at our institution, investigates a CAR-T cell product of defined composition targeting the orphan tyrosine-protein kinase transmembrane receptor (ROR1) for advanced ROR1+ malignancies including MCL.

SUMMARY

MCL is a rare and aggressive type of lymphoma with poor prognosis in the relapsed or refractory setting, particularly in patients relapsing after ibrutinib treatment. Allo-HCT remains the only option to achieve long-term remission in patients with R/R MCL. Despite being well-established, randomized trials comparing distinct allo-HCT modalities, or evaluating its use versus alternative approaches are lacking. Recent retrospective data proposed ibrutinib as a promising bridge to allo-HCT, with PFS probabilities of 60% at 1 year. Pretransplant ibrutinib failure was associated with poor outcomes after allo-HCT. We recommend that patients responding to ibrutinib, but at high risk of disease progression should be referred timely to a transplant center for evaluation and discussion of the risks to benefits. The development of HAPLO PT-Cy allo-HCT now permits the identification of a suitable related donor in many more patients. HAPLO PT-CY allo-HCT after RIC is becoming an established approach, associated with comparable OS, PFS, and significantly lower rates of chronic GVHD in patients with R/R lymphomas, including MCL.

Despite its curative potential, allo-HCT remains overall hindered by high treatment-related mortality and high relapse rates limiting its benefits. In addition, the risk of extensive chronic GVHD also makes the decision difficult. Complicating this is the promising results that have been recently reported using CAR-T cells targeting the CD19 antigen. Preliminary data from 2 pivotal clinical trials (ZUMA-2, KTE-X19; TRANSCEND-NHL-001, liso-cel) are showing promise with an acceptable toxicity profile and very high response rates. It is likely that this approach could be FDA approved in the next year or so. In addition, a large number of clinical trials investigating CAR-T cell therapies for a range of additional cell targets are currently ongoing. In our opinion, CAR-T cell therapies will likely transform the therapeutic landscape of relapsed refractory MCL in the future, and may further decrease the need for consideration of allo-HCT.

DISCLOSURE

J. Gauthier has no conflict of interest to disclose. D.G. Maloney has received research funding from Kite Pharma, Juno Therapeutics, Celgene; and has received honoraria for participation in advisory boards meetings with Kite Pharma, Celgene, Juno Therapeutics, Novartis and Pharmacyclics.

REFERENCES

1. Vose JM. Mantle cell lymphoma: 2017 update on diagnosis, risk-stratification, and clinical management. Am J Hematol 2017;92(8):806–13.

2. Hoster E, Dreyling M, Klapper W, et al. A new prognostic index (MIPI) for patients with advanced-stage mantle cell lymphoma. Blood 2008;111(2):558–65.

3. Bernard M, Gressin R, Lefrère F, et al. Blastic variant of mantle cell lymphoma: a rare but highly aggressive subtype. Leukemia 2001;15(11):1785–91.
4. Gouill S, Thieblemont C, Oberic L, et al. Rituximab after Autologous Stem-Cell Transplantation in Mantle-Cell Lymphoma. N Engl J Med 2017;377(13):1250–60.
5. Wang ML, Rule S, Martin P, et al. Targeting BTK with ibrutinib in relapsed or refractory mantle-cell lymphoma. N Engl J Med 2013;369(6):507–16.
6. Jain P, Romaguera J, Srour SA, et al. Four-year follow-up of a single arm, phase II clinical trial of ibrutinib with rituximab (IR) in patients with relapsed/refractory mantle cell lymphoma (MCL). Br J Haematol 2018;182(3):404–11.
7. Rule S, Dreyling M, Goy A, et al. Ibrutinib for the treatment of relapsed/refractory mantle cell lymphoma: extended 3.5-year follow up from a pooled analysis. Haematologica 2018;104(5):e211–4.
8. Rule S, Cook G, Russell NH, et al. Allogeneic stem cell transplantation as part of front line therapy for Mantle cell lymphoma. Br J Haematol 2018;184(6): 999–1005.
9. Cheah CY, Chihara D, Romaguera JE, et al. Patients with mantle cell lymphoma failing ibrutinib are unlikely to respond to salvage chemotherapy and have poor outcomes. Ann Oncol 2015;26(6):1175–9.
10. Martin P, Maddocks K, Leonard JP, et al. Postibrutinib outcomes in patients with mantle cell lymphoma. Blood 2016;127(12):1559–63.
11. Urbano-Ispizua A, Pavletic SZ, Flowers ME, et al. The impact of graft-versus-host disease on the relapse rate in patients with lymphoma depends on the histological subtype and the intensity of the conditioning regimen. Biol Blood Marrow Transplant 2015;21(10):1746–53.
12. Robinson S, Dreger P, Caballero D, et al. The EBMT/EMCL consensus project on the role of autologous and allogeneic stem cell transplantation in mantle cell lymphoma. Leukemia 2014;29(2):464–73.
13. Gauthier J, Chantepie S, Bouabdallah K, et al. Allogreffe de cellules souches hématopoïétiques dans la lymphome de Hodgkin, le lymphome du manteau et autres hémopathies lymphoïdes rares : recommandations de la Société francophone de greffe de moelle et de thérapie cellulaire (SFGM-TC). Bull Cancer 2017;104(12S):S112–20.
14. Tam CS, Bassett R, Ledesma C, et al. Mature results of the M. D. Anderson Cancer Center risk-adapted transplantation strategy in mantle cell lymphoma. Blood 2009;113(18):4144–52.
15. Fenske TS, Zhang M-J, Carreras J, et al. Autologous or reduced-intensity conditioning allogeneic hematopoietic cell transplantation for chemotherapy-sensitive mantle-cell lymphoma: analysis of transplantation timing and modality. J Clin Oncol 2014;32(4):273–81.
16. Dreger P, Michallet M, Bosman P, et al. Ibrutinib for bridging to allogeneic hematopoietic cell transplantation in patients with chronic lymphocytic leukemia or mantle cell lymphoma: a study by the EBMT Chronic Malignancies and Lymphoma Working Parties. Bone Marrow Transplant 2018;54(1):44–52.
17. Kharfan-Dabaja MA, Reljic T, El-Asmar J, et al. Reduced-intensity or myeloablative allogeneic hematopoietic cell transplantation for mantle cell lymphoma: a systematic review. Future Oncol 2016;12(22):2631–42.
18. Kanakry JA, Gocke CD, Bolaños-Meade J, et al. Phase II study of nonmyeloablative allogeneic bone marrow transplantation for B cell lymphoma with post-transplantation rituximab and donor selection based first on non-HLA factors. Biol Blood Marrow Transplant 2015;21(12):2115–22.

19. Maris MB, Sandmaier BM, Storer BE, et al. Allogeneic hematopoietic cell transplantation after fludarabine and 2 Gy total body irradiation for relapsed and refractory mantle cell lymphoma. Blood 2004;104(12):3535–42.

20. Vaughn JE, Sorror ML, Storer BE, et al. Long-term sustained disease control in patients with mantle cell lymphoma with or without active disease after treatment with allogeneic hematopoietic cell transplantation after nonmyeloablative conditioning. Cancer 2015;121(20):3709–16.

21. Mussetti A, Devlin SM, Castro-Malaspina HR, et al. Non-myeloablative allogeneic hematopoietic stem cell transplantation for adults with relapsed and refractory mantle cell lymphoma: a single-center analysis in the rituximab era. Bone Marrow Transplant 2015;50(10):1293–8.

22. Lin RJ, Ho C, Hilden PD, et al. Allogeneic haematopoietic cell transplantation impacts on outcomes of mantle cell lymphoma with TP53 alterations. Br J Haematol 2018;184(6):1006–10.

23. Luznik L, O'Donnell PV, Symons HJ, et al. HLA-haploidentical bone marrow transplantation for hematologic malignancies using nonmyeloablative conditioning and high-dose, posttransplantation cyclophosphamide. Biol Blood Marrow Transplant 2008;14(6):641–50.

24. Ghosh N, Karmali R, Rocha V, et al. Reduced-intensity transplantation for lymphomas using haploidentical related donors versus HLA-matched sibling donors: a center for international blood and marrow transplant research analysis. J Clin Oncol 2016;34(26):3141–9.

25. Kanate AS, Mussetti A, Kharfan-Dabaja MA, et al. Reduced-intensity transplantation for lymphomas using haploidentical related donors vs HLA-matched unrelated donors. Blood 2016;127(7):938–47.

26. Turtle CJ, Hanafi L-A, Berger C, et al. Immunotherapy of non-Hodgkin's lymphoma with a defined ratio of CD8+ and CD4+ CD19-specific chimeric antigen receptor–modified T cells. Sci Transl Med 2016;8(355):355ra116.

27. Neelapu SS, Locke FL, Bartlett NL, et al. Axicabtagene Ciloleucel CAR T-cell therapy in refractory large B-cell lymphoma. N Engl J Med 2017;377(26):2531–44.

28. Locke FL, Ghobadi A, Jacobson CA, et al. Long-term safety and activity of axicabtagene ciloleucel in refractory large B-cell lymphoma (ZUMA-1): a single-arm, multicentre, phase 1–2 trial. Lancet Oncol 2018;20:31–42.

29. Schuster SJ, Bishop MR, Tam CS, et al. Tisagenlecleucel in adult relapsed or refractory diffuse large B-cell lymphoma. N Engl J Med 2018;380(1):45–56.

30. Turtle CJ, Hanafi L-A, Berger C, et al. CD19 CAR–T cells of defined CD4+:CD8+ composition in adult B cell ALL patients. J Clin Invest 2016;126(6):2123–38.

31. Turtle CJ, Hay KA, Hanafi L-A, et al. Durable molecular remissions in chronic lymphocytic leukemia treated with CD19-specific chimeric antigen receptor–modified T cells after failure of ibrutinib. J Clin Oncol 2017;35(26):3010–20.

32. Abramson JS, Palomba ML, Gordon LI, et al. Pivotal safety and efficacy results from Transcend NHL 001, a multicenter phase 1 study of lisocabtagene maraleucel (liso-cel) in relapsed/refractory (R/R) large B cell lymphomas. Washington, DC: American Society of Hematology; 2019.

33. Weinkove R, George P, Dasyam N, et al. Selecting costimulatory domains for chimeric antigen receptors: functional and clinical considerations. Clinical & Translational Immunology 2019;8(5):e1049.

34. Wang ML, Munoz, Goy A, et al. 754 KTE-X19, an anti-CD19 chimeric antigen receptor (CAR) T cell therapy, in patients (Pts) with relapsed/refractory (R/R) mantle cell lymphoma (MCL): results of the Phase 2 ZUMA-2 study. Blood 2019; 134(suppl 1) (ASH Abstract).

35. Lee DW, Gardner R, Porter DL, et al. Current concepts in the diagnosis and management of cytokine release syndrome. Blood 2014;124(2):188–95.
36. Hay KA, Hanafi L-A, Li D, et al. Kinetics and biomarkers of severe cytokine release syndrome after CD19 chimeric antigen receptor–modified T-cell therapy. Blood 2017;130(21):2295–306.
37. Wang M, Gordon LI, Palomba ML, et al. Safety and preliminary efficacy in patients (pts) with relapsed/refractory (R/R) mantle cell lymphoma (MCL) receiving lisocabtagene maraleucel (Liso-cel) in TRANSCEND NHL 001. J Clin Oncol (ASCO Abstract) 2019;37(15):7516.

Understanding Health-Related Quality of Life in Patients with Mantle Cell Lymphoma

Priyanka A. Pophali, MD[a], Gita Thanarajasingam, MD[b],*

KEYWORDS

- Mantle cell lymphoma • HRQOL • Toxicity • Chronic therapy • Adverse events
- Patient-reported outcomes

KEY POINTS

- Understanding health-related quality of life is important for patients with mantle cell lymphoma, an incurable malignancy managed with a spectrum of approaches, from observation to aggressive immunochemotherapy to chronic targeted therapies.
- Optimal, consensus management strategies for mantle cell lymphoma are not clearly defined.
- Health-related quality of life data can provide important complementary information to individualize the treatment selection for a given patient.
- Existing data on health-related quality of life in patients with mantle cell lymphoma are limited and many unanswered questions remain.
- Clinical trials in development for mantle cell lymphoma should routinely incorporate health-related quality of life end points in their study design.

INTRODUCTION

Mantle cell lymphoma (MCL) is a unique non-Hodgkin lymphoma (NHL) subtype characterized by heterogeneous clinical behavior with features of both aggressive and indolent disease. Historically felt to be incurable, treatment of MCL is directed at inducing prolonged remission and/or achieving optimal disease and symptom control.

Funding sources: Dr G. Thanarajasingam receives grant funding from a Mayo Clinic Center for Clinical and Translational Science KL2 Mentored Career Development Award, which is funded by the National Center for Advancing Translational Science (NCATS), US National Institutes of Health (NIH) (KL2 TR002379).

[a] Division of Hematology, Oncology and Palliative Care, Department of Medicine, University of Wisconsin, 1111 Highland Avenue, Room 4031, Madison, WI 53705, USA; [b] Division of Hematology, Department of Medicine, Mayo Clinic, 200 1st Street Southwest, Rochester, MN 55905, USA
* Corresponding author.
E-mail address: thanarajasingam.gita@mayo.edu

Hematol Oncol Clin N Am 34 (2020) 971–982
https://doi.org/10.1016/j.hoc.2020.06.011
0889-8588/20/© 2020 Elsevier Inc. All rights reserved.

Numerous controversies exist with no firmly established standards for treatment in the frontline or relapsed/refractory setting, underscoring the relevance of accounting for health-related quality of life (HRQOL) in treatment decision making. In the frontline setting, for young, fit patients, it remains to be established if the most aggressive induction approaches (such as R-HyperCVAD or Nordic MCL2 regimen) are superior to less aggressive chemotherapy (such as bendamustine and rituximab [BR]) with or without consolidative autologous stem cell transplant (ASCT) and/or maintenance anti-CD20 antibody therapy. In this population, where superiority of survival outcomes with one approach has not been clearly established, illuminating HRQOL among disparate treatment approaches would be beneficial, although data are lacking. In the relapsed or refractory disease setting, exciting scientific progress in therapeutic options, including the development of first- and second-generation Bruton tyrosine kinase (BTK) inhibitors, immunomodulators, proteasome inhibitors, B-cell lymphoma 2 inhibitors, has led to improved outcomes and a variety of potential management strategies for patients on and off study. Patients with MCL are now living longer with their disease, many on chronically administered treatments in various stages of remission or stable disease. In this population, treatment tolerability including the impact of adverse events over months to years of continuous treatment on a patients' HRQOL, is relevant, although once again, bears limited existing data.

This review highlights why HRQOL in patients with MCL matters, revisits what is known about HRQOL and other patient-centered outcomes in this disease, and explores the numerous unanswered questions that remain. We first discuss these issues as applied to frontline therapy for newly diagnosed disease, then in the relapsed/refractory setting, drawing knowledge from other types of NHL where relevant. We conclude by exploring challenges and future directions in understanding the patient experience through better evaluation of the patient perspective and HRQOL in MCL.

WHY IS UNDERSTANDING HEALTH-RELATED QUALITY OF LIFE PARTICULARLY RELEVANT IN PATIENTS WITH MANTLE CELL LYMPHOMA?

Before exploring the particular importance of HRQOL in patients with MCL, it is valuable to clarify terminology. Patient-reported outcomes (PRO) are evaluations that come directly from a patient about the status of their health without amendment or interpretation of their response by a clinician or anyone else.[1] PROs are an assessment method, designed to provide the patient's perspective on functional outcomes, adverse events, and symptoms over time, treatment preferences, and other aspects. Meanwhile, the terms quality of life (QOL) and HRQOL are specific clinical outcomes assessed using one (or several) PRO measures. QOL is a broad multidimensional concept that covers all aspects of life even beyond health (but is sometimes used interchangeably with HRQOL), complicating its measurement. HRQOL maintains a narrower focus on the effects of illness and treatment, and has been defined as the subjective perception of the effect of health (including disease and treatment) on domains including physical, psychological, and social functioning and overall well-being.[2] The goal of evaluating HRQOL in cancer clinical trials is to evaluate the effects of cancer and its treatment together on the patient's subjective perception of his or her well-being; these data are intended to complement the usual primary outcomes (response rate, survival).[3]

It is possible to assess HRQOL generally and by domain with a variety of validated instruments, such as the Functional Assessment of Chronic Illness and Functional Assessment of Cancer Therapy (FACT) scales[4,5] (including the lymphoma-specific scale FACT-Lym),[6] European Organization for Research and Treatment of Cancer

(EORTC) questionnaires,[7] EuroQOL EQ-5D instruments,[8] among others.[9] For the purposes of this article, we focus not on detailed data from specific instruments, but rather on trends in HRQOL data evaluating the perspectives of patients with MCL on their disease and treatment experience.

HRQOL assessment is relevant in newly diagnosed as well as in patients with relapsed or refractory MCL. In frontline therapy, when there is no clearly defined approach that offers a superior overall survival based on current randomized clinical trial data, HRQOL data can help to guide the best choice of regimen for a given patient. Evaluation of HRQOL and adverse events from the patient perspective is also crucial in patients with MCL in the relapsed and refractory setting. As opposed to frontline treatment which typically involves finite-duration cytotoxic approaches (with or without maintenance anti-CD20 antibody therapy), treatments for relapsed and refractory MCL in the modern era include the use of several chronic or continuously administered oral therapies. The toxicity profile of these novel agents is starkly different from that of shorter duration conventional cytotoxic therapy and, when treatment is prolonged, in addition to treatment safety, evaluation of both tolerability and toxicity over time from the patient's perspective becomes even more important.

HEALTH-RELATED QUALITY OF LIFE IN PATIENTS WITH NEWLY DIAGNOSED MANTLE CELL LYMPHOMA

With an understanding of the relevance of HRQOL assessment in patients with MCL, we now explore what is known about HRQOL in patients with newly diagnosed MCL based on existing studies. MCL is a heterogeneous disease where some patients presenting with asymptomatic, low burden, often incidentally identified, leukemic-phase MCL can defer therapy at diagnosis.[10] Data from trials on patients with follicular lymphoma suggest that observation (vs treatment with rituximab) may have a negative impact on HRQOL, related to coping with the illness.[11] However, no HRQOL data for watchful waiting in MCL are available.

For patients who require treatment at diagnosis, multiple therapy options bear similar efficacy (primary outcomes) and a different toxicity profile. Therefore, evaluation of HRQOL and the patient perspective becomes crucial. Attempts to elucidate HRQOL differences between intensive treatment regimens for young, fit patients newly diagnosed with MCL have been made, but are limited in the ability to provide clinically meaningful evidence. Widmer and colleagues[12] reported a single-center retrospective study comparing the outcome and therapy tolerance of 43 young, fit patients with MCL treated with R-CHOP/ASCT versus R-HyperCVAD/MTX-AraC without ASCT. They found no difference in progression-free survival or overall survival between the 2 groups. However, the hospitalization rate, hematologic toxicity, and economic burden were significantly higher in the R-HyperCVAD group. HRQOL was measured using EORTC QLQ-C30, a standardized questionnaire that incorporates global health status, functional assessment, and symptom assessment. In this study, EORTC QLQ-C30 data were evaluable for 24 patients and reportedly better in the R-HyperCVAD group, although these results are indeterminate because only 5 patients with QLQ-C30 data received R-HyperCVAD. The authors recommend R-CHOP/ASCT over R-HyperCVAD given the significant toxicity and attribute the contradictory HRQOL data to discrepancy in physician-observed adverse events and patient experience. The major limitation of the study design was that the HRQOL surveys were administered retrospectively and likely subject to recall bias.[12]

For patients who are not candidates for intensive frontline therapy, the results from 2 phase III randomized trials of first-line therapy for indolent NHL and MCL established the noninferiority of BR to R-CHOP/R-CVP in terms of response rates and progression-free survival.[13,14] In one of these studies, the BRIGHT trial, HRQOL was a secondary end point systematically collected using the EORTC QLQ-C30.[15] The study included 74 patients with MCL (17% of total study participants), 36 in the BR arm and 38 in the R-CHOP/R-CVP arm. By conventional clinician-based common terminology criteria for adverse event[16] assessment, BR had different adverse events with little alopecia and neuropathy, but more nausea (potentially owing to differences in prophylactic antiemetic regimens between arms) and hypersensitivity reactions. This study also identified that, from the patient perspective, fatigue was improved at several time points in the BR group compared with standard therapy. In contrast, physician common terminology criteria for adverse event reporting reported rates of fatigue as similar between arms, a difference that underscores the value of including PROs for adverse event assessment in trials and confirms a large body of research affirming systematic underreporting of clinician-rated adverse events as compared with patient reports.[17–19] Like the primary analysis, HRQOL was not evaluated by tumor type (MCL) specifically, but among all patients, treatment with BR was associated with improved scores for cognitive, physical, social, and emotional functioning for at least 1 time point, and with improved physical functioning throughout therapy. The BRIGHT study provides valuable PRO and HRQOL data on regimens that can assist patients and their physicians with decision making. Although in the current era most patients not fit enough for an aggressive frontline approach undergo BR (rather than R-CHOP or R-CVP), the principle remains that in this malignancy, HRQOL assessment and measurement of other PROs can offer valuable patient-centered perspectives on the treatment experience to assist patients and their clinicians in an individualized treatment choice when multiple approaches are possible.

HRQOL data specifically for ASCT in first remission for MCL are lacking. With a median age at diagnosis of 68 years, a majority of patients with MCL are elderly. A single-center cross-sectional study evaluated the impact of ASCT in older patients (>60 years) with lymphoma (19% with MCL) on HRQOL using 2 different instruments (Euroqol EQ-5D and FACT-BMT[20]) at a median of 49 months (range, 17–96 months) after ASCT. They found that HRQOL was well-preserved after ASCT compared with an age-matched general population.[21] Similar results were reported by Farooq and colleagues,[22] who assessed HRQOL using FACT-G longitudinally in lymphoma patients who underwent ASCT versus those who did not. This study evaluated several different lymphoma histologies. Of the patients with MCL included, 28 received ASCT and 51 did not. Thirty-nine percent of all autologous transplants were performed in first remission. They reported no difference in HRQOL at 3 and 6 years after lymphoma diagnosis among patients treated with or without ASCT.[22]

Rituximab maintenance has become the standard of care in newly diagnosed patients after induction therapy followed by autologous transplant.[23] Patients with MCL who are ineligible for ASCT are often placed on maintenance rituximab based on evidence that it improves outcomes, although this conclusion remains controversial.[24–26] HRQOL in patients receiving rituximab maintenance has been evaluated in a single-center randomized study of 122 patients with CD20+ B-cell NHL (only 8 patients with MCL). This study showed that HRQOL, as measured by EORTC-QLQ-C30 and Euroqol EQ-5D, was not affected by maintenance rituximab therapy administered every 3 months for 2 years compared with observation.[27]

For patients who are unfit or elderly and determined to be ineligible for transplantation or cytotoxic chemotherapy for newly diagnosed disease, there is no consensus on management and little HRQOL data. Ruan and colleagues[28] conducted a single-arm phase II study of lenalidomide-rituximab induction and maintenance and did evaluate

HRQOL with FACT-Lym and FACT-Lym Trial Outcome Index[5] (which provides a composite of physical and functional well-being along with FACT-Lym). Trends toward improvement were noted in patient HRQOL scores, but these changes were not statistically or clinically significant.[28]

HEALTH-RELATED QUALITY OF LIFE IN PATIENTS WITH RELAPSED/REFRACTORY MANTLE CELL LYMPHOMA

As opposed to frontline treatment where standard approaches typically include conventional cytotoxic chemotherapy, chronically administered targeted agents are often used in the second-line treatment of patients with relapsed or refractory MCL. Many of these drugs have been approved based on single-arm phase II study results. In the absence of data establishing superiority of one treatment approach over another, HRQOL data may be valuable in making therapy decisions for individual patients. Additionally, the toxicity profile, burden of adverse events and impact on the patient of continuously administered targeted therapies or immunomodulators is entirely different compared with cytotoxic chemotherapy, and the concept of not just safety but tolerability is particularly relevant when a therapy is continuous or chronic. A recent multistakeholder group including clinicians and patients established that the tolerability of a cancer treatment is defined as "the degree to which symptomatic and non-symptomatic adverse events associated with the product's administration affect the ability or desire of the patient to adhere to the dose or intensity of therapy."[29] By definition, understanding tolerability requires the patient perspective, in addition to safety data and knowledge about dose modifications, discontinuation, and interruptions.[30] There exist limited data on some agents to guide us in this regard in the relapsed/refractory MCL population.

Three BTK inhibitors—ibrutinib, acalabrutinib, and zanubrutinib are currently approved by the US Food and Drug Administration for relapsed MCL. No head-to-head comparisons of these drugs are available and therefore choice of BTK inhibitor is often based on the anticipated toxicity and tolerability of the drug in individual patient situations. There are no published data on HRQOL with the second-generation BTK inhibitors acalabrutinib and zanubrutinib. However, HRQOL data were reported from RAY (MCL3001), a phase III international randomized trial of ibrutinib versus temsirolimus in previously treated MCL.[31] This trial used FACT-Lym and EQ-5D-5 L to provide longitudinal assessments of HRQOL on day 1 of the first 6 cycles, then every 9 weeks for 15 months and then every 24 weeks until disease progression, death, or clinical cutoff. Results showed that patients treated with ibrutinib had substantial improvements in FACT-Lym subscale and total scores, EQ-5D-5 L scores from baseline as well as compared with temsirolimus patients. It is interesting to note that the positive changes initially observed in physical well-being decreased with time and even dropped below the baseline after about 20 cycles of ibrutinib. For reference, the median progression-free survival for the ibrutinib arm in this trial was 14.6 months (95% confidence interval, 10.4–not estimable). This raises the question of whether cumulative toxicity or adverse events over time from ibrutinib may have affected physical well-being after long-term chronic therapy, even though there was an improvement at the beginning of therapy owing to a decrease in disease symptom burden.

As discussed elsewhere in this article, the use of lenalidomide has been explored in elderly or unfit patients in the frontline. However, lenalidomide is more commonly used in patients with relapsed or refractory MCL. Rule and colleagues[32] presented data from the MCL-002 (SPRINT) trial that did collect HRQOL data using the EORTC QLQ-C30. Patients with relapsed/refractory MCL in this trial were randomized 2:1 to lenalidomide as a single agent versus investigator's choice chemotherapy. HRQOL was measured at baseline, alternate cycles from 2 to 8, and at the end of treatment. They found that HRQOL was maintained with lenalidomide from baseline through the last treatment cycle. HRQOL was similar among patients treated with lenalidomide versus chemotherapy, except for higher rates of clinically meaningful improvement in HRQOL for physical function and pain in the lenalidomide group.[32]

To our knowledge, HRQOL data, if available, for many of the other targeted agents approved and in the pipeline for MCL such as acalabrutinib, zanubrutinib, venetoclax, and bortezomib have not been published to date and are often not systematically collected in trials. This lack is especially concerning because these therapies, given for months to years in the relapsed setting, can have chronic, and at times cumulative, toxicities. For example, although no long-term studies of bortezomib specifically in patients with MCL are available, neuropathy is a well-known and established adverse event of bortezomib use that can severely affect physical and functional well-being domains of HRQOL. Because targeted agents typically reserved for the relapsed/refractory setting are now being brought forth to the front-line setting, including HRQOL as a predefined end point for clinical trials is increasingly important. Establishing the impact of these novel therapies on HRQOL in patients with MCL specifically may help to guide treatment decisions and patient counseling.

Allogeneic stem cell transplantation is sometimes offered as a potentially curative intent therapy for young, fit patients with MCL who have relapsed after multiple lines of therapy or have poor prognostic markers such as p53 mutations. The short- and long-term impacts of allogeneic stem cell transplant on HRQOL in other hematologic malignancies are well-established.[33] Although no studies specific to allogeneic transplantation in MCL are reported, allogeneic transplantation is expected to lead to early moderate declines in HRQOL, which largely return to baseline at 100 days after transplantation. The long-term impact on HRQOL is largely driven by acute and chronic graft-versus-host disease.

Chimeric antigen receptor T-cell (CAR-T) therapy is upcoming as a treatment option for patients with relapsed MCL.[34] Early data on HRQOL changes during the first few weeks after CAR-T therapy show that HRQOL decreases in the first 2 weeks after CAR-T therapy, similar to autologous transplantation, but recovers after week 2, unlike allogeneic transplantation where the trend toward decrease in HRQOL is deeper and sustained.[35] Although there were no patients with MCL among this cohort, it is encouraging to have some helpful HRQOL data on CAR-T therapy because it represents an exciting potential therapeutic modality for patients with MCL whose disease has progressed through multiple lines of therapy.

CHALLENGES IN THE EVALUATION OF HEALTH-RELATED QUALITY OF LIFE IN MANTLE CELL LYMPHOMA

The existing literature of HRQOL assessments in patients with MCL demonstrates findings of interest, but mainly highlights the need for further systematic, consensus evaluation of PROs evaluating HRQOL to understand better the MCL patient experience specifically in both newly diagnosed and relapsed/refractory disease. Many therapeutic clinical trials group MCL with indolent NHL histologies making it difficult to interpret HRQOL results in the specific context of MCL, which has a unique biology and disease course. Routine inclusion of HRQOL measures as a secondary, key, or at least exploratory end points in MCL specific trials is the best way to address this knowledge gap. However, there are challenges inherent to instrument selection and data analysis for PROs in MCL trials. Yost and colleagues[36] prospectively validated the FACT-G as a tool in patients with NHL and included about 5% MCL. The FACT-Lym has been validated as an instrument to assess HRQOL in patients with relapsed/refractory MCL and was shown to differentiate patients based on performance status and worsening health status.[37] Most instruments have not been validated in a lymphoma population specifically, but this should not be a barrier to their use. Previously discussed instruments such as the EORTC QLQ-C30 and the EQ-5D-5 L, many of which have been used in the research reviewed elsewhere in this article, are also appropriate choices for assessment of HRQOL in patients with MCL.

HRQOL is a composite outcome that is influenced by multiple other variables, including social support and lifestyle factors such as physical activity, diet, body weight, tobacco, and alcohol use,[38-40] each of which is relevant in MCL and other types of NHL. These factors are likely both determinants as well as effects of an individual's HRQOL, which adds complexity. HRQOL is impacted by treatment-related adverse events and disease-related symptoms, which can also be more specifically addressed by tools such as the Patient Reported Outcomes Version of the Common Terminology Criteria for Adverse Events,[41] whereby patients self-report the frequency, severity, and interference of multiple symptomatic adverse events that can be graded similarly to clinician reported adverse events per the Common Terminology Criteria for Adverse Events. Tools such as the FACT-GP5 item that asks patients to rate the "overall burden of side effects" over time may elucidate a more global impact of adverse events on HRQOL in patients on chronic therapy.[42] Patient reporting of adverse events may improve the accuracy toxicity assessment and constitutes a key element of tolerability evaluation.[43] Knowing which instrument to use, how often to administer it, and what data results is not always straightforward. In the future, it would be optimal to have consensus on which tools should be used in which types of studies or for which type of Hodgkin and NHL, but for now investigators should involve health outcomes research specific colleagues, including biostatisticians for expertise on the selection of the tool and analysis of data during protocol development where possible. If not, it is reasonable to select tools based on the level of comfort with the implementation of the instrument.

Collecting the right PROs at the right frequency is only part of the challenge to understanding HRQOL in patients with MCL. Knowing how to analyze and present the PRO data in a clinically meaningful way is another.[44,45] Longitudinal PRO analysis and display is important. Adverse events influence HRQOL, and understanding them better is vital for patients on long-term therapy for MCL. To understand the experience of a patient with MCL on a chronically administered targeted agent, a conventional maximum grade table demonstrating incidence of high grade cytopenias and clinician-rated adverse events, is insufficient for evaluation of tolerability and the time profile of adverse events.[3] For example, common terminology criteria for adverse event defines grade 2 diarrhea as more than 4 to 6 stools per day above baseline. Although this may be a tolerable side effect in the short term and is often not reported in conventional toxicity tables, over months to years of treatment this adverse event may become intolerable and have substantial ramifications on multiple domains of a patient's HRQOL. Knowing that headache from acalabrutinib may come on early and dissipate in the first couple of weeks or that neuropathy from bortezomib has a late onset and cumulative burden, is relevant to patients, yet there are often few data on toxicity over time, including burden of chronic low-grade adverse events over time.[46] Simple approaches to analysis of common terminology criteria for adverse events, PRO adverse events, and HRQOL data over time are available.[47] Additionally, there has been recent emphasis on understanding the burden of adverse events overall on the patient and their HRQOL, which may provide greater insights, to better understand the MCL patient's treatment experience over time.[48–50]

FUTURE DIRECTIONS AND SUMMARY

In the future, the goal should be systematic real-time collection of PROs in patients with MCL on and off clinical studies to understand HRQOL better. In addition to being important end points in clinical trials of therapeutic agents for MCL, the ultimate goal of HRQOL data is to improve the experience of patients with MCL in the real world. Mobile technology, electronic platforms, and wearable devices are all being investigated and implemented to facilitate the collection of PROs from patients.[51] This process will make improved understanding of HRQOL in MCL and other cancers more feasible in the near future in patients on trials and those in routine practice. HRQOL data can guide treatment selection for patients in the clinic and be part of shared decision making on a treatment strategy. Understanding adverse events, including their time profile and overall burden from the patient perspective, can guide education on a treatment regimen so patients know what to anticipate. This knowledge can help to optimize the selection and timing of symptom control for toxicities in which an adverse event intervention is available. There is increasing evidence for supportive interventions such as physical activity programs during and after treatment to help with adverse events such as peripheral neuropathy and fatigue and thus to improve HRQOL.[52,53] Better knowledge of adverse event data from patient perspective could prevent the development of late, longer term, or cumulative toxicity because it could guide clinicians on the appropriate time for dose reductions, treatment holidays, or dose discontinuation where necessary to improve HRQOL while maintaining disease control.

Ultimately, there is substantial room for improvement in understanding the patient experience with treatment for MCL. In this disease with distinct biological features and a heterogeneous clinical course among patients, understanding HRQOL is particularly relevant. For patients with newly diagnosed MCL, without clearly established strategies for optimal induction and frontline treatment, further knowledge about HRQOL could equip patients and clinicians with tools to individualize treatment decisions. In the relapsed, refractory setting, the use of numerous chronically administered agents to treat disease sometimes for months to years at a time highlights the relevance of understanding treatment tolerability and its impact on HRQOL in this population. Limited data on HRQOL in MCL, which we have reviewed here, exist but many unanswered questions remain. Broad, systematic, and scientifically rigorous implementation of HRQOL assessment in mantle cell studies in development has the potential to provide better understanding of and improvement in the experience of MCL patient at the bedside.

DISCLOSURE

The authors have no commercial or financial conflicts of interest.

REFERENCES

1. United States Food and Drug Administration. Guidance for industry: patient-reported outcome measures: use in medical product development to support labeling claims. 2009. Available at: http://www.fda.gov/downloads/Drugs/GuidanceComplianceRegulatoryInformation/Guidances/UCM193282.pdf. Accessed August 31, 2017.

2. Wilson IB, Cleary PD. Linking clinical variables with health-related quality of life. A conceptual model of patient outcomes. JAMA 1995;273(1):59–65.

3. Thanarajasingam G, Minasian LM, Baron F, et al. Beyond maximum grade: modernising the assessment and reporting of adverse events in haematological malignancies. Lancet Haematol 2018;5(11):e563–98.

4. FACIT. Functional Assessment of Chronic Illness Therapy (FACIT). Available at: https://www.facit.org/FACITOrg/Questionnaires. Accessed January 29, 2020.

5. Webster K, Cella D, Yost K. The Functional Assessment of Chronic Illness Therapy (FACIT) measurement system: properties, applications, and interpretation. Health Qual Life Outcomes 2003;1:79.

6. Hlubocky FJ, Webster K, Beaumont J, et al. A preliminary study of a health related quality of life assessment of priority symptoms in advanced lymphoma: the National Comprehensive Cancer Network-Functional Assessment of Cancer Therapy - Lymphoma Symptom Index. Leuk Lymphoma 2013;54(9):1942–6.

7. EORTC. European Organisation for Research and Treatment of Cancer (EORTC). Quality of Life in Cancer Patients Core 30 (QLQ-C30). 2020. Available at: http://groups.eortc.be/qol. Accessed January 29, 2020.

8. Balestroni G, Bertolotti G. EuroQol-5D (EQ-5D): an instrument for measuring quality of life. Monaldi Arch Chest Dis 2012;78(3):155–9.

9. Georgakopoulos A, Kontodimopoulos N, Chatziioannou S, et al. EORTC QLQ-C30 and FACT-Lym for the assessment of health-related quality of life of newly diagnosed lymphoma patients undergoing chemotherapy. Eur J Oncol Nurs 2013;17(6):849–55.

10. Martin P, Chadburn A, Christos P, et al. Outcome of deferred initial therapy in mantle-cell lymphoma. J Clin Oncol 2009;27(8):1209–13.

11. Ardeshna KM, Qian W, Smith P, et al. Rituximab versus a watch-and-wait approach in patients with advanced-stage, asymptomatic, non-bulky follicular lymphoma: an open-label randomised phase 3 trial. Lancet Oncol 2014;15(4):424–35.

12. Widmer F, Balabanov S, Soldini D, et al. R-hyper-CVAD versus R-CHOP/cytarabine with high-dose therapy and autologous haematopoietic stem cell support in fit patients with mantle cell lymphoma: 20 years of single-center experience. Ann Hematol 2018;97(2):277–87.

13. Flinn IW, van der Jagt R, Kahl BS, et al. Randomized trial of bendamustine-rituximab or R-CHOP/R-CVP in first-line treatment of indolent NHL or MCL: the BRIGHT study. Blood 2014;123(19):2944–52.

14. Rummel MJ, Niederle N, Maschmeyer G, et al. Bendamustine plus rituximab versus CHOP plus rituximab as first-line treatment for patients with indolent and mantle-cell lymphomas: an open-label, multicentre, randomised, phase 3 non-inferiority trial. Lancet 2013;381(9873):1203–10.

15. Burke JM, van der Jagt RH, Kahl BS, et al. Differences in quality of life between bendamustine-rituximab and R-CHOP/R-CVP in patients with previously untreated advanced indolent non-Hodgkin lymphoma or mantle cell lymphoma. Clin Lymphoma Myeloma Leuk 2016;16(4):182–90.e1.

16. National Cancer Institute. Common terminology criteria for adverse events (CTCAE) version 5.0. Bethesda (MD): U.S. Department of Health and Human Services; 2017.

17. Fromme EK, Eilers KM, Mori M, et al. How accurate is clinician reporting of chemotherapy adverse effects? A comparison with patient-reported symptoms from the Quality-of-Life Questionnaire C30. J Clin Oncol 2004;22(17):3485–90.

18. Basch E, Iasonos A, McDonough T, et al. Patient versus clinician symptom reporting using the National Cancer Institute Common Terminology Criteria for Adverse Events: results of a questionnaire-based study. Lancet Oncol 2006;7(11):903–9.
19. Basch E, Bennett A, Pietanza MC. Use of patient-reported outcomes to improve the predictive accuracy of clinician-reported adverse events. J Natl Cancer Inst 2011;103(24):1808–10.
20. McQuellon RP, Russell GB, Cella DF, et al. Quality of life measurement in bone marrow transplantation: development of the Functional Assessment of Cancer Therapy-Bone Marrow Transplant (FACT-BMT) scale. Bone Marrow Transplant 1997;19(4):357–68.
21. Lemieux C, Ahmad I, Bambace NM, et al. Evaluation of the impact of autologous hematopoietic stem cell transplantation on the quality of life of older patients with lymphoma. Biol Blood Marrow Transplant 2020;26(1):157–61.
22. Farooq U, Larson M, Maurer M, et al. Long term quality of life in lymphoma patients after autologous hematopoietic cell transplantation. Biol Blood Marrow Transpl 2018;24:S25–118.
23. Le Gouill S, Thieblemont C, Oberic L, et al. Rituximab after autologous stem-cell transplantation in mantle-cell lymphoma. N Engl J Med 2017;377(13):1250–60.
24. Vidal L, Gafter-Gvili A, Dreyling M, et al. Maintenance treatment for patients with mantle cell lymphoma: a systematic review and meta-analysis of randomized trials. Hemasphere 2018;2(4):e136.
25. Hill BT, Switchenko JM, Martin P, et al. Maintenance rituximab improves outcomes in mantle cell lymphoma patients who respond to induction therapy with bendamustine + rituximab without autologous transplant. Blood 2019; 134(Supplement_1):1525.
26. Rummel MJ, Knauf W, Goerner M, et al. Two years rituximab maintenance vs. observation after first-line treatment with bendamustine plus rituximab (B-R) in patients with mantle cell lymphoma: first results of a prospective, randomized, multicenter phase II study (a subgroup study of the StiL NHL7-2008 MAINTAIN trial). J Clin Oncol 2016;34(15_suppl):7503.
27. Witzens-Harig M, Reiz M, Heiss C, et al. Quality of life during maintenance therapy with the anti-CD20 antibody rituximab in patients with B cell non-Hodgkin's lymphoma: results of a prospective randomized controlled trial. Ann Hematol 2009;88(1):51–7.
28. Ruan J, Martin P, Shah B, et al. Lenalidomide plus rituximab as initial treatment for mantle-cell lymphoma. N Engl J Med 2015;373(19):1835–44.
29. Basch E, Campbell A, Hudgens S, et al. Broadening the definition of tolerability in cancer clinical trials to better measure the patient experience. 2018. Availabe at: https://www.focr.org/sites/default/files/Comparative%20Tolerability%20Whitepaper_FINAL.pdf. Accessed April 7, 2020.
30. Kluetz PG, Kanapuru B, Lemery S, et al. Informing the tolerability of cancer treatments using patient-reported outcome measures: summary of an FDA and Critical Path Institute Workshop. Value in Health 2018;21(6):742-7.
31. Hess G, Rule S, Jurczak W, et al. Health-related quality of life data from a phase 3, international, randomized, open-label, multicenter study in patients with previously treated mantle cell lymphoma treated with ibrutinib versus temsirolimus. Leuk Lymphoma 2017;58(12):2824–32.
32. Rule S, Arcaini L, Jan W, et al. Quality of life in relapsed/refractory mantle cell lymphoma patients treated with lenalidomide vs investigator's choice: MCL-002 (SPRINT) trial. European Haematology Association. Vienna, June 11-14, 2015.

33. Pidala J, Anasetti C, Jim H. Quality of life after allogeneic hematopoietic cell transplantation. Blood 2009;114(1):7–19.
34. Michael L, Wang JM, Goy A, et al. KTE-X19, an anti-CD19 chimeric antigen receptor (CAR) T cell therapy, in patients (Pts) with relapsed/refractory (R/R) mantle cell lymphoma (MCL): results of the phase 2 ZUMA-2 study. Blood 2019; 134(Supplement_1):754.
35. Sidana S, Thanarajasingam G, Griffin J, et al. Patient experience of chimeric antigen receptor (CAR)-T cell therapy vs. stem cell transplant: longitudinal patient reported adverse events, cognition and quality of life. Blood 2019; 134(Supplement_1):794.
36. Yost KJ, Thompson CA, Eton DT, et al. The Functional Assessment of Cancer Therapy - general (FACT-G) is valid for monitoring quality of life in patients with non-Hodgkin lymphoma. Leuk Lymphoma 2013;54(2):290–7.
37. Carter GC, Liepa AM, Zimmermann AH, et al. Validation of the Functional Assessment of Cancer Therapy–Lymphoma (FACT-LYM) in patients with relapsed/refractory mantle cell lymphoma. Blood 2008;112(11):2376.
38. Courneya KS, Sellar CM, Stevinson C, et al. Randomized controlled trial of the effects of aerobic exercise on physical functioning and quality of life in lymphoma patients. J Clin Oncol 2009;27(27):4605–12.
39. Soares A, Biasoli I, Scheliga A, et al. Association of social network and social support with health-related quality of life and fatigue in long-term survivors of Hodgkin lymphoma. Support Care Cancer 2013;21(8):2153–9.
40. Spector DJ, Noonan D, Mayer DK, et al. Are lifestyle behavioral factors associated with health-related quality of life in long-term survivors of non-Hodgkin lymphoma? Cancer 2015;121(18):3343–51.
41. Dueck AC, Mendoza TR, Mitchell SA, et al. Validity and Reliability of the US National Cancer Institute's Patient-Reported Outcomes Version of the common terminology criteria for adverse events (PRO-CTCAE). JAMA Oncol 2015;1(8): 1051–9.
42. Pearman TP, Beaumont JL, Mroczek D, et al. Validity and usefulness of a single-item measure of patient-reported bother from side effects of cancer therapy. Cancer 2018;124(5):991–7.
43. Kluetz PG, Chingos DT, Basch EM, et al. Patient-reported outcomes in cancer clinical trials: measuring symptomatic adverse events with the National Cancer Institute's patient-reported outcomes version of the common terminology criteria for adverse events (PRO-CTCAE). Am Soc Clin Oncol Educ Book 2016;35:67–73.
44. Calvert M, Kyte D, Mercieca-Bebber R, et al. Guidelines for inclusion of patient-reported outcomes in clinical trial protocols: the SPIRIT-PRO extension. JAMA 2018;319(5):483–94.
45. Coens C, Pe M, Dueck AC, et al. International standards for the analysis of quality-of-life and patient-reported outcome endpoints in cancer randomised controlled trials: recommendations of the SISAQOL Consortium. Lancet Oncol 2020;21(2):e83–96.
46. Thanarajasingam G, Hubbard JM, Sloan JA, et al. The imperative for a new approach to toxicity analysis in oncology clinical trials. J Natl Cancer Inst 2015; 107(10).
47. Thanarajasingam G, Atherton PJ, Novotny PJ, et al. Longitudinal adverse event assessment in oncology clinical trials: the Toxicity over Time (ToxT) analysis of Alliance trials NCCTG N9741 and 979254. Lancet Oncol 2016;17(5):663–70.
48. Lee SM, Hershman DL, Martin P, et al. Toxicity burden score: a novel approach to summarize multiple toxic effects. Ann Oncol 2012;23(2):537–41.

49. Cabarrou B, Boher JM, Bogart E, et al. How to report toxicity associated with targeted therapies? Ann Oncol 2016;27(8):1633–8.
50. Tabernero J, Van Cutsem E, Ohtsu A, et al. QTWiST analysis of the RECOURSE trial of trifluridine/tipiracil in metastatic colorectal cancer. ESMO Open 2017; 2(5):e000284.
51. Thompson CA, Yost KJ, Bartz A, et al. Patient-reported outcomes, emoji, and activity measured on the Apple Watch in cancer patients. J Clin Oncol 2018; 36(15_suppl):6501.
52. Kim BJ, Park HR, Roh HJ, et al. Chemotherapy-related polyneuropathy may deteriorate quality of life in patients with B-cell lymphoma. Qual Life Res 2010;19(8): 1097–103.
53. Streckmann F, Kneis S, Leifert JA, et al. Exercise program improves therapy-related side-effects and quality of life in lymphoma patients undergoing therapy. Ann Oncol 2014;25(2):493–9.

Key Clinical and Translational Research Questions to Address Unmet Needs in Mantle Cell Lymphoma

Thomas D. Rodgers Jr, MD*, Jonathan W. Friedberg, MD, MMSc

KEYWORDS

- Mantle cell lymphoma • Chimeric antigen receptor T-cell (CAR-T)
- Minimal residual disease (MRD) • Novel agents • Precision therapy
- Mantle cell lymphoma international prognostic index (MIPI)

KEY POINTS

- Recent advancements in mantle cell lymphoma have led to significant improvements in patients outcomes and new clinical and translations questions.
- Previously dominated by intensive regimens, novel agents and combinations challenge the need for high-dose and intense regimens for young fit patients with mantle cell lymphoma.
- The use of minimal residual disease testing has increased in mantle cell lymphoma, and new evidence demonstrates the potential usefulness of minimal residual disease status as response-adapted therapy.
- Recent evidence demonstrates the efficacy of chimeric antigen receptor T-cell therapy; however, questions remain, including the durability of remissions and the possibility of a cure.
- Prognostic indices take into consideration patient characteristics and laboratory studies. Future studies should prioritize genetic and biologic markers, particularly when considering treatment decisions.

INTRODUCTION

It is an exciting time in the treatment of mantle cell lymphoma (MCL). Our understanding of disease heterogeneity, along with new treatment strategies and novel agents, has led to a marked improvement in patient outcomes. Although incurable, the median overall survival (OS) has doubled over the last 20 years owing to treatment regimens

James P. Wilmot Cancer Institute, University of Rochester Medical Center, 601 Elmwood Avenue, Box 704, Rochester, NY 14642, USA
* Corresponding author.
E-mail address: Thomas_Rodgers@URMC.Rochester.edu

Hematol Oncol Clin N Am 34 (2020) 983–996
https://doi.org/10.1016/j.hoc.2020.06.012
0889-8588/20/© 2020 Elsevier Inc. All rights reserved.

with improved efficacy and more tolerable toxicity profiles.[1] As in any area of science, growing knowledge has produced new uncertainty. We are now poised to ask questions that challenge old treatment paradigms, involve novel therapies, and use new technologies.

In this article, we highlight a selection of questions that we believe will drive the future of MCL. These are not meant to be all inclusive, and it is essential to note that the answers to these questions will not apply to all patients. Beyond disease heterogeneity, many patients continue to be underrepresented in our current clinical trials owing to factors such as disease tempo, along with advancing patient age or frailty. In asking these questions, we aim to highlight the unmet needs that exist today while also outlining clinical studies positioned to change future treatment decisions. Based on the available literature and with clinical experience, we provide expert opinion on how to proceed until further studies are available (**Table 1**).

QUESTION 1: FOR YOUNG FIT PATIENTS, CAN WE REPLACE INTENSIVE INDUCTION REGIMENS WITH ALTERNATIVES INCORPORATING LESS TOXIC, MORE EFFECTIVE NOVEL AGENTS?

MCL is a heterogeneous disease affecting varied segments of the population. Although most patients require therapy soon after their diagnosis, it is known that a minority can harbor an indolent disease, often safely observed for several years.[2] Adding to the complexity, although the average age at diagnosis is 68 years, younger and older patients are frequently diagnosed with differing comorbidity profiles and performance statuses.[3] These variations in disease course and presentation have led to multiple treatment strategies with contrasting intensity and toxicity profiles.

For younger fit patients, more aggressive strategies have been used in an attempt to prolong progression-free survival (PFS) and OS. It is important to note that these treatment regimens are not considered to be curable, because most patients will ultimately experience disease relapse.[4,5] Currently, there is no single standard of care in the upfront treatment of patients with MCL. Given modest OS compared with other indolent lymphomas, strategies have been deployed, including the use of high-dose cytarabine and autologous stem cell transplantation (ASCT). As we discuss elsewhere in this article, although the toxicity profile is understood, the comparative usefulness of these regimens is not yet clear. It is crucial in the era of novel therapies to know whether the long-term outcomes are improved for young fit patients with the use of intensive regimens in the light of varied toxicity profiles.

Current treatment patterns vary, including chemoimmunotherapy regimens similar to those used in follicular and diffuse large B-cell lymphoma (DLBCL) compared with strategies used in Burkitt's and lymphoblastic lymphoma. The STiL and BRIGHT trials investigated the less intense regimen bendamustine and rituximab (BR) versus rituximab, cyclophosphamide, doxorubicin, vincristine, and prednisone (R-CHOP) in MCL. compared with R-CHOP, BR had an improved PFS and a more tolerable toxicity profile.[6,7] The objective response rate was near 90%, although the PFS was a modest 3 years.

Akin to treatment paradigms in aggressive lymphomas such as Burkitt's and lymphoblastic lymphoma, a consolidative ASCT and high-dose cytarabine containing regimens have been studied in an attempt to prolong responses. The only study in which randomized patients to ASCT or no ASCT after upfront CHOP therapy demonstrated improved OS of 7.5 years versus 5.3 years with this treatment modality compared with maintenance therapy alone.[8] It is important to note that this study was conducted was before the introduction of rituximab or other novel agents.

Table 1
Selection of key ongoing clinical trials in MCL

Trial or Regimen	Phase	Treatment	Clinicaltrial.gov Identification
TRIANGLE	3	Arm 1: R-CHOP/RDHAP to ASCT Arm 2: R-CHOP/ibrutinib + RDHAP to ASCT with ibrutinib maintenance Arm 3: R-CHOP/ibrutinib + RDHAP to ibrutinib maintenance	NCT02858258
EA4151	3	Induction with MRD assessment: Positive: ASCT + rituximab maintenance Negative: ASCT + rituximab maintenance vs maintenance alone	NCT03267433
SYMPATICO	3	Ibrutinib + venetoclax or placebo in R/R, cohort of first-line ibrutinib + venetoclax in patients with TP53 mutations	NCT03112174
ENRICH	2/3	Ibrutinib and rituximab in R/R patients or first-line in patients >65 y	NCT01880567
E1411	2	First line: 4 arms bendamustine and rituximab with or without bortezomib followed by maintenance of rituximab or rituximab/lenalidomide. Initial data presented.	NCT01415752
WINDOW-1	2	R-HCVAD/methotrexate-ara-C combined after ibrutinib/rituximab	NCT02427620
WINDOW-2	2	R-HCVAD/methotrexate-ara-C combined after venetoclax/rituximab	NCT03710772
ALR	2	First-line acalabrutinib, lenalidomide, and rituximab	NCT03863184
ZUMA-2	2	CAR-T (KTE-C19) in R/R, initial data published	NCT02601313
VLR	1	First-line venetoclax, lenalidomide and rituximab	NCT03523975

Abbreviation: R-CHOP, rituximab, cyclophosphamide, doxorubicin, vincristine, and prednisone.

The inclusion of high-dose cytarabine in upfront therapy has been studied in multiple different regimens. Most notably, these include hyperfractionated cyclophosphamide, vincristine, doxorubicin, and dexamethasone (HyperCVAD), dose intensified R-CHOP (NORDIC regimen), and other combinations with BR/R-CHOP.[9] HyperCVAD combined with methotrexate and cytarabine (HCVAD/methotrexate-ara-C) was first studied in 1998. Compared with CHOP, PFS and OS were increased with the intensive regimen.[10] In 2005, rituximab was added to hyperCVAD alternating with high-dose cytarabine and methotrexate (R-HCVAD/methotrexate-ara-C) with a 97% objective response rate and a 3-year OS of 82%.[11]

Further expanding the use of cytarabine, the NORDIC regimen used high doses of CHOP alternating with rituximab and cytarabine before ASCT. The 6-year PFS and OS were 66% and 70%, respectively.[12] Long-term OS data from the NORDIC and R-HCVAD/methotrexate-ara-C studies revealed a median OS of 8.5 and 10.7 years, respectively.[13,14] Although survival data are encouraging from these studies, toxicities were pronounced. The single-center phase II study with R-HCVAD/methotrexate-ara-C had an 8% treatment-related mortality.[11] Additionally, under the Nordic regimen, which incorporated a consolidative ASCT, nearly 20% of chemotherapy cycles administered led to a hospitalization.[12]

The toxicity and efficacy of upfront cytarabine-containing regimens followed by ASCT have also been further studied in 2 prospective trials. The first investigated R-CHOP versus R-CHOP alternating with rituximab plus dexamethasone, high-dose cytarabine, and cisplatin (R-DHAP) for 6 cycles. Time to treatment failure was significantly longer in the cytarabine containing arm at 9.1 years versus 3.9 years. That being said, hematologic toxicities were pronounced, and OS has not been shown to be significantly different.[15] Another study (S1106) investigated R-HCVAD/methotrexate-ara-C versus BR, both followed by ASCT. The trial was ultimately closed early owing to increased toxicity and difficult stem cell mobilization in the hyperCVAD arm. After 5 years of follow-up, there was no difference in PFS, OS, or minimal residual disease (MRD) negativity between the 2 treatment groups. That being said, the cohort receiving R-HCVAD/methotrexate-ara-C experienced higher rates of adverse events.[16,17]

Beyond chemotherapy-based regimens, additional combinations have been investigated using novel agents such as the immunomodulatory drug lenalidomide, anti-CD20 antibodies, Bruton's tyrosine kinase inhibitors, and the BCL-2 inhibitor venetoclax. These studies have primarily investigated patient populations with contraindications to standard chemotherapy. A multicenter phase II study evaluated the efficacy of combined therapy with lenalidomide and rituximab in the upfront setting, with the median age of participants being 65 years. The 5-year PFS and OS were 64% and 77%, respectively. Additionally, 8 of 10 patients that completed more than 3 years of treatment were MRD negative, demonstrating the durability of response.[18,19] Other novel regimens, such as ibrutinib, venetoclax, and the CD20 antibody obinutuzumab, have early safety data with notable efficacy.[20] Ongoing studies are evaluating additional combinations such as acalabrutinib or venetoclax with lenalidomide, rituximab (NCT03863184 and NCT03523975) in addition to the ENRICH trial with ibrutinib and rituximab (NCT01880567).

Based on these data, the role of cytarabine and ASCT in the upfront treatment of patients with MCL is quite nuanced. Although it seems that more aggressive treatment options such as an ASCT or cytarabine-containing regimens lead to improved outcomes, their toxicities likely limit their combination in the upfront setting. It is also not clear that either option leads to an improvement in OS in the era of rituximab and novel therapies.[8]

Future studies will help to clarify the inclusion of these aggressive treatments in the upfront setting. Although not an exhaustive list, 2 phase III studies are positioned to further refine the role of these intensive modalities, namely, the ECOG-ACRIN E4151 study (NCR03267433) and the TRIANGLE study (NCT02858258). EA4151 will primarily investigate the role of MRD negativity in informing the need for ASCT (discussed elsewhere in this article), although it will include patients who underwent different induction regimens. The TRIANGLE study is a 3-arm trial investigating ibrutinib's inclusion into upfront therapy along with the usefulness of an ASCT. The study randomizes patients to 6 cycles of R-CHOP/R-DHAP followed by ASCT, 6 cycles of R-CHOP/ibrutinib-R-DHAP followed by ASCT, and 2 years of ibrutinib maintenance or 6 cycles of RCHOP + ibrutinib/R-DHAP without an ASCT and 2 years of ibrutinib maintenance. Shorter courses of R-HCVAD/methotrexate-ara-C combined after ibrutinib/rituximab or venetoclax/rituximab are also being studied in WINDOW-1 and -2 trials (NCT02427620 and NCT03710772).

Beyond current trials, longer follow-up and comparative studies of less intense regimens before an ASCT are needed, such as bendamustine containing regimens.[9] Recently, the E1411 study demonstrated that BR induced MRD negativity in nearly 90% of patients before ASCT.[21] Further follow-up will help to clarify the long-term efficacy of less aggressive induction therapies.

Until additional studies reveal further details, and if a clinical trial is not available, we feel that BR is a reasonable comparative standard, although we appreciate that considerable debate remains. The regimen is superior to R-CHOP, well-tolerated, and induces high rates of MRD negativity (importance discussed elsewhere in this article). If patients obtain a partial or complete response to therapy, an ASCT should be considered if the patient is otherwise young and fit. We anticipate that with the inclusion of novel agents in upfront and maintenance settings will further limit the use of intensive cytarabine regimens and perhaps in a select group of patients the need for an ASCT.

QUESTION 2: CAN WE USE MINIMAL RESIDUAL DISEASE STATUS AS RESPONSE-ADAPTED THERAPY FOR MANTLE CELL LYMPHOMA?

An autologous stem cell transplant is often pursued in young fit patients who have an adequate response to upfront therapy. This concept has been a standard based on pre-rituximab data conducted by the European MCL network, which began enrolling patients in 1996. Patients were enrolled in their first remission after CHOP-like inductions and randomized to either ASCT with cyclophosphamide and total body irradiation or alpha-interferon maintenance.[22] Prolonged follow-up (median, 6.1 years) revealed an OS of 7.5 years in the ASCT group compared with 5.4 years in the interferon group.[8]

There have not been additional prospective studies confirming this benefit in the age of novel therapies. In a retrospective study, using a propensity score-weighted analysis of more than 1000 patients from 25 academic centers, no OS benefit was found with the use of ASCT consolidation.[23] It is critical to understand the usefulness and benefit of an ASCT in light of known toxicities, particularly in patients of more advanced age and increasing comorbidities. Beyond patient characteristics, MCL is a biologically heterogeneous disease with aggressive and indolent forms. To better identify the patients who would benefit from additional intensive therapies, MRD analysis has been used in MCL.

Studies using quantitative real-time polymerase chain reaction to test clonal immunoglobulin heavy chain (IgH) rearrangements reveal that MRD positivity is an independent risk factor of early relapse after initial induction therapy. This has been shown in those patients after an ASCT and in older adults or those ineligible for an ASCT.[24–26] Using the cytarabine containing Nordic regimen, those patients who were MRD positive after ASCT had a PFS of 20 months compared with 142 months in those who were MRD negative. Preemptive rituximab maintenance was able to convert to MRD negativity in 87% of the MRD positive patients after ASCT.[26] Rituximab maintenance was later shown to prolong PFS and OS after ASCT with an R-DHAP induction.[27] A single-center retrospective review suggested that pretransplant MRD status was also informative. For those patients who were MRD negative before ASCT, PFS, and OS at 5 years were 75% and 82%, respectively. Patients who were MRD positive before ASCT had a median PFS of 2.38 years and an OS of 3.0 years.[28]

Given the unclear benefit across all populations in the rituximab era and with known disease heterogeneity, the benefit of an ASCT may be unevenly distributed across risk groups. As previously demonstrated, MRD positivity after induction therapy (with or without consolidative ASCT) predicts for worse outcomes and maintenance therapies seem to be able to augment this status. For this reason, it has been hypothesized that low-risk groups such as those able to achieve MRD negativity after induction therapy, may benefit less from a consolidative ASCT. This finding invites the question: is an ASCT necessary in patients who can achieve MRD negativity?

The ECOG-ACRIN 4151 study is poised to answer the question of whether or not we can apply a risk-stratified approach to ASCT in MCL. The study will be open to adult patients up to the age of 70 years who would otherwise be candidates for an ASCT. Induction therapy will be per investigator's choice. Patients who are MRD negative (as determined by next-generation evaluation of circulating tumor DNA) at the end of therapy will be randomized to 3 years of maintenance with rituximab without ASCT or ASCT alone. Those who are MRD positive or indeterminate will proceed to ASCT with rituximab maintenance. This study could demonstrate that low-risk patients can defer consolidative ASCT.

We acknowledge challenges with the use of MRD testing. It is expensive, not widely available, and variation in target/tissue types make broad use challenging. That being said, the ability to risk stratify patients, and more precisely use an ASCT or maintenance therapy, would be a significant step forward in the care of patients with MCL. We anticipate that undetectable MRD status will continue to be a benchmark for future studies.

QUESTION 3: WILL CHIMERIC ANTIGEN RECEPTOR T-CELL THERAPY REPRESENT A CURE FOR MANTLE CELL LYMPHOMA?

Unfortunately, nearly all patients will have a recurrence of their disease, mainly secondary to the development of chemotherapy resistance. Based on the introduction of several nonchemotherapy options, including the proteasome inhibitor bortezomib, the immunomodulatory agent lenalidomide, and the Bruton's tyrosine kinase inhibitors ibrutinib, acalabarutinib and zanubrutinib, outcomes for patients with relapsed/refractory disease have improved.[29–33]

There is no one standard of care option for patients with relapsed/refractory disease, and the choice is often based on the prior regimens used. Outcomes vary based on prior therapy and patient fitness, although those who relapse after ibrutinib have a median OS of 5.8 months.[34] Stem cell transplantation with either an autologous or allogeneic transplant can be pursued, although it may have diminished efficacy in the second or beyond complete response and if the patients are not in a complete response at the time of transplantation.[35,36]

Recently, anti-CD19 chimeric antigen receptor T-cell (CAR-T) therapy has been investigated in non-Hodgkin lymphomas (NHL). This process has led to the approval of this modality in refractory large cell lymphoma after 2 or more prior lines of therapy.[37,38] Its use has also been investigated in indolent NHLs such as follicular lymphoma (FL) and MCL. Recently, results from the ZUMA-2 study investigating the CAR-T agent KTE-X19 were presented. For MCL, the study included patients relapsed/refractory to an anthracycline-based regimen, anti-CD20 monoclonal antibody therapy, and either ibrutinib or acalabrutinib. As in other CAR-T studies, patients received conditioning chemotherapy with cyclophosphamide and fludarabine. At a median follow-up of 13.2 months, the objective response rate was 86%, with a complete response of 57%. At 1 year, the PFS and OS were 71% and 86%, respectively. Common grade 3 or higher adverse events were primarily hematologic with anemia, thrombocytopenia, and neutropenia occurring in 54%, 39%, and 36% of patients, respectively. Grade 3 or greater cytokine release syndrome occurred in 18% of patients, with 46% of patients having a grade 3 or greater neurologic event.[39]

CAR-T therapy will likely be approved in MCL, although several questions remain. Most notably, it is not clear whether this modality represents a possible cure for a subset of patients with MCL. Given the typical disease course, prolonged patient follow-up will be critical to assess such a benefit. That being said, comparisons can be made to other hematologic malignancies where longer follow-up does exist. For example, in

DLBCL and FL, 3- and 4-year experiences have been published. For patients with DLBCL and FL receiving the CAR-T product tisagenlecleucel at a single center, the median duration of response for responding patients was not reached at nearly 49 months.[40] Similar data were recently presented from the ZUMA-1 trial, where almost 50% of the patients remained alive at 3 years, the majority without evidence of relapse.[41] These data demonstrate durable remissions with the potential of a cure in DLBCL and FL. Although promising, long-term follow-up from the ZUMA-2 trial in MCL is necessary to understand the duration of response in MCL.

Relapses after CAR-T therapy are likely mediated by different resistance patterns such as T-cell exhaustion or antigen loss, downregulation, alternative splicing, or masking.[41–44] Different approaches are being developed to address resistance, such as combining CAR-T with other therapies or including maintenance treatments after CAR-T.[45,46] A further understanding of these mechanisms in MCL will help to better craft CAR-T regimens. Other questions are currently being asked in other forms of NHL, such as DLBCL. These include but are not limited to, the proper timing of CAR-T therapy, determining a risk-stratified approach to its use, and developing CAR-T options with decreased toxicity.

The ZUMA 7 trial (NCT03391466) is investigating axicabtagene ciloleucel (Axi-Cel) versus salvage chemotherapy followed by an ASCT in patients who are refractory or relapsed after first-line therapy in DLBCL.[47] Although the treatment paradigms differ between DLBCL and MCL, in high-risk groups (such as those with TP53 mutations), CAR-T therapy may be able to be used earlier in treatment strategies. Other agents, such as JCAR017, are being studied in MCL through the TRANSCEND-NHL-001 study (NCT02621044). Initial data from 9 patients have been presented in MCL, although long-term follow-up is pending.[48] That being said, recently presented data from the DLBCL patients revealed low rates (2%) of grade 3 or greater cytokine release syndrome.[49] Finally, given the significant heterogeneity of MCL, further studies will be able to discern which groups benefit the most from this treatment modality.

CAR-T therapy is a promising treatment option for patients with relapsed MCL. Recently published data demonstrate response rates of more than 80%, with the majority of patients being disease free at 1 year. Although the duration of follow-up remains short, if long-term outcomes mirror those of DLBCL or FL, a segment of the population will likely have durable remissions or a potential cure. Apart from long-term follow-up, additional trials should focus on resistance patterns, combination therapy, and patient risk stratification.

QUESTION 4: CAN GENOMIC AND MOLECULAR INFORMATION REPLACE THE MANTLE CELL LYMPHOMA INTERNATIONAL PROGNOSTIC INDEX FOR PROGNOSIS, AND HOW CAN WE INCORPORATE THIS INFORMATION INTO A PRECISION APPROACH TO THERAPY?

As mentioned elsewhere in this article, MCL is a heterogeneous malignancy. Although a segment of the population is known to have a more indolent course, many patients will, unfortunately, experience rapidly progressing disease, often poorly responsive to available therapies. The World Health Organization divides MCL into 2 main clinical subtypes, conventional MCL and nonmodal MCL, which have distinct clinical courses. In 2008, the Mantle Cell Lymphoma International Prognostic Index (MIPI) score was developed to help identify prognostic factors that could be used in the clinic and research trials for MCL. The analysis included data from 3 randomized trials investigating advanced MCL (GLSG1996, GLSG2000, and the European MCL Trial 1) and classified patients as having low, intermediate, or high risk disease based on age, lactate dehydrogenase, leukocyte count, and performance status. Using this system, the median OS was not reached for low-risk disease, although those with an intermediate- and high-risk MIPI score had a median OS of 51 and 29 months, respectively.[50]

In an attempt to assess prognosis using tumor histology, further iterations of the MIPI score (known as MIPI-b and MIPI-c) defined risk groups using the addition of the proliferation index Ki-67[51,52] (**Table 2**). These combinations better described low and intermediate-risk disease. Although informative, these indices have significant limitations. In addition to a paucity of prospectively assessed data, it is unclear how they apply in the era of novel combinations. Finally, with advancing technologies, other markers independent of the MIPI score have been identified and associated with outcome. These markers include an array of biologic factors in addition to genetic and epigenetic profiling with prognostic and predictive implications for our expanding armamentarium of novel agents.

Independent of the Ki67 index and MIPI score, evaluation of DNA extracted from MCL samples from patients in the European MCL Younger trial, identified the deletion of CDKN2A and TP53 as poor prognostic factors. In the trial, patients received upfront chemotherapy with cytarabine followed by an ASCT. Despite this aggressive regimen, patients with simultaneous deletions of CDKN2A and TP53 had an OS of 1.8 years compared with 7.0 years without either deletion.[53] Similar outcomes were seen when analyzing samples from the Nordic MCL2 and MCL3 studies. Mutations of TP53 were identified as an independent adverse prognostic factor. Those patients with mutations had a median OS of 1.7 years compared with 12.7 years in patients without a TP53 mutation.[54] More recently, TP53 mutational load was evaluated and found to stratify patients further.[55] Based on the previously mentioned Nordic trials and more recently published experiences, patients with TP53 mutations have significantly worse outcomes. This finding is primarily owing to the fact that they do not seem to benefit from aggressive treatment modalities such as high-dose cytarabine-containing regimens and consolidative ASCT.[54,56]

Table 2
Iterations of the MIPI

Name	Included Factors	Risk Stratification
MIPI[50]	Age, ECOG performance status, LDH, and WBC counts	*Low risk*: OS not reached *Intermediate risk*: OS 51 mo *High risk*: OS 29 mo
s-MIPI (simplified)[66]	Age, ECOG performance status, LDH, and WBC counts Developed for ease of bedside use	*Low risk*: 81% 5-y OS *Intermediate risk*: 63% 5-y OS *High risk*: 35% 5-y OS
MIPI-b[66]	Age, ECOG performance status, LDH, WBC counts, and Ki67%	*Low risk*: 81% 5-y OS *Intermediate risk*: 83% 5-y OS *High risk*: 37% 5-y OS
MIPI-c[52]	Age, ECOG performance status, LDH, WBC counts, and Ki67	*Low risk*: 85% 5-y OS *Low to intermediate risk*: 72% 5-y OS *High to intermediate Risk*: 43% 5-y OS *High risk*: 17% 5-y OS
MIPI + TP53/NOTCH1[59]	Age, ECOG performance status, LDH, WBC counts, and Ki67% with *TP53* and *NOTCH*	TP53 status added prognostic value to MIPI

Abbreviation: WBC, white blood cell.
   Data from Refs.[50,52,59,66]

Beyond TP53, NOTCH1 mutations have also been associated with inferior outcomes with a median OS of 1.4 years in patients with NOTCH1 mutations compared with 3.9 years in those without such a mutation.[57] Genetic markers such as KMT2D, MLL2, MEF2B, and WHSC1 mutations have been found to have prognostic importance in MCL, outlining patients with more rapidly progressing disease and decreased OS.[58] Other factors have been evaluated and associated with improved outcomes after treatment including high SOX11 expression and the presence of unmutated immunoglobulin heavy chain variable region genes.[59,60] Adding to the complexity, these mutations infrequently occur in isolation with varied prognostic significance when occurring in combination with other mutations.

Gene expression and epigenetic profiling have also been investigated in MCL. Multiple gene expression assays have been developed, including a variable number of genes analyzed. High-risk groups were identified as having worse outcomes and shorter time to first treatment. Overall, they were also able to differentiate between the 2 World Health Organization types, nonmodal MCL and conventional MCL.[61–63] Finally, methylation patterns are also able to demonstrate distinct subgroups, with a range of clinical outcomes.[64]

These data demonstrate the importance of factors beyond those assessed in the MIPI. Although the MIPI identifies risk groups, it is not typically used to guide therapeutic decisions regarding the intensity or inclusion of novel agents. Advancing technology reveals important markers independent of the MIPI and may be able to better guide future therapies. Although retrospective analyses have demonstrated the usefulness of combining TP53 and NOTCH1 expression with the standard MIPI score,[59] further studies are needed to evaluate the importance of genetic and other biologic markers prospectively. The previously mentioned WINDOW and TRIANGLE studies will assess patient's NOTCH1 and TP53 mutation status and thus may be able to further clarify their prognostic importance in patients treated with novel combinations. The SYMPATICO trial (NCT03112174) is investigating venetoclax and ibrutinib in a cohort of high-risk older adults as defined by TP53 status. Mutational analysis is also being conducted in a similar population treated with venetoclax after upfront BR and cytarabine in older adults (NCT03567876). Although providing prognostic data, the MIPI score has considerable limitations in the age of novel agents and varied treatment regimens and modalities.

The inclusion of more advanced genetic and gene expression profiling should be prioritized in clinical trials, replacing or combined with the standard MIPI. Beyond prognostic information, our expanding knowledge of MCL heterogeneity should be used to craft a precision approach to treatment. For example, patients in the relapsed setting with TP53 mutations have similar responses to certain novel agents compared with a patient without mutated disease.[65] We suggest that novel agents should be prioritized in these high-risk populations with particular consideration of alternative cellular therapies, such as CAR-T or allogeneic stem cell transplant. Patients with lower risk profiles may additionally benefit from shorter courses of treatment, sparing unneeded toxicity. Although the MIPI clearly defines prognosis, in the era of expanding technologies and understanding of heterogeneity, we believe the future MCL therapies will be tailored to the distinct patient given their unique disease profile.

SUMMARY

Our understanding of disease heterogeneity, along with more effective and less toxic treatment regimens, has led to significant improvements in patient care. Patients with MCL are now living longer with an expanding list of effect novel agents. That being said, MCL is still considered to be an incurable illness, and many questions remain. As we have highlighted above, these questions can only be answered with ongoing research, including well designed clinical trials. It is critical for the advancement of care for patients today and in the future that we prioritize clinical trials across the spectrum of MCL, including patients with high-risk disease and those typically restricted from clinical trials owing to age or comorbidities. In doing so, we can answer critical questions that face our patients in everyday practice.

REFERENCES

1. Herrmann A, Hoster E, Zwingers T, et al. Improvement of overall survival in advanced stage mantle cell lymphoma. J Clin Oncol 2009;27:511–8.
2. Martin P, Chadburn A, Christos P, et al. Outcome of deferred initial therapy in mantle-cell lymphoma. J Clin Oncol 2009;27:1209–13.
3. Zhou Y, Wang H, Fang W, et al. Incidence trends of mantle cell lymphoma in the United States between 1992 and 2004. Cancer 2008;113:791–8.
4. Schulz H, Bohlius JF, Trelle S, et al. Immunochemotherapy with rituximab and overall survival in patients with indolent or mantle cell lymphoma: a systematic review and meta-analysis. J Natl Cancer Inst 2007;99:706–14.
5. Freedman AS, Neuberg D, Gribben JG, et al. High-dose chemoradiotherapy and anti-B-cell monoclonal antibody-purged autologous bone marrow transplantation in mantle-cell lymphoma: no evidence for long-term remission. J Clin Oncol 1998; 16:13–8.
6. Flinn IW, van der Jagt R, Kahl BS, et al. Randomized trial of bendamustine-rituximab or R-CHOP/R-CVP in first-line treatment of indolent NHL or MCL: the BRIGHT study. Blood 2014;123:2944–52.
7. Rummel MJ, Niederle N, Maschmeyer G, et al. Bendamustine plus rituximab versus CHOP plus rituximab as first-line treatment for patients with indolent and mantle-cell lymphomas: an open-label, multicentre, randomised, phase 3 non-inferiority trial. Lancet 2013;381:1203–10.
8. Dreyling MH, Hoster E, Van Hoof A, et al. Early consolidation with myeloablative radiochemotherapy followed by autologous stem cell transplantation in first remission in mantle cell lymphoma: long term follow up of a randomized trial of the European MCL Network. Blood 2008;112:769.
9. Armand P, Redd R, Bsat J, et al. A phase 2 study of rituximab-bendamustine and rituximab-cytarabine for transplant-eligible patients with mantle cell lymphoma. Br J Haematol 2016;173:89–95.
10. Khouri IF, Romaguera J, Kantarjian H, et al. Hyper-CVAD and high-dose methotrexate/cytarabine followed by stem-cell transplantation: an active regimen for aggressive mantle-cell lymphoma. J Clin Oncol 1998;16:3803–9.
11. Romaguera JE, Fayad L, Rodriguez MA, et al. High rate of durable remissions after treatment of newly diagnosed aggressive mantle-cell lymphoma with rituximab plus hyper-CVAD alternating with rituximab plus high-dose methotrexate and cytarabine. J Clin Oncol 2005;23:7013–23.
12. Geisler CH, Kolstad A, Laurell A, et al. Long-term progression-free survival of mantle cell lymphoma after intensive front-line immunochemotherapy with in vivo-purged stem cell rescue: a nonrandomized phase 2 multicenter study by the Nordic Lymphoma Group. Blood 2008;112:2687–93.
13. Eskelund CW, Kolstad A, Jerkeman M, et al. 15-year follow-up of the second Nordic mantle cell lymphoma trial (MCL2): prolonged remissions without survival plateau. Br J Haematol 2016;175:410–8.

14. Chihara D, Cheah CY, Westin JR, et al. Rituximab plus hyper-CVAD alternating with MTX/Ara-C in patients with newly diagnosed mantle cell lymphoma: 15-year follow-up of a phase II study from the MD Anderson Cancer Center. Br J Haematol 2016;172:80–8.

15. Hermine O, Hoster E, Walewski J, et al. Addition of high-dose cytarabine to immunochemotherapy before autologous stem-cell transplantation in patients aged 65 years or younger with mantle cell lymphoma (MCL Younger): a randomised, open-label, phase 3 trial of the European Mantle Cell Lymphoma Network. Lancet 2016;388:565–75.

16. Chen RW, Li H, Bernstein SH, et al. RB but not R-HCVAD is a feasible induction regimen prior to auto-HCT in frontline MCL: results of SWOG Study S1106. Br J Haematol 2017;176:759–69.

17. Kamdar M, Li H, Chen RW, et al. Five-year outcomes of the S1106 study of R-hyper-CVAD vs R-bendamustine in transplant-eligible patients with mantle cell lymphoma. Blood Adv 2019;3:3132–5.

18. Ruan J, Martin P, Shah B, et al. Lenalidomide plus rituximab as initial treatment for mantle-cell lymphoma. N Engl J Med 2015;373:1835–44.

19. Ruan J, Martin P, Christos P, et al. Five-year follow-up of lenalidomide plus rituximab as initial treatment of mantle cell lymphoma. Blood 2018;132:2016–25.

20. Le Gouill S, Morschhauser F, Bouabdallah K, et al. Ibrutinib, venetoclax plus obinutuzumab in newly diagnosed mantle cell lymphoma patients. Blood 2019;134:1530.

21. Smith M, Jegede O, Parekh S, et al. Minimal residual disease (MRD) assessment in the ECOG1411 randomized phase 2 trial of front-line bendamustine-rituximab (BR)-based induction followed by rituximab (R) ± lenalidomide (L) consolidation for mantle cell lymphoma (MCL). Blood 2019;134:751.

22. Dreyling M, Lenz G, Hoster E, et al. Early consolidation by myeloablative radio-chemotherapy followed by autologous stem cell transplantation in first remission significantly prolongs progression-free survival in mantle-cell lymphoma: results of a prospective randomized trial of the European MCL Network. Blood 2005;105:2677–84.

23. Gerson JN, Handorf E, Villa D, et al. Survival outcomes of younger patients with mantle cell lymphoma treated in the rituximab era. J Clin Oncol 2019;37:471–80.

24. Pott C, Schrader C, Gesk S, et al. Quantitative assessment of molecular remission after high-dose therapy with autologous stem cell transplantation predicts long-term remission in mantle cell lymphoma. Blood 2006;107:2271–8.

25. Liu H, Johnson JL, Koval G, et al. Detection of minimal residual disease following induction immunochemotherapy predicts progression free survival in mantle cell lymphoma: final results of CALGB 59909. Haematologica 2012;97:579–85.

26. Kolstad A, Pedersen LB, Eskelund CW, et al. Molecular monitoring after autologous stem cell transplantation and preemptive rituximab treatment of molecular relapse; results from the Nordic mantle cell lymphoma studies (MCL2 and MCL3) with median follow-up of 8.5 years. Biol Blood Marrow Transplant 2017;23:428–35.

27. Le Gouill S, Thieblemont C, Oberic L, et al. Rituximab after autologous stem-cell transplantation in mantle-cell lymphoma. N Engl J Med 2017;377:1250–60.

28. Cowan AJ, Stevenson PA, Cassaday RD, et al. Pretransplantation minimal residual disease predicts survival in patients with mantle cell lymphoma undergoing autologous stem cell transplantation in complete remission. Biol Blood Marrow Transplant 2016;22:380–5.

29. Goy A, Bernstein SH, Kahl BS, et al. Bortezomib in patients with relapsed or refractory mantle cell lymphoma: updated time-to-event analyses of the multicenter phase 2 PINNACLE study. Ann Oncol 2009;20:520–5.
30. Trneny M, Lamy T, Walewski J, et al. Lenalidomide versus investigator's choice in relapsed or refractory mantle cell lymphoma (MCL-002; SPRINT): a phase 2, randomised, multicentre trial. Lancet Oncol 2016;17:319–31.
31. Dreyling M, Jurczak W, Jerkeman M, et al. Ibrutinib versus temsirolimus in patients with relapsed or refractory mantle-cell lymphoma: an international, randomised, open-label, phase 3 study. Lancet 2016;387:770–8.
32. Wang M, Rule S, Zinzani PL, et al. Acalabrutinib in relapsed or refractory mantle cell lymphoma (ACE-LY-004): a single-arm, multicentre, phase 2 trial. Lancet 2018;391:659–67.
33. Song Y, Zhou K, Zou D, et al. Safety and activity of the investigational Bruton tyrosine kinase inhibitor zanubrutinib (BGB-3111) in patients with mantle cell lymphoma from a phase 2 trial. Blood 2018;132:148.
34. Martin P, Maddocks K, Leonard JP, et al. Postibrutinib outcomes in patients with mantle cell lymphoma. Blood 2016;127:1559–63.
35. Fenske TS, Zhang MJ, Carreras J, et al. Autologous or reduced-intensity conditioning allogeneic hematopoietic cell transplantation for chemotherapy-sensitive mantle-cell lymphoma: analysis of transplantation timing and modality. J Clin Oncol 2014;32:273–81.
36. Rajabi B, Sweetenham JW. Mantle cell lymphoma: observation to transplantation. Ther Adv Hematol 2015;6:37–48.
37. Neelapu SS, Locke FL, Bartlett NL, et al. Axicabtagene ciloleucel CAR T-cell therapy in refractory large B-cell lymphoma. N Engl J Med 2017;377:2531–44.
38. Schuster SJ, Bishop MR, Tam CS, et al. Tisagenlecleucel in adult relapsed or refractory diffuse large B-cell lymphoma. N Engl J Med 2019;380:45–56.
39. Wang ML, Munoz J, Goy A, et al. KTE-X19, an anti-CD19 chimeric antigen receptor (CAR) T cell therapy, in patients (Pts) with relapsed/refractory (R/R) mantle cell lymphoma (MCL): results of the phase 2 ZUMA-2 study. Blood 2019;134:754.
40. Chong EA, Svoboda J, Nasta SD, et al. CD19-directed car T cell therapy (CTL019) for relapsed/refractory diffuse large B-cell and follicular lymphomas: four year outcomes. Hematol Oncol 2019;37:137–8.
41. Neelapu SS, Rossi JM, Jacobson CA, et al. CD19-loss with preservation of other B cell lineage features in patients with large B cell lymphoma who relapsed post-axi-cel. Blood 2019;134:203.
42. Long AH, Haso WM, Shern JF, et al. 4-1BB costimulation ameliorates T cell exhaustion induced by tonic signaling of chimeric antigen receptors. Nat Med 2015;21:581–90.
43. Ruella M, Xu J, Barrett DM, et al. Induction of resistance to chimeric antigen receptor T cell therapy by transduction of a single leukemic B cell. Nat Med 2018;24:1499–503.
44. Sotillo E, Barrett DM, Black KL, et al. Convergence of acquired mutations and alternative splicing of CD19 enables resistance to CART-19 immunotherapy. Cancer Discov 2015;5:1282–95.
45. Ardeshna KM, Marzolini MAV, Norman J, et al. Phase 1/2 study of AUTO3 the first bicistronic chimeric antigen receptor (CAR) targeting CD19 and CD22 followed by an anti-PD1 in patients with relapsed/refractory (r/r) diffuse large b cell lymphoma (DLBCL): results of cohort 1 and 2 of the Alexander Study. Blood 2019;134:246.

46. Neelapu SS, Kharfan-Dabaja MA, Oluwole OO, et al. A phase 2, open-label, multicenter study evaluating the safety and efficacy of axicabtagene ciloleucel in combination with either rituximab or lenalidomide in patients with refractory large B-cell lymphoma (ZUMA-14). Blood 2019;134:4093.

47. Oluwole OO, Bishop MR, Gisselbrecht C, et al. ZUMA-7: a phase 3 randomized trial of axicabtagene ciloleucel (Axi-Cel) versus standard-of-care (SOC) therapy in patients with relapsed/refractory diffuse large B cell lymphoma (R/R DLBCL). J Clin Oncol 2018;36:TPS7585.

48. Wang M, Gordon LI, Palomba ML, et al. Safety and preliminary efficacy in patients (pts) with relapsed/refractory (R/R) mantle cell lymphoma (MCL) receiving lisocabtagene maraleucel (Liso-cel) in TRANSCEND NHL 001. J Clin Oncol 2019; 37:7516.

49. Abramson JS, Palomba ML, Gordon LI, et al. Pivotal safety and efficacy results from transcend NHL 001, a multicenter phase 1 study of Lisocabtagene Maraleucel (liso-cel) in Relapsed/Refractory (R/R) large B cell lymphomas. Blood 2019; 134:241.

50. Hoster E, Dreyling M, Klapper W, et al. A new prognostic index (MIPI) for patients with advanced-stage mantle cell lymphoma. Blood 2008;111:558–65.

51. Salek D, Vesela P, Boudova L, et al. Retrospective analysis of 235 unselected patients with mantle cell lymphoma confirms prognostic relevance of Mantle Cell Lymphoma International Prognostic Index and Ki-67 in the era of rituximab: long-term data from the Czech Lymphoma Project Database. Leuk Lymphoma 2014;55:802–10.

52. Hoster E, Rosenwald A, Berger F, et al. Prognostic value of Ki-67 index, cytology, and growth pattern in mantle-cell lymphoma: results from randomized trials of the European Mantle Cell Lymphoma Network. J Clin Oncol 2016;34:1386–94.

53. Delfau-Larue MH, Klapper W, Berger F, et al. High-dose cytarabine does not overcome the adverse prognostic value of CDKN2A and TP53 deletions in mantle cell lymphoma. Blood 2015;126:604–11.

54. Eskelund CW, Dahl C, Hansen JW, et al. TP53 mutations identify younger mantle cell lymphoma patients who do not benefit from intensive chemoimmunotherapy. Blood 2017;130:1903–10.

55. Obr A, Klener P Jr, Kriegova E, et al. High TP53 mutation load predicts primary refractory mantle cell lymphoma. Blood 2019;134:3995.

56. Ferrero S, Rossi D, Rinaldi A, et al. KMT2D mutations and TP53 disruptions are poor prognostic biomarkers in mantle cell lymphoma receiving high-dose therapy: a FIL study. Haematologica 2020;105(6):1604–12.

57. Kridel R, Meissner B, Rogic S, et al. Whole transcriptome sequencing reveals recurrent NOTCH1 mutations in mantle cell lymphoma. Blood 2012;119:1963–71.

58. Yang P, Zhang W, Wang J, et al. Genomic landscape and prognostic analysis of mantle cell lymphoma. Cancer Gene Ther 2018;25:129–40.

59. Nordstrom L, Sernbo S, Eden P, et al. SOX11 and TP53 add prognostic information to MIPI in a homogenously treated cohort of mantle cell lymphoma–a Nordic Lymphoma Group study. Br J Haematol 2014;166:98–108.

60. Navarro A, Clot G, Royo C, et al. Molecular subsets of mantle cell lymphoma defined by the IGHV mutational status and SOX11 expression have distinct biologic and clinical features. Cancer Res 2012;72:5307–16.

61. Rosenwald A, Wright G, Wiestner A, et al. The proliferation gene expression signature is a quantitative integrator of oncogenic events that predicts survival in mantle cell lymphoma. Cancer Cell 2003;3:185–97.

62. Scott DW, Abrisqueta P, Wright GW, et al. New molecular assay for the proliferation signature in mantle cell lymphoma applicable to formalin-fixed paraffin-embedded biopsies. J Clin Oncol 2017;35:1668–77.

63. Clot G, Jares P, Gine E, et al. A gene signature that distinguishes conventional and leukemic nonnodal mantle cell lymphoma helps predict outcome. Blood 2018;132:413–22.

64. Queiros AC, Beekman R, Vilarrasa-Blasi R, et al. Decoding the DNA methylome of mantle cell lymphoma in the light of the entire B cell lineage. Cancer Cell 2016;30: 806–21.

65. Jerkeman M, Eskelund CW, Hutchings M, et al. Ibrutinib, lenalidomide, and rituximab in relapsed or refractory mantle cell lymphoma (PHILEMON): a multicentre, open-label, single-arm, phase 2 trial. Lancet Haematol 2018;5:e109–16.

66. Hoster E, Klapper W, Hermine O, et al. Confirmation of the mantle-cell lymphoma international prognostic index in randomized trials of the European Mantle-Cell Lymphoma Network. J Clin Oncol 2014;32:1338–46.

UNITED STATES POSTAL SERVICE ®

Statement of Ownership, Management, and Circulation
(All Periodicals Publications Except Requester Publications)

1. Publication Title	2. Publication Number	3. Filing Date
HEMATOLOGY/ONCOLOGY CLINICS OF NORTH AMERICA	002 – 473	9/18/2020

4. Issue Frequency	5. Number of Issues Published Annually	6. Annual Subscription Price
FEB, APR, JUN, AUG, OCT, DEC	6	$443.00

7. Complete Mailing Address of Known Office of Publication (Not printer) (Street, city, county, state, and ZIP+4®)

ELSEVIER INC.
230 Park Avenue, Suite 800
New York, NY 10169

Contact Person
Malathi Samayan

Telephone (Include area code)
91-44-4299-4507

8. Complete Mailing Address of Headquarters or General Business Office of Publisher (Not printer)

ELSEVIER INC.
230 Park Avenue, Suite 800
New York, NY 10169

9. Full Names and Complete Mailing Addresses of Publisher, Editor, and Managing Editor (Do not leave blank)

Publisher (Name and complete mailing address)

DOLORES MELONI, ELSEVIER INC.
1600 JOHN F KENNEDY BLVD. SUITE 1800
PHILADELPHIA, PA 19103-2899

Editor (Name and complete mailing address)

STACY EASTMAN, ELSEVIER INC.
1600 JOHN F KENNEDY BLVD. SUITE 1800
PHILADELPHIA, PA 19103-2899

Managing Editor (Name and complete mailing address)

PATRICK MANLEY, ELSEVIER INC.
1600 JOHN F KENNEDY BLVD. SUITE 1800
PHILADELPHIA, PA 19103-2899

10. Owner (Do not leave blank. If the publication is owned by a corporation, give the name and address of the corporation immediately followed by the names and addresses of all stockholders owning or holding 1 percent or more of the total amount of stock. If not owned by a corporation, give the names and addresses of the individual owners. If owned by a partnership or other unincorporated firm, give its name and address as well as those of each individual owner. If the publication is published by a nonprofit organization, give its name and address.)

Full Name	Complete Mailing Address
WHOLLY OWNED SUBSIDIARY OF REED/ELSEVIER, US HOLDINGS	1600 JOHN F KENNEDY BLVD. SUITE 1800 PHILADELPHIA, PA 19103-2899

11. Known Bondholders, Mortgagees, and Other Security Holders Owning or Holding 1 Percent or More of Total Amount of Bonds, Mortgages, or Other Securities. If none, check box → ☐ None

Full Name	Complete Mailing Address
N/A	

12. Tax Status (For completion by nonprofit organizations authorized to mail at nonprofit rates) (Check one)
The purpose, function, and nonprofit status of this organization and the exempt status for federal income tax purposes:
☒ Has Not Changed During Preceding 12 Months
☐ Has Changed During Preceding 12 Months (Publisher must submit explanation of change with this statement)

PS Form **3526**, July 2014 [Page 1 of 4 (see instructions page 4)] PSN: 7530-01-000-9931   PRIVACY NOTICE: See our privacy policy on www.usps.com.

---

13. Publication Title	14. Issue Date for Circulation Data Below
HEMATOLOGY/ONCOLOGY CLINICS OF NORTH AMERICA	JUNE 2020

15. Extent and Nature of Circulation			Average No. Copies Each Issue During Preceding 12 Months	No. Copies of Single Issue Published Nearest to Filing Date
a. Total Number of Copies (Net press run)			157	137
b. Paid Circulation (By Mail and Outside the Mail)	(1)	Mailed Outside-County Paid Subscriptions Stated on PS Form 3541 (Include paid distribution above nominal rate, advertiser's proof copies, and exchange copies)	62	49
	(2)	Mailed In-County Paid Subscriptions Stated on PS Form 3541 (Include paid distribution above nominal rate, advertiser's proof copies, and exchange copies)	0	0
	(3)	Paid Distribution Outside the Mails Including Sales Through Dealers and Carriers, Street Vendors, Counter Sales, and Other Paid Distribution Outside USPS®	48	40
	(4)	Paid Distribution by Other Classes of Mail Through the USPS (e.g., First-Class Mail®)	0	0
c. Total Paid Distribution (Sum of 15b (1), (2), (3), and (4))		►	110	89
d. Free or Nominal Rate Distribution (By Mail and Outside the Mail)	(1)	Free or Nominal Rate Outside-County Copies included on PS Form 3541	31	29
	(2)	Free or Nominal Rate In-County Copies Included on PS Form 3541	0	0
	(3)	Free or Nominal Rate Copies Mailed at Other Classes Through the USPS (e.g., First-Class Mail)	0	0
	(4)	Free or Nominal Rate Distribution Outside the Mail (Carriers or other means)	0	0
e. Total Free or Nominal Rate Distribution (Sum of 15d (1), (2), (3) and (4))		►	31	29
f. Total Distribution (Sum of 15c and 15e)		►	141	118
g. Copies not Distributed (See Instructions to Publishers #4 (page #3))		►	16	19
h. Total (Sum of 15f and g)		►	157	137
i. Percent Paid (15c divided by 15f times 100)		►	78.01%	75.42%

* If you are claiming electronic copies, go to line 16 on page 3. If you are not claiming electronic copies, skip to line 17 on page 3.

16. Electronic Copy Circulation	Average No. Copies Each Issue During Preceding 12 Months	No. Copies of Single Issue Published Nearest to Filing Date
a. Paid Electronic Copies ►		
b. Total Paid Print Copies (Line 15c) + Paid Electronic Copies (Line 16a) ►		
c. Total Print Distribution (Line 15f) + Paid Electronic Copies (Line 16a) ►		
d. Percent Paid (Both Print & Electronic Copies) (16b divided by 16c × 100) ►		

☒ I certify that 50% of all my distributed copies (electronic and print) are paid above a nominal price.

17. Publication of Statement of Ownership
☒ If the publication is a general publication, publication of this statement is required. Will be printed in the OCTOBER 2020 issue of this publication.
☐ Publication not required.

18. Signature and Title of Editor, Publisher, Business Manager, or Owner

Malathi Samayan

Malathi Samayan Distribution Controller

Date 9/18/2020

I certify that all information furnished on this form is true and complete. I understand that anyone who furnishes false or misleading information on this form or who omits material or information requested on the form may be subject to criminal sanctions (including fines and imprisonment) and/or civil sanctions (including civil penalties).

PS Form **3526**, July 2014 (Page 3 of 4) PRIVACY NOTICE: See our privacy policy on www.usps.com

Moving?

Make sure your subscription moves with you!

To notify us of your new address, find your **Clinics Account Number** (located on your mailing label above your name), and contact customer service at:

Email: **journalscustomerservice-usa@elsevier.com**

800-654-2452 (subscribers in the U.S. & Canada)
314-447-8871 (subscribers outside of the U.S. & Canada)

Fax number: 314-447-8029

Elsevier Health Sciences Division
Subscription Customer Service
3251 Riverport Lane
Maryland Heights, MO 63043

*To ensure uninterrupted delivery of your subscription, please notify us at least 4 weeks in advance of move.

Printed and bound by CPI Group (UK) Ltd, Croydon, CR0 4YY

03/10/2024

01040483-0002

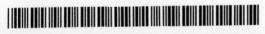